CRITICALLY ILL ADULTS: NURSING CARE PLANNING GUIDES

CRITICALLY ILL ADULTS: NURSING CARE PLANNING GUIDES

Edited by

RANDY MARION CAINE, RN, MS, CS, CCRN

Associate Professor of Nursing
Director, Trauma/Emergency Clinical Nurse Specialist Program
California State University, Long Beach
Long Beach, California

PATRICIA McKAY BUFALINO, RN, MN

Assistant Professor of Nursing
Riverside Community College
Riverside, California

WILLIAMS & WILKINS
Baltimore • Hong Kong • London • Sydney

Editors: Margo Neal, Rose Mary Carroll-Johnson
Associate Editor: Linda Napora
Copy Editor: Nora Galvin
Design: Joanne Janowiak
Production: Anne G. Seitz

428 East Preston Street
Baltimore, MD 21202, U.S.A.

Accurate indications, adverse reactions, and dosage schedules for drugs are provided in this book, but it is possible that they may change. The reader is urged to review the package information data of the manufacturers of the medications mentioned.

Printed in the United States of America

Library of Congress Cataloging-in-Publication Data

Critically ill adults: nursing care planning guides / edited by Randy Marion Caine, Patricia McKay Bufalino,
p. cm.—(Applying nursing diagnosis)
Bibliography: p.
ISBN 0-683-01351-3
1. Intensive care nursing—Outlines, syllabi, etc. 2. Psychiatric nursing—Outlines, syllabi, etc. 3. Nursing care plans—Outlines, syllabi, etc. I. Caine, Randy Marion. II. Bufalino, Patricia McKay. III. Series.
[DNLM: 1. Critical Care—methods—outlines. 2. Nursing Assessment—methods—outlines. 3. Patient Care Planning—outlines.
WY 18 C9347]
RT120.15C79 1988
610.73'61—dc19
DNLM/DLC
for Library of Congress

88 89 90 91 92
1 2 3 4 5 6 7 8 9 10

Foreword

Since the inception of critical care, there has not been a time more challenging than that facing critical care nurses today. The health care industry is going through revolutionary changes resulting in an unstable and unpredictable hospital system. Technological, pharmaceutical, and medical innovations are being introduced daily, creating a tremendous challenge to keep informed and current. Patient stays in the critical care unit are getting shorter and shorter, requiring increased acuity and complexity of care. And finally, the current nursing shortage has a strong impact on efforts at continuity of care and the increasing stress felt by critical care nurses.

In order to maintain quality care in the current environment, it is imperative that critical care nurses strive to provide continuity in patient care and increase the efficiency of patient care. *Critically Ill Adults: Nursing Care Planning Guides* is a valuable resource to help accomplish both of these objectives.

This text provides an in-depth discussion of the nursing process as it applies to critically ill adults with medical and surgical problems. The content for each patient problem addresses an overview of the condition, assessment criteria and guidelines, potential nursing diagnoses with rationale statements, selected interventions, and evaluation criteria. The patient as an individual with social and family roles is considered throughout.

The authors have presented an excellent resource for nurses who provide care in a variety of acute care settings. Nurses can utilize various aspects of this content to facilitate care provided. Applying the information as it fits the patient situation encourages creative, individualized and comprehensive care for the critically ill adult.

Randy Caine and Patti Bufalino have provided a needed tool to enhance patient care within the critical care unit. This book offers the critical care nurse the knowledge necessary to plan, communicate, and coordinate care utilizing the nursing process in a manner consistent with meeting the challenge of critical care nursing today.

Chris Breu, RN, MN
Assistant Director of Nursing/Critical Care
Humana Hospital-Suburban
Louisville, Kentucky

Preface

Nurses in practice, and nursing students faced with the task of preparing for clinical laboratory, reported finding our *Nursing Care Planning Guides for Adults* very helpful. Critical care nurses commented that a more compact version specifically designed for their practice would be even more helpful. This book is our response to those comments.

Critically Ill Adults: Nursing Care Planning Guides is intended as a reference for planning the nursing care of patients who are acutely ill and/or require specialized nursing care. We recognize that some of the guides that have been selected for inclusion may not seem as "critical" in large specialized medical centers, but we have chosen to include them to assist nurses in smaller critical care facilities to plan nursing care. Indeed, with the current economic environment in acute health care settings and the nursing shortage, many patients require more care than usual staffing patterns permit and thus are placed in critical care units.

The nursing process has been used as a framework for this text. The reader will find assessment data; long-term goals; nursing diagnoses with rationales for their selection; short-term goals for each diagnosis; nursing actions that address the independent, interdependent, and dependent domains of nursing care; and otucome criteria by which to evaluate the short-term goals. The outline style used allows the nurse to quickly choose and identify assessment findings, nursing diagnoses, and implementations appropriate to the individualized care of critically ill patients.

These guides should be used in conjunction with other resources. At times, it may be necessary to select strategies from several guides rather than concentrating solely on the reason for the patient's hospitalization. The reader is encouraged to select those appropriate to the care of the individual patient and family.

In summary, *Critically Ill Adults: Nursing Care Planning Guides* should be used by nurses who require a handy reference for planning care for adult patients in critical care or specialty units. It will also be beneficial to nurses who find themselves responsible for planning care for a diverse population of critically ill patients.

R.M.C.
P.M.B.

Acknowledgments

The preparation of any lengthy manuscript requires the assistance, guidance, and support of many people. The authors particularly thank the contributors for their tolerance of revisions, schedules, and deadlines.

In addition, no book is published without the patient and expert guidance of editorial staff and so the authors would sincerely like to thank Rose Mary Carroll-Johnson and Margo Neal of Williams & Wilkins.

Finally, the support of one's family is also necessary, and the authors wish to express their love and thanks, respectively, to Donald and Joshua Caine and Chuck, Charles, Michael, and Jeanne Bufalino.

R.M.C.
P.M.B.

Contributors

Pamela Bellefeuille, RN, CS, MN
Assistant Professor of Nursing
California State University, Long Beach
Long Beach, CA

Patricia McKay Bufalino, RN, MN
Assistant Professor of Nursing
Riverside Community College
Riverside, CA

Randy Marion Caine, RN, MS, CS, CCRN
Associate Professor of Nursing
Director, Trauma/Emergency Clinical Nurse Specialist Program
California State University, Long Beach
Long Beach, CA

Suzette Cardin, RN, MS, CCRN
Nurse Manager, Coronary Care Unit/Coronary Observation Unit
UCLA Medical Center
Los Angeles, CA

JoAnn Chasteen, RN, MN
Associate Professor of Nursing
Riverside Community College
Riverside, CA

Marie Thonis Colucci, RN, MN
Associate Professor of Nursing
Riverside Community College
Riverside, CA

Sharon J. Evans, RN, MSN
Associate Professor of Nursing
Riverside Community College
Riverside, CA

Susan B. Fowler, RN, MS, CCRN, CNRN
Clinical Nurse Specialist
Luther Hospital
Eau Claire, WI

Wendy W. Hollis, RN, MN
Assistant Professor of Nursing
Los Angeles Harbor College
Wilmington, CA

Retha Vornholt Keenan, RN, MSN, NP
Instructor, Mental Health Nursing
Los Angeles Community College
Los Angeles, CA
El Camino Community College
Torrance, CA

Carolyn Sue Kross, RN, MSN
Associate Professor of Nursing
Riverside Community College
Riverside, CA

C. J. Marshak, RN, MN, CCRN
Clinical Nurse Specialist/Educational Consultant
Culver City, CA

Mary Beth Navas, RN, MN, CCRN
Clinical Nurse Specialist, Critical Care
Riverside Community Hospital-Medical Center
Riverside, CA

Joan W. Reighley, RN, MN
Assistant Professor of Nursing
West Los Angeles College
Los Angeles, CA

Joanne Kraenzle Schneider, RN, MN, CCRN
Nursing Diagnosis Resource Person
St. Francis Regional Medical Center
Wichita, KS

Ann M. Schofield, RN, MS
Lecturer in Nursing
California State University, Los Angeles
Los Angeles, CA

Kathleen Templin, RN, MN, CCRN
Assistant Professor of Nursing
California State University, Long Beach
Long Beach, CA

Mary Catherine Tennies-Moseley, RN, MN
Assistant Professor of Nursing
Riverside Community College
Riverside, CA

Jane C. Walton, RN, MS
Coordinator, Practical Nursing Program
Arizona Western College
Yuma, AZ

Bethany K. Worgess, RN, BSN, ANP
Graduate Student in Nursing
California State University, Long Beach
Emergency Room Staff Nurse
Memorial Medical Center
Long Beach, CA

Contents

Introduction

Nursing process is the method by which the professional nurse acts to improve the health status of patients. It is applied in the context of the patient's medical diagnosis but leads the nurse to develop strategies individual to the particular patient's needs.

There are five steps to the process:

1. Assessment
2. Analysis
3. Plan
4. Implementation
5. Evaluation

The guides developed in this book detail each of these steps for commonly encountered medical conditions. By extrapolating from each section the information pertinent to the particular client and by adapting the nursing plan in light of patient needs and the physician's orders, the reader can arrive at a plan of care designed to enhance the patient's chances of attaining maximum health.

Each part of the nursing process builds on and grows out of the preceding step. In addition, the process is cyclical and ongoing. In this context, then, specific information is presented for specific kinds of patient problems.

Assessment, the organized, systematic, and purposeful gathering of information about a patient's current or future health, is essential to permit grouping or clustering of data for analysis leading to identification of nursing concerns or nursing diagnosis. Assessment data are compiled from the patient record, through physical examination, and by interviews with the patient, family members, and/or other health care professionals; however, the most important source of information is the patient.

To assist the nurse in clustering data, four components of a nursing assessment have been identified. They are *pertinent history, physical findings, psychosocial concerns and developmental factors,* and *patient and family knowledge* about the condition and its treatment.

Pertinent history includes the precipitating events and/or illnesses leading to the patient's current condition. This information may already be documented in the patient record or the nurse may have to structure the nursing interview to ensure gathering of meaningful data. Knowing the patient's history enables the nurse to better interpret other aspects of the nursing assessment, leading to more valid nursing diagnoses and appropriate selection of specific strategies likely to be effective in assisting the patient in achieving desired goals.

The nursing physical examination, routinely performed on patients at the time of admission, provides a physical overview of the patient from head to toe. In the physical findings section of each nursing care planning guide, you will find key physical assessment data especially significant for the condition under discussion. Sometimes this will be specific manifestations or abnormalities you may expect to find. In other cases it was more appropriate to list specific parameters needing assessment. Additionally, many guides include laboratory findings that aid the physician in making a diagnosis and that the nurse can expect to monitor while caring for a patient with that specific condition.

Understanding the ways in which a person has been influenced by society, cultural heritage, and the expected developmental tasks for a person of a given age are helpful in predicting patient responses and in planning specific nursing interventions to achieve desired goals. Information about previous coping strategies and existing functional support systems provides clues to identifying psychosocial nursing diagnoses. Additionally, certain patient conditions are more likely to be manifested in specific ethnic or age groups. For these reasons, the psychosocial concerns and developmental variations likely to be associated with the condition described in the nursing care planning guide are highlighted.

In current nursing practice, it is imperative that discharge planning begin at the time of admission to the health care agency. To help the nurse assess the learning needs of patients and families, important aspects of the condition and treatment plan that the patient needs to promote compliance after discharge are listed. Each nursing care planning guide includes the nursing diagnosis "Knowledge deficit." The nurse's choice to use the suggested diagnosis, to adapt it to the specific learning needs of the patient/family, or identify a more relevant diagnosis depends upon the interpretation of the assessment data obtained concerning the patient's and family's baseline knowledge.

Just as nursing diagnosis provides a framework for nursing practice, an organized nursing assessment is essential to identifying valid nursing diagnoses for a particular patient. An incomplete or incorrect database will interfere with the identification of actual or potential problems. Therefore, by systematically reviewing or obtaining information about the patient's pertinent history, physical findings, psychosocial concerns and developmental variations, and the patient's and family's knowledge of the condition and treatment, the nurse ensures that a complete database is collected. The stage is set for competent analysis leading to identification of pertinent nursing diagnoses as a framework for providing care.

A **nursing diagnosis** is a statement of a nursing problem based on a critical appraisal and analysis of the assessment data. It represents those activities the nurse performs that acknowledge her/his independent functioning. Nursing diagnosis is an ongoing process, not restricted only to the written nursing care plan.

Within the scope of individual state nurse practice law there are important aspects of both dependent and independent functions. The dependent dimensions of nursing practice describe those interventions the nurse cannot legally prescribe. For example, the nurse cannot prescribe nitroglycerin to a patient admitted with acute chest pain. The nurse requires an order from the physician prior to the administration of that medication. This represents the dependent domain of nursing. The independent dimension of nursing practice on the other hand describes those interventions the nurse can legally prescribe. An example of this is a patient in traction who complains of boredom and frustration because of confinement to bed. The nurse may in this situation prescribe diversional activities such as television or referral to volunteer services to obtain books or magazines.

The important aspect to consider when identifying nursing diagnoses is that the diagnostic statement describes an actual or potential problem that nurses, because of their education and experience, are licensed and legally responsible and accountable to treat. Therefore, nursing diagnoses are different from other patient-related problems that are the responsibility of other health care providers.

The nursing diagnosis is written as a two-part statement, the nursing diagnostic statement and the etiology/contributing factors. For example:

Ineffective individual coping related to chronicity of disease condition, effect on usual roles and responsibilities, inadequate support system.

The nursing diagnosis directs the nurse in terms of her/his goals and interventions. Nursing diagnoses may apply to either individuals or groups. That is, not all diagnostic statements refer only to the patient. The family member or significant other may also require nursing actions in order to ensure a successful patient outcome.

Nursing diagnoses utilized in this book have been established and approved by the North American Nursing Diagnosis Association. A complete list can be found in the Appendix.

Planning is the third step in the nursing process and follows patient-specific assessment and diagnosis of nursing problems. Planning allows nursing care to be delivered in a logical, organized, goal-directed, patient-centered manner and directs the implementation and evaluation of nursing care. Planning always occurs prior to implementation of nursing actions. In emergency situations planning may occur simultaneously with implementation because of the acuity of the situation.

Planning involves

- prioritizing patient problems
- establishing patient-centered goals
- stating specific nursing actions/interventions for each problem

The changing environment of the health care setting necessitates that the nurse set priorities to allow for appropriate delivery of care to the patient in a time-efficient, cost-effective manner, thus enabling one to address the patient's biopsychosocial needs more completely. Prioritization is influenced by patient status, the degree of urgency with which the patient views the problem, the treatment plan, and potential complications. The nursing care section of each care plan has been organized in order of decreasing priority to assist the reader in this process.

When establishing goals, the nurse collaborates with the patient, when possible. Mutually agreed-upon goals foster patient compliance and motivation. The best goals reflect the prior nursing assessment and diagnosis. Included in each plan are both short- and long-term goals to promote optimal wellness. Goals need to reflect observable behaviors so that the nurse can measure progress toward the goal or lack thereof.

Implementation is the fourth step in the nursing process. It is during this step that the plan of care is put into action through ongoing assessment, actual performance of bedside nursing actions, appropriate charting of nursing care that has been given, and communication with other health team members. Nursing actions need to be individualized for each patient. They are developed to meet the established goals and should direct care to answer the questions who, where, what, when, how, and how often. The need for assessment of changing patient status is invaluable in providing current and relevant information to maintain a plan of care. As the client moves along the health-illness continuum, the nursing role increasingly focuses on patient/family education and maximizing self-care abilities. The need for quality care and equally good documentation is essential to maintain a care plan reflective of the patient's changing status.

Evaluation, the last step of the nursing process, includes observing the patient's response to the nursing actions; determining the patient's progress towards the goals, objectives, expected outcomes; and revising or modifying the written care plan accordingly.

The patient's estimation of progress towards the goal and degree of satisfaction with the outcome is an essential part of the evaluation process. In addition, family or significant others, the chart, and appropriate health team members are also consulted. Data from each source should confirm and validate the data from other sources; inconsistent findings require further investigation to determine reasons for discrepancies.

When the patient's response to the nursing actions and progress towards the goals are evaluated, a number of outcomes are possible. If the goal has been achieved and the identified need/problem has been resolved, the nurse determines the next priority. If progress is being made but the goal has not been reached, nursing interventions can be continued, discontinued, or modified. If there has been no progress toward the goal, the nurse asks the following questions:

1. Is the goal realistic for this patient and this situation? Does it need to be changed? Does the critical time need to be changed? What factors were involved in progress or lack of progress towards goal?
2. Was the nursing diagnosis accurate? Were data overlooked or is there new data to include? Have new problems emerged that need attention? Is this the patient's priority or is there some other need/problem that seems more important to the patient?
3. Are the nursing actions effective/ineffective? Are there other options to try? Consult with peers, supervisors, and current professional literature.

Revise or modify the care plan as necessary according to answers to these questions. The nursing process is dynamic and cyclic; ongoing evaluation provides valuable information to keep nursing process effective and nursing practice accountable.

The act of planning patient care by using the nursing process is an integral part of modern professional nursing care. The user of this book, whether a nursing student or an experienced nurse, will find it to be an invaluable reference not just to nursing process but to the dynamic, ever-changing arena of individualized nursing care plans.

Bibliography

Carpenito, L. (1984). *Handbook of nursing diagnosis.* Philadelphia: Lippincott.

Carpenito, L. (1983). *Nursing diagnosis: Application to clinical practice.* Philadelphia: Lippincott.

Gordon, M. (1982). *Nursing diagnosis: Process and application.* New York: McGraw-Hill.

Section 1

Nursing Care for Selected Medical and Surgical Problems

The Patient with Acquired Immune Deficiency Syndrome

Definition/Discussion

Acquired immune deficiency syndrome (AIDS) is a poorly understood impairment of the body's immune system occurring in previously healthy individuals. This impairment makes these individuals vulnerable to a variety of infectious agents that might not otherwise cause disease. AIDS is defined by the Centers for Disease Control (CDC) in Atlanta as either biopsy- or autopsy-proven Kaposi's sarcoma in persons less than 60 years old, or life-threatening or fatal opportunistic infections that are highly predictive of cell-mediated immunodeficiency in persons who are not immunosuppressed for some other reason.

The extremely grave prognosis of AIDS (50%-100% mortality, depending on the underlying opportunistic disease), its relative newness (first identified in 1981), accelerating incidence, and the connotation of being associated with minority social groups (homosexuals and IV drug users) all combine to make AIDS a psychosocial problem as well as a medical disorder. The public is fearfully distrustful of AIDS patients, resulting in social isolation. This social isolation is distressing for all AIDS patients, but particularly for the so-called "innocent" victims of AIDS, the children who were born to high-risk women (sexual partners of high-risk males) and those who contracted AIDS after receiving contaminated blood products. CDC investigators do not know of any patient with AIDS who has regained lost immunity.

Nursing Assessment

☐ PERTINENT HISTORY

Weight loss of more than 10 lb during a period of less than 2 months, unrelated to diet or increased activity; prolonged loss of appetite; unexplained, persistent, or recurrent fevers, chills, or night sweats; profound fatigue that is not transient or explained by physical activity, substance abuse, or a psychologic disorder; persistent and unexplained diarrhea or bloody stools; inclusion in a high-risk group (e.g., sexually active homosexual or bisexual men, intravenous drug users, Haitian immigrants, hemophiliacs and other frequent transfusion recipients)

☐ PHYSICAL FINDINGS

Lymphadenopathy in neck, axillae, and groin unexplained by other illness; whitish coating or spotting on the throat or tongue associated with painful swallowing; dry, persistent cough unrelated to smoking; purplish skin lesions or other new growths on top of or beneath the skin, on oral, nasal, or anal mucous membranes, or beneath the eyelids (Kaposi's sarcoma); herpetic lesions; general debility; laboratory studies indicating immunosuppression and presence of microorganisms

☐ PSYCHOSOCIAL CONCERNS/ DEVELOPMENTAL FACTORS

Expressed or denied anxiety about uncertain etiology and grave prognosis; physical limitations imposed as disease progresses likely to interfere with ability to continue usual occupational role, possibly resulting in increased dependency in social and familial roles; effects of societal attitudes (e.g., fear, distrust, condemnation, pity, ostracism) on attainment of developmental tasks, self-esteem, social isolation, and control

PATIENT AND FAMILY KNOWLEDGE

Level of knowledge, readiness and willingness to learn, disease process, associated risk factors, treatments, precautions, screening tests, fears, coping strategies

Nursing Care

LONG-TERM GOAL

The patient will be maintained in a state of biopsychosocial integrity with as much independence and community contact as possible, adhering to treatment regimen, living within restrictions, and adjusting to actual/potential losses.

NURSING DIAGNOSIS #1

Potential for infection related to immunosuppression

Rationale: *Current investigations into the etiology of AIDS suggest it is initiated by a viral agent. Because of the body's inability to fight off disease, the AIDS patient is particularly vulnerable to opportunistic infections caused by protozoa (e.g.,* Pneumocystis carinii, Toxoplasma gondii, *and* Enamoeba histolytica*), viruses (e.g., cytomegalovirus [CMV], herpes simplex, and herpes zoster), bacteria (e.g.,* Mycobacterium tuberculosis, Klebsiella pneumonia, *and* Salmonella enteritidis*), and fungi (e.g.,* Candida albicans *and* Cryptococcus neoformans*).*

GOAL

The patient will be maintained in appropriate isolation; will be monitored for early signs of infection; staff, other patients, and visitors will be free from contagion.

IMPLEMENTATION

- Maintain isolation as per hospital protocol; precautions include
  - gloving whenever the care giver anticipates contact with the patient's body fluids, secretions, or excretions
  - wearing a gown if the patient has copious secretions or excretions
  - wearing a mask if performing a procedure in which secretions or excretions might splatter inadvertently
- It is not necessary to use isolation techniques when entering the room to talk with the patient or to administer an oral medication.
- Arrange for a private room; do not place two AIDS patients in the same room since they may have different organisms involved and may acquire others through cross-contamination.
- Routinely clean patient-care surfaces with soap and water.
- Take extraordinary care to avoid self-wounds from sharp instruments contaminated with potentially infectious material (e.g., blood, excreta).
- Use disposable needles and syringes only, if feasible; if reusable syringes must be used, terminally decontaminate them before cleaning and repackaging.
- Do not bend needles after use, but promptly place in a puncture-resistant container used solely for such disposal; do not reinsert needles into their original sheaths before discarding them (a common cause of needle injury).
- Use only Luer-Lok syringes or one-piece needle-syringe units to aspirate fluids from patients, so that collected fluid can be safely discharged through the needle.
- Maintain meticulous sterile technique; ensure used instruments are cleaned and sterilized.
- Carefully monitor vital signs and laboratory tests ordered for signs of infection.
- Administer antimicrobial therapy as ordered, carefully monitoring for side effects/toxicity.
- Caution visitors about exposing the patient to infections; teach them to observe isolation precautions, especially good handwashing, before and after entering patient's room.
- Advise pregnant women (visitors and staff) to avoid contact with the patient because of the possibility of exposure to CMV.
- Avoid unnecessary exaggeration of isolation precautions or avoiding the patient to prevent physical and emotional isolation.

EVALUATION CRITERIA/DESIRED OUTCOMES

The Patient

- Maintains isolation precautions
- Has signs and symptoms of new infection detected early
- Is protected from cross-contamination from other patients, visitors, or staff

NURSING DIAGNOSIS #2

a. **Impairment of skin integrity** (perineal) related to immunosuppression
b. **Alteration in oral mucous membranes** related to immunosuppression

Rationale: *The patient's immune deficiency increases the risk for skin and mucous membrane lesions. Common skin problems include Kaposi's sarcoma, herpetic lesions, or candidiasis.*

☐ GOAL

The patient will experience maximum possible comfort; will maintain integrity of skin and mucous membranes.

☐ IMPLEMENTATION

- Provide skin care at least every 4 hours or more frequently if needed (diaphoresis and diarrhea are extremely irritating to the skin).
- Change linen frequently and give sponge baths when fever is present.
- Clean skin lesions with warm, soapy water; rinse and apply dressing and antimicrobial ointment if ordered, covering with a nonadherent pad.
- Cleanse rectal area after each bowel movement with warm, soapy water; when herpetic lesions are present, rinse and pat dry with soft cloth, not toilet paper.
- Brush teeth with soft toothbrush to treat oral candida; follow with half-strength peroxide mouthwash; offer oral care every 2-4 hours.
- Ensure position change at least every 2 hours; obtain an egg-crate or alternating pressure mattress when indicated.

☐ EVALUATION CRITERIA/DESIRED OUTCOMES

The Patient

- Expresses a feeling of comfort
- Is free from skin breakdown, oral pain or lesions

NURSING DIAGNOSIS #3

a. **Ineffective airway clearance** related to viscous secretions, ineffective cough, fatigue
b. **Ineffective breathing patterns** related to severe, nonrelieved cough
c. **Impaired gas exchange** related to loss of functioning lung tissue secondary to opportunistic respiratory infection (specify causative agent if known)

Rationale: *Pneumonia secondary to* Pneumocystis carnii *or CMV is a common complication of AIDS. If not successfully treated, respiratory failure may contribute to the cause(s) of death. A nonproductive, chronic cough may be one of the presenting symptoms that causes the person to seek medical attention initially.*

☐ GOAL

The patient will maintain pulmonary function; will have a decreased risk of aspiration; will demonstrate improved gas exchange; will experience relief from symptoms of pain, weakness, and dyspnea; will demonstrate effective coughing and energy conservation.

☐ IMPLEMENTATION

- Obtain a baseline assessment of respiratory function including relevant history, respiratory rate and character, use of accessory muscles, breath sounds, skin color, general appearance, and arterial blood gases.
- Monitor use and effectiveness of ordered therapies such as oxygen, mechanical ventilation, humidification, chest tubes, and pharmaceuticals.
- Reassess respiratory status every 2 hours or as necessary for signs and symptoms of respiratory insufficiency/failure (e.g., tachypnea, tachycardia, dyspnea, apprehension, irritability, or confusion); refer to *The Patient with Pneumonia,* page 194.
- Administer antitussives/expectorants as ordered; note effectiveness.
- Suction at least every 2 hours; obtain specimens as ordered; carefully monitor lab results.
- Administer antimicrobials on time as or-

dered; observe carefully for side effects/toxicity.

- Administer antipyretic to control temperature; note effect on fever.
- Monitor blood gases; report significant changes and modify ventilatory settings as ordered.
- Provide humidification and intermittent positive pressure breathing with postural drainage as ordered; turn, cough, deep breathe, and encourage inspirometer use at least every 2 hours.
- Organize nursing care to permit periods of uninterrupted rest.
- Administer narcotic analgesics and sedatives cautiously; evaluate response.

☐ EVALUATION CRITERIA/DESIRED OUTCOMES

The Patient

- Has decreased dyspnea on exertion
- Expectorates secretions
- Expresses relief from symptoms causing discomfort
- Demonstrates improved respiratory functioning
- Has blood gas values within normal limits

NURSING DIAGNOSIS #4

a. **Alteration in nutrition: less than body requirements** related to catabolic state, anorexia, difficulty swallowing

b. **Impaired swallowing** related to esophagitis

Rationale: *In the presence of infection, metabolic requirements are increased. Preexisting mouth lesions or esophageal lesions may make chewing or swallowing painful, decreasing the patient's incentive to eat and further compromising the immune status.*

☐ GOAL

The patient will receive adequate intake to meet metabolic requirements.

☐ IMPLEMENTATION

- Carefully record daily weights, oral intake, and calorie counts.
- Encourage full consumption of prescribed diet; give soft foods and liquids; have family and friends bring in favorite foods; provide small high-protein, high-calorie supplements between meals.
- Administer supplemental vitamins and minerals.
- Initiate referral to dietician as needed.
- If patient is unable to maintain sufficient oral intake, consult with physician about starting tube feedings. (Hyperalimentation is not advised because of the associated risk of infection.)

☐ EVALUATION CRITERIA/DESIRED OUTCOMES

The Patient

- Increases intake with resultant gain or stabilization of weight
- Improves skin turgor and condition of skin, hair, nails, and mucous membranes

NURSING DIAGNOSIS #5

Alteration in bowel elimination: diarrhea related to opportunistic bowel infection (specify agent if known), prescribed medication (specify drug), tube feeding intolerance

Rationale: *Protozoan and bacterial infections of the bowel will likely present as diarrhea. Antimicrobial medications and tube feedings may be poorly tolerated by individual patients with the intolerance manifested as diarrhea.*

☐ GOAL

The patient will experience maximum comfort and control of diarrhea.

☐ IMPLEMENTATION

- Encourage fluids, maintaining an oral intake of 3,000 cc/day to prevent dehydration.
- Cleanse and carefully dry rectal area after each bowel movement.
- Administer antidiarrheal agents as ordered.
- If causative factor is thought to be medication or tube feeding, consult with physician about the possibility of changing prescribed medication or tube-feeding formula.

☐ EVALUATION CRITERIA/DESIRED OUTCOMES

The Patient

- Has decreased number of stools/day
- Expresses a feeling of comfort
- Has a balanced intake and output

NURSING DIAGNOSIS #6

a. **Grieving** related to diagnosis, loss of healthy status
b. **Ineffective individual/family coping** related to diagnosis, life-style choices
c. **Impaired social interaction** related to isolation precautions, grieving over diagnosis
d. **Social isolation** related to societal nonacceptance of disease

Rationale: *The seriousness of an AIDS diagnosis challenges the coping resources of the strongest individuals and family units. For some families the time of diagnosis also necessitates adjustment to the patient's sexual orientation, thus compounding the necessary coping tasks. The physical distancing required by isolation precautions may foster social isolation if the disease process and the reasons for the required precautions are poorly understood, as is the case with AIDS.*

☐ GOAL

The patient will deal adaptively with changes in usual social interactions; will devise new coping strategies; patient and family/friends will be able to express feelings, concerns, and fears; support systems intact prior to hospitalization will be continued.

☐ IMPLEMENTATION

- Assess patient and family/friends for stage of grieving; refer to *The Patient Experiencing Grief and Loss,* page 272.
- Support adaptive responses, remembering that in the initial stage any response may be adaptive except homicidal or suicidal behavior.
- Encourage realistic assessment of the situation by providing information, answering questions, and gentle truth telling.
- Recognize and support the patient's need for unique, personal adjustments to change.
- Be aware that patient's friends may withdraw out of fear of catching the disease; educate as necessary.
- Encourage family, friends, and staff to visit with the patient, avoiding unnecessary exaggeration of isolation precautions.
- Recognize the need for privacy when sexual partner is visiting, honoring wishes for confidentiality and assisting others (family, friends, and staff) to cope with patient's preference.
- Initiate referrals to mental health nurse or clinician as appropriate.

☐ EVALUATION CRITERIA/DESIRED OUTCOMES

The Patient

- Maintains social interaction with family, friends, and staff
- Verbalizes satisfaction with emotional support provided by staff/family/friends

NURSING DIAGNOSIS #7

Altered sexuality patterns related to physiologic limitations and life-style changes imposed by disease process

Rationale: *Because transmission of AIDS is believed to be through direct contact with contaminated body fluids through intimate sexual contact (as well as through sharing of contaminated needles, transfusions of blood products, and percutaneous blood exposure), intimate contact is discouraged for the patient. Since sexuality is an integral part of the patient's identity, alternate means of expression may need to be developed.*

☐ GOAL

The patient will explore/use alternate ways to meet sexual needs.

☐ IMPLEMENTATION

- Plan nursing care to permit time to encourage the patient to express feelings or concerns about sexual activity and the spread of AIDS; let the patient set the pace.
- Support the patient's partner who may feel a threat to own life because of the mode of transmission.
- Educate regarding safe sexual activity

- abstaining from sex with partners with a known infection
- select partners from a small group of known friends
- avoid combination of oral and anal sex
- use a condom during sex

• Use the word "partner" rather than "wife" or "husband" and regard the patient's partner as a "significant other" worthy of receiving information usually given to family only, if appropriate.
• Refrain from moralizing about or judging sexual choices; prevent misunderstandings about homosexuals by educating staff and holding team conferences to express feelings.
• Maintain confidentiality of homosexual patients who have not openly revealed their sexual orientation and fear the rejections of others if this information becomes known.

☐ EVALUATION CRITERIA/DESIRED OUTCOMES

The Patient

• Expresses satisfaction with close relationships and methods of sexual expression

NURSING DIAGNOSIS #8

Powerlessness related to grave prognosis

Rationale: *The patient with AIDS confronts living with a chronic disease that is poorly understood and for which there is no known cure and little hope for improvement. Powerlessness may be manifested by expressed dissatisfaction in ability to control the disease process; reluctance or refusal to participate in decision making; apathetic, aggressive, actingout, or violent behavior; uneasiness or anxiety; or depression.*

☐ GOAL

The patient will be able to identify those aspects of AIDS and its treatment that can be controlled; will participate in decision making concerning treatment.

☐ IMPLEMENTATION

• Assess specific aspects of AIDS that are most distressing; review initial psychosocial assessment for information about usual coping patterns and identified support persons; use this information in refining planned interventions.
• Allow the patient to express fears and concerns; listen attentively without minimizing the patient's feelings; offer suggestions without directly telling the patient what to do; when possible, offer alternative solutions to patient problems and encourage the patient to make the final decision.
• Keep informed about condition, treatments, and test results.
• Provide opportunities for patient to control as many decisions as possible such as physical set-up of room and daily activities.
• Do not offer choices that do not exist; respect and follow the patient's choices when you have given the option of making a choice.
• Record preferences on care plan to ensure that others will acknowledge preferences.

☐ EVALUATION CRITERIA/DESIRED OUTCOMES

The Patient

• Expresses feelings of increased control over some aspects of own life
• Participates in the decision-making process regarding treatment

NURSING DIAGNOSIS #9

Knowledge deficit regarding safe hygiene practices in the home, indications for seeking additional medical attention

Rationale: *To decrease the risks of recurrent infection in the patient and transfer of AIDS to care giver(s), the patient and family need guidelines for safe care in the home and reminders of when to contact the physician.*

☐ GOAL

The patient will receive safe, adequate care at home, posing a minimal risk to healthy family members.

☐ IMPLEMENTATION

• Emphasize to family and friends that AIDS is spread by intimate contact with bodily fluids and that casual, nonintimate contact is thought to be safe.
• Teach the patient/family good handwashing techniques.

- Advise disinfecting the patient's bathroom and toilet with a 1:10 solution of 5.25% bleach and water.
- Tell patient/family to wash soiled linens in a washing machine with hot water, detergent, and bleach.
- Instruct patient/family to wash eating utensils in hot soapy water.
- Demonstrate how to dispose of soiled tissues, dressings, and gloves in plastic bags, securing the closure tightly before discarding; ask for return demonstration.
- Caution patient/family to restrict visitors to those who are healthy and not susceptible to illness.
- Instruct the patient/family/significant other about the signs of AIDS and encourage them to seek medical attention should these signs become evident.
- Ensure the patient has a written list of prescribed medications with times, dosages, and possible side effects; explain measures to minimize toxic effects and ask patient to repeat this information at another time; reinforce correct explanations and correct misinformation.
- Explain cross-infection and the signs of infection; stress the need to contact the physician immediately should these signs be noticed.
- Provide information about available community services and initial referrals as necessary; explain that relapses are possible and likely and encourage follow-up care; give the toll-free number (800/221-9044) of the National Gay Task Force crisis line, which has up-to-date information about AIDS. (The number in New York is 212/807-6016).

☐ EVALUATION CRITERIA/DESIRED OUTCOMES

The Patient

- Lists signs of AIDS, necessary precautions for providing home care, and indications for contacting physician
- Verbalizes plans to receive continuing care at home from family/significant others.

The Patient with Acute Renal Failure

Definition/Discussion

Acute renal failure (ARF) is a sudden loss of the kidney's ability to excrete the waste products of cell metabolism. It is frequently associated with another disease process.

ARF is characterized by insufficient production of urine (less than 400 cc/day) and a loss of internal homeostasis, resulting in a rise in nitrogenous waste products and a hypervolemic state. ARF may result from drugs, surgical procedures, trauma, obstruction of the urinary system, transfusion reactions, and a variety of medical diseases. Prognosis is guarded (mortality rate is 50%), but ARF is reversible if the disease process is recognized early and treatment is initiated immediately.

Nursing Assessment

☐ **PERTINENT HISTORY**

Kidney or urinary tract infections; major abdominal or vascular surgery; critical illness; family history of renal disease; current medications; recent flu episode; sepsis; recent, unexplained weight gain; hypertension; respiratory, cardiac, or liver disease; usual pattern and amount of voiding

☐ **PHYSICAL FINDINGS**

Hematuria, oliguria, or anuria; bruising, petechiae; edema, swollen eyelids, pallor, pruritus, dry skin; dyspnea, increased rate and depth of respirations; hyper/hypotension; lethargy, drowsiness, headache, muscle twitching, restless leg syndrome, convulsions; nausea, anorexia, taste of ammonia in mouth or urine odor on breath, stomatitis, diarrhea; laboratory studies: elevated sediment, osmolarity, and creatinine on urinalysis; elevated serum ammonia, albumin, creatinine, bilirubin, and uric acid; elevated BUN; electrolyte disturbances and resultant ECG changes; anemia, prolonged coagulation studies

☐ **PSYCHOSOCIAL CONCERNS/ DEVELOPMENTAL FACTORS**

Anxiety, fear of death or the unknown precipitated by the critical-care environment; associated changes in physical appearance precipitating body-image disturbance

☐ **PATIENT AND FAMILY KNOWLEGE**

Possible course of episode prognosis, level of knowledge, readiness and willingness to learn

Nursing Care

☐ **LONG-TERM GOAL**

The patient will regain normal kidney function and resume usual activities and roles.

NURSING DIAGNOSIS #1

a. **Alteration in fluid volume: excess** related to decreased kidney function
b. **Alteration in cardiac output: decreased** related to fluid volume excess, disturbances in renin-angiotensin system

Rationale: *Damaged renal tissue is not able to maintain homeostasis. Fluid, sodium, potassium, magnesium, and phosphates are retained and an abnormal amount of calcium is excreted. Disturbances in the renin-angiotensin system result in hypertension, which may increase cardiac afterload and contribute to the development of heart failure with resultant decreased cardiac output and the possibility of pulmonary edema. Cardiac dysrhythmias sec-*

ondary to electrolyte imbalances can be life threatening.

GOAL

The patient will receive a fluid intake adjusted to body need during the acute phase of illness; will maintain electrolyte balance and normal blood pressure; will be relieved of chest pain or discomfort; will be free from cardiac failure/tamponade.

IMPLEMENTATION

- Record intake and output accurately every hour initially, then every 4 hours; daily intake should equal output plus 500 cc (average daily insensible loss thorough skin and lungs).
- Monitor vital signs, neurologic status (level of consciousness, headache, visual or pupillary changes, restlessness, seizures) every hour initially, then every 4 hours or as directed; report significant changes.
- Monitor cardiac rhythm continuously; record a rhythm strip every 4 hours or more frequently if irregular pattern develops; measure pulmonary artery pressure, and cardiac output every 1-2 hours; report changes to physician.
- Regulate IVs carefully; maintain fluid restrictions; check with the pharmacist to determine if medications may be mixed in less than usual amounts of fluid.
- Administer antihypertensive medications titrating them to systolic blood pressure specified by physician or hospital protocol; monitor effects.
- Monitor serum electrolyte levels, ammonia, creatinine, BUN; report abnormal values; refer to Table 1, *Common Fluid and Electrolyte Imbalances*, page 17.
- Auscultate breath and heart sounds at least every 8 hours.
- Assess peripheral pulses, check for peripheral edema or distended neck veins every 4 hours; note skin turgor at least every 8 hours.
- Weigh patient daily, at same time, on same scale, in the same clothes (1 kg = 1,000 cc fluid); use bed scale if necessary.
- Administer diuretics, carefully monitoring toxic effects and urinary output after administration.
- Encourage intake of diet low in sodium; restrict oral intake of fluids within imposed limits.
- Promote rest by keeping environment as quiet as possible and by organizing care to allow patient uninterrupted periods of rest.
- Prepare patient for dialysis if necessary; refer to *The Patient Requiring Peritoneal Dialysis*, page 188, or *The Patient Requiring Hemodialysis*, page 111.

EVALUATION CRITERIA/DESIRED OUTCOMES

The Patient

- Has normal serum electrolytes
- Is free from peripheral edema, respiratory difficulty, increase in body weight
- Maintains/regains urinary output
- Has a balanced intake and output
- Has vital signs within normal limits

NURSING DIAGNOSIS #2

Alteration in comfort: pain related to effects of pericarditis

Rationale: *Increased levels of ammonia present in renal failure are toxic to the pericardial sac and may produce pericarditis with possible tamponade.*

GOAL

The patient will experience relief from pain.

IMPLEMENTATION

- Assess for presence of chest pain (cardiac or pleuritic), dyspnea, paradoxical pulse (weaker with inspiration), pericardial friction rub, narrowing pulse pressure, distended neck veins, peripheral edema, rales, cardiac dysrhythmias, and faver.
- Medicate for pain as needed; monitor effects; consult with physician for changed order if relief not obtained.
- Position for comfort with head of bed elevated 30°-40°; administer oxygen as ordered.
- If tamponade presents, assist with emergency pericardiocentesis; provide emotional support to patient/family.

☐ EVALUATION CRITERIA/DESIRED OUTCOMES

The Patient

- Is free from chest pain or discomfort
- Will receive prompt emergency treatment should cardiac tamponade develop

NURSING DIAGNOSIS #3

a. **Potential for infection** related to decreased functioning of immune system
b. **Potential for injury** (bleeding) related to anemia and increased coagulation times

Rationale: *Renal failure causes decreased inflammatory response and a reduction in antibody production. Wound healing is delayed, precipitating the development of infections. Renal failure causes decreased production of erythropoietin, resulting in a decrease in the production of red blood cells. Coagulation factor production is also decreased. Prolonged clotting times may result in excessive bleeding from what might normally be considered minimal trauma, especially in the presence of sepsis or disseminated intravascular clotting (progressive stages of shock).*

☐ GOAL

The patient will be free from infection and bleeding.

☐ IMPLEMENTATION

- Assess patient closely for any signs of overt or covert bleeding (frank blood, fluid "weeping" around sites of penetration of the skin, weakness, pallor); know that a narrowing pulse pressure combined with increased heart and respiratory rates suggests covert bleeding.
- Monitor for signs of infection (malaise, elevated temperature, abnormal white blood cell count, redness or inflammation, drainage or secretions with positive bacterial cultures); know that sepsis may be present without febrile response.
- Change patient's position, encourage use of blow bottles or incentive inspirometer, and have patient cough and deep breathe every 2 hours to prevent pulmonary complications; in patients unable to expectorate use nasaltracheal suction every 2 hours or as needed; for patients requiring mechanical ventilation suction the endotracheal tube every 2 hours or as needed.
- Protect patient from chilling and drafts; provide extra covers as needed.
- If indwelling urinary catheter is used, ensure maintenance of a closed drainage system; empty collection bag at least every 8 hours and measure carefully; observe urinary drainage for color, odor, and particles; record specific gravity; report highly concentrated or very dilute urine.
- Provide care to all wound and puncture sites using strict aseptic technique; rotate IV sites every 48-72 hours and change tubing every 48 hours or according to hospital protocol.
- Administer prophylactic antibiotics in a timely manner to ensure maintenance of therapeutic blood levels; monitor for signs of toxicity.
- Monitor hematologic studies; administer blood components as ordered; refer to Table 2, *Blood and Blood Components*, page 17.

☐ EVALUATION CRITERIA/DESIRED OUTCOMES

The Patient

- Is afebrile, has other vital signs within normal limits
- Is free from overt bleeding
- Has negative urine and sputum cultures
- Maintains/regains normal hematology studies

NURSING DIAGNOSIS #4

a. **Alteration in nutrition: less than body requirements** related to anorexia, stomatitis, dislike of dietary restrictions
b. **Impairment of skin integrity** related to poor nutritional status, immobility

Rationale: *Symptoms of anorexia, metallic taste, nausea, vomiting, stomatitis, gastrointestinal ulcers, diarrhea, and a dislike for restricted diet may result in inadequate nutritional intake leading to breakdown of body protein and negative nitrogen balance, with resultant impaired skin integrity.*

☐ GOAL

The patient will ingest adequate amounts of prescribed diet; will maintain positive nitrogen balance.

IMPLEMENTATION

- Provide a diet high in carbohydrates, vitamins, and fat, and low in sodium, potassium, and protein (allowed protein should be high in essential amino acids); consult with dietician if patient refuses foods provided; give frequent, small feedings and provide dietary supplements if individual dietary regimen permits.
- Record daily food intake; monitor serum protein levels.
- If patient is unable to tolerate oral intake, administer tube feedings, total parenteral nutrition, intralipids as ordered; refer to *The Patient Receiving Total Parenteral Nutrition,* page 229.
- If antacids are prescribed, ensure they are low in magnesium.
- Change patient position every 2 hours; support and protect bony prominences; provide preventive skin care (e.g., back rub/massage, application of lotion); encourage ambulation as tolerated.

EVALUATION CRITERIA/DESIRED OUTCOMES

The Patient

- Ingests 90% of prescribed diet
- Maintains body weight
- Has normal muscle tone, serum protein levels
- Maintains skin integrity

NURSING DIAGNOSIS #5

Anxiety related to unexpected serious illness and uncertain prognosis

Rationale: *Since ARF can lead to chronic renal failure or death, the patient/family is likely to experience feelings of anxiety about outcome of acute situation.*

GOAL

The patient/family will experience only a moderate amount of anxiety; will understand condition and treatments as necessary and desired.

IMPLEMENTATION

- Plan supportive care and explanations according to family anxiety levels.
- Ask the patient what s/he is feeling and explain that patients usually have a variety of feelings, often similar to those just expressed; provide adequate time to permit patient free expression.
- Communicate progress to patient/family; interpret lab results, vital signs, urinary output, etc., as requested.
- Answer all questions as honestly as possible including fears and questions about death.
- Explain the purpose and sequence of all procedures and treatments; allow the patient to participate in decision making as much as possible.
- Allow control over daily schedule as possible.

EVALUATION CRITERIA/DESIRED OUTCOMES

The Patient/family

- Describes specific condition and likely prognosis accurately
- Participates in decision-making process
- Exhibits decreased anxiety through calm facial expression, relaxed posturing, normal respiratory and heart rates

NURSING DIAGNOSIS #6

Knowledge deficit regarding care after acute episode

Rationale: *The patient/family needs to understand the importance of continued vigilance to preserve existing renal function and to prevent recurrence or progression to chronic renal insufficiency. Depending on readiness to learn, some clients will ask for this information while the patient is still in the critical care unit.*

GOAL

The patient/family will understand the prescribed convalescent regimen.

IMPLEMENTATION

- Assess specific learning needs of patient/family; modify teaching plan accordingly.
- Teach about normal kidney function and discuss alterations that the patient experienced.
- Provide patient with written guidelines for prescribed medications, diet and fluid restric-

tions; review these several times prior to discharge; provide opportunities for questions.
- Review toxic effects of medications; instruct patient to inform physician if toxicity is evident.
- Explain the importance of rest during the recovery phase; assist the patient in planning for exercise as tolerated.
- Review signs of infection; instruct patient to report their occurrence to physician.
- Tell patient/family that full recovery may take up to a year; emphasize importance of obtaining follow-up care as scheduled.

☐ EVALUATION CRITERIA/DESIRED OUTCOMES

The Patient/family
- Describes acute renal failure and prescribed treatment during convalescent phase
- Lists toxic effects of medications, signs of infection, and indications for contacting physician
- Expresses awareness of time required for healing and measures designed to facilitate full recovery.

Table 1 Common Fluid and Electrolyte Imbalances

Imbalance	Precipitating Factors	Signs and Symptoms	Lab Findings
ECF excess (fluid volume excess or overload, hypervolemia)	Excessive IV/oral fluid intake; occurs most commonly because of kidney dysfunction as a result of CHF, liver, or renal disease	Dyspnea, shortness of breath, acute weight gain (more than 5% of body weight), pitting edema, moist rales (crackles) on auscultation of breath sounds, increased BP and CVP, JVD	Decreased RBC, Hct, and Hbg; urine specific gravity less than 1.010
ECF excess (fluid volume excess or overload, hypervolemia)	Excessive IV/oral fluid intake; occurs most commonly because of kidney dysfunction as a result of CHF, liver, or renal disease	Dyspnea, shortness of breath, acute weight gain (more than 5% of body weight), pitting edema, moist rales (crackles) on auscultation of breath sounds, increased BP and CVP, IVD	Decreased RBC, Hct, and Hbg; urine specific gravity less than 1.010
ECF deficit (dehydration, hypovolemia)	GI losses (e.g., vomiting, diarrhea, NG and fistulous drainage, excessive tap water enemas, loss of intestinal juices, intestinal obstruction) decreased oral fluid intake, systemic infection, fever, conditions resulting in plasma-to-interstitial fluid shifts (e.g., burns, ascites), excessive use of diuretics	Dry skin and mucous membranes, poor skin turgor, longitudinal wrinkles or furrows on tongue, weight loss of more than 5% of usual body weight, decreased BP and CVP, nausea and vomiting, anorexia, oliguria	Increased RBC, Hct, Hgb; urine specific gravity greater than 1.030
Hypernatremia (sodium excess)	Excessive water losses that do not change the amount of sodium within the body (thus increasing sodium concentration), decreased oral water intake, excessive ingestion	Vary according to causative factor. *Water deficits:* fatigue and lethargy progressing to seizures and coma, dry and sticky mucous membranes, flushed	Serum Na^+ greater than 145 mEg/liter; urine specific gravity greater than 1.030 (with water deficit); urine Na^+ greater than 40 mEg/liter; elevated BUN, plasma protein,

Table 1 Common Fluid and Electrolyte Imbalances, Cont.

Imbalance	Precipitating Factors	Signs and Symptoms	Lab Findings
	of table salt or bicarbonate soda, prolonged and profuse diarrhea, fever, excessive IV infusion of hypertonic solution, excessive oral protein intake without accompanying increased oral water intake (e.g., fad diets)	skin, poor skin turgor, intense thirst, elevated temparature, tachycardia, decreased BP *Excess sodium intake:* (see signs and symptoms of ECF excess)	serum/urine osmolarity
Hyponatremia (sodium deficit)	Decreased intake or increased output of sodium; increased intake or decreased concentrate output of water, excessive sweating, drinking of plain (electrolyte-free) water, infusion of electrolyte-free IVs, GI losses, repeated water enemas, heat exhaustion, renal disease, burns, Addison's disease, syndrome of inappropriate secretion of antidiuretic hormone (SIADH), psychogenic polydipsia	Vary according to causative factor. *Sodium loss greater than water loss:* signs of dehydration (e.g., dry mucous membranes poor skin turgor, decreased CVP, elevated pulse, malaise, muscle weakness, abdominal cramps, headache, convulsions, oliguria) *Sodium loss and water retention:* signs of water intoxication (e.g., increased CVP, weight gain, headache, apathy, seizures, nausea and vomiting, diarrhea, muscle cramps)	Serum Na^+ less than 136 mEg/liter (with Na+ loss only, normal values if both Na^+ and water lost), urine Na+ less than 20 mEg/liter (with Na^+ loss greater than water loss) or normal to high (with water retention), decreased BUN, Hct, serum and urine osmolarity
Hyperkalemia (potassium excess)	Excessive oral (e.g., salt substitutes) or IV (e.g., too rapid or excess administration) intake, renal disease, adrenal insufficiency, conditions where cellular activity is breaking down or destroying tissues (e.g., MI, burns, crushing injuries, chemotherapy), conditions associated with metabolic acidosis (e.g., shock, renal failure, diabetic ketoacidosis), insulin deficiency (insulin augments entrance of potassium ions into the ICF), digitalis overdose, Addison's disease, massive blood transfusions	Muscle weakness/flaccidity, expecially in lower extremities; intestinal colic/diarrhea; pulse slower than normal; cardiac dysrhythmias, leading to possible cardiac arrest	Serum K^+ greater than 5.5 mEg/liter

Table 1 Common Fluid and Electrolyte Imbalances, Cont.

Imbalance	Precipitating Factors	Signs and Symptoms	Lab Findings
Hypokalemia (potassium deficit)	Decreased dietary intake or excessive losses (e.g., excessive perspiration, prolonged diarrhea, intestinal drainage, polyuria), conditions that cause a shift of potassium from the ECF to the ICF (e.g., alkalosis, increased insulin levels), use of potent diuretics, CHF, pulmonary edema, hypertension, cirrhosis, alcoholism, acute myelogenous leukemia, excess corticosteroids (e.g., stress situations, Cushing's syndrome), sodium retention (e.g., as in edema), hyperaldosteronism	General malaise and apathy; decreased tone in skeletal and smooth muscles (e.g., paralytic ileus, difficulty in voiding); respiratory depression leading to respiratory arrest; muscle cramps; abdominal distension; dizziness on rising; mental confusion; ECG changes: ST segment depression, inverted T waves; cardiac dysrhythmias leading to cardiac arrest	Serum K^+ less than 3.5 mEg/liter
Hypercalcemia (calcium excess)	Inability to excrete excess calcium, demineralization of bones, hyperparathyroidism, malignant neoplastic disease, Paget's disease, overuse of calcium-containing antacids, urinary tract infections, excessive vitamin D supplements, digitalis toxicity, hypophosphatemia (phosphorus and calcium are reciprocally related)	Hypotonicity of muscles, muscle fatigue, weakness, malaise, confusion, headache, lethargy, depression, anorexia, vomiting, thirst, constipation, polyuria, kidney stones, flank pain, pain in deep bones and bone cavities, pathologic fractures, dysrhythmias	Serum Ca^{++} level greater than 5.8 mEg/liter (10.5 mg%); heavy precipitates in urine
Hypocalcemia (calcium deficit)	Insufficient intake of calcium and vitamin D, malabsorption of calcium, excess calcium losses (e.g., with renal insufficiency or hypoparathyroidism), surgical removal of parathyroid glands, hyperphosphatemia, hypomagnesemia (interferes with calcium-elevating effects of parathyoid hormone), peritonitis, pancreatic disease, stress, diuretic phase or renal failure	Tetany, tingling of ends of fingers, carpopedal spasms, convulsions, abdominal/muscle cramps, prolonged QT interval on ECG	Serum Ca^{++} less than 4.5 mEg/liter (8.5 mg%)

Table 1 Common Fluid and Electrolyte Imbalances, Cont.

Imbalance	Precipitating Factors	Signs and Symptoms	Lab Findings
Hypermagnesemia (magnesium excess)	Excess oral intake of magnesium-containing antacids, excess IV magnesium administration, renal failure, hypothyroidism, hyperparathyroidism, Addison's disease	Flushed skin, sense of warmth, drowsiness, lethargy, mental confusion, coma, hypoactive reflexes, depressed respirations, sinus bradycardia, heart block, cardiac arrest	Serum Mg^{++} greater than 2.5 mEg/liter
Hypomagnesemia (magnesium deficit)	Chronic alcoholism (with or without cirrhosis), inadequate dietary intake, prolonged gastric suction; impaired renal conservation of magnesium; intestinal malabsorption syndrome (e.g., after small bowel bypass surgery); prolonged diarrhea; diuretics; primary aldosteronism; hyperthyroidism; acute pancreatitis; gentamicin and cisplatin toxicities	Confusion, dizziness, convulsions, muscle twitching, hyperactive reflexes, parasthesias of feet and legs, pain associated with cold hands and feet, premature ventricular contractions and ventricular fibrillation	Serum Mg^{++} less than 1.5 mEg/liter
Hyperphosphatemia (phosphate excess)	Renal insufficiency, hypoparathyroidism, hypocalcemia, increased catabolism, vitamin D intoxication, myelogenous leukemia, lymphoma	As for hypocalcemia (inverse relationship between calcium and phosphorus within the body); tetany, soft tissue calcification	Serum phosphorus level greater than 3.0 mEg/liter (4.5 mg/dl)
Hypophosphatemia (phosphate deficit)	Hyperparathyroidism, hypercalcemia, respiratory alkalosis, hyperalimentation, malabsorption syndrome, excessive use of antacids that bind phosphorus (e.g., Amphojel, Basaljel), alcoholism	As for hypercalcemia; paresthesias; tremors, ataxia, incoordination, shallow respirations, disorientation, confusion, convulsions, coma	Serum phosphorus level less than 1.2 mEg/liter (2.8 mg/dl)

Table 2 Blood and Blood Components

Blood/Blood Component	Indications	Administration Information
Whole Blood		
• Cellular and plasma constituents plus anticoagulant • Type and crossmatch ABO *identical*	Acute massive hemorrhage with hypovolemia	1 unit = 500 cc IV piggybacked with NS infuse over 2 hr; first 50 cc at 50 gtts/min to test for reaction; continue at 60-80 gtts/min *Expiration:* 35 days after collection *Storage:* 1°-6°C

Table 2 Blood and Blood Components, Cont.

Blood/Blood Component	Indications	Administration Information
Red Blood Cells • Packed red blood cells (PRBC) • Type and crossmatch ABO *identical*	Elderly, debilitated; congestive heart failure; chronic anemia; replace blood loss from surgery; treat chemotherapy-induced erythrocytopenia; 1 unit will increase hemotocrit 3% (average adult)	1 unit = 250-300 cc IV piggybacked with NS over 1½-2 hr *Expiration:* 35 days after collection *Storage:* 1°-6°C
Saline Washed Red Cells • Red cells washed with saline to remove leukocytes, cellular debris, plasma • Type and crossmatch ABO *compatible*	IgA deficiencies; history of multiple severe urticarial/febrile reactions to blood; renal patients; hyperkalemia; bone-marrow transplant patients; paroxysmal nocturnal hemoglobinuria	1 unit = 270 cc IV piggybacked with NS over 2 hr *Expiration:* 24 hr after washing *Storage:* 1°-6°C
Irradiated Red Blood Cells • RBCs exposed to 1,500 rad to eliminate viable lymphocytes • Type and crossmatch ABO *compatible*	Bone-marrow transplant patients; neonates; AIDS patients	Same as Whole Blood
Granulocytes • WBCs extracted from unit of while blood • Type and crossmatch ABO *compatible* • Effectiveness questionable	Septic patients with low WBC not responding to antibiotics; oncology patients with severe bone-marrow depression and progressive infection	1 unit = 300 cc Use within 24 hr of collection IV piggybacked with NS; infuse at 50 gtts/min to test for reaction (first 5 min); continue at 60-80 gtts/min for 2 hr
Platelets • Platelet component harvested from whole blood • No typing required • May be single or multiple donors	Patients actively bleeding withthrombocytopenia/coagulopathies; nonbleeding patients with platelet count less than 10,000 mm^3; platelets may not be as effective if patient is febrile, has infection, DIC or active bleeding, splenomegaly; becomes refractory to random donors	1 unit = 50 cc Usually administered in multiple units IV piggybacked with NS, infuse rapidly (1 unit over 10 min) *Expiration:* 3-5 days (2 hr after pooling) *Storage:* room temperature
Fresh Frozen Plasma (FFP) • Plasma separated from whole blood and frozen • Contains all plasma-clotting factors • Type and crossmatch ABO *compatible*	Bleeding patients with coagulation deficiencies; unknown type of hemophilia	1 unit = 180-275 cc IV piggybacked with NS at 10 cc/min *Expiration:* 1 year (frozen); 24 hr (thawed) *Storage:* 1°-6°C (thawed)
Cryoprecipitated Antihemolytic Factor (AHF) (Factor VIII; fibrinogen)	Treatment of hemophilia A (Factor VIII deficiency); von	1 unit = 10 cc IV at rapid rate (1 unit/min)

Table 2 Blood and Blood Components, Cont.

Blood/Blood Component	Indications	Administration Information
• Prepared by thawing FFP and collecting precipitated protein • No typing required (ABO compatibility preferred but not essential)	Willebrand's disease	*Expiration:* 1 year (frozen) 2 hr (thawed) *Storage:* −18°C
Factor VIII AHF Concentrate (Profilate, Factorate, Koate, Hemofil, Humafac)	Hemophilia A	1 unit = 10 cc *Storage:* 4°C for 2 yr as dry crystals; 3 hr room temperature after reconstitution
Factor IX (Koynex Concentrate, Problex) • Comes from pooled plasma, may be thousands of donors/unit	Hemophilia B; hemophilia A with inhibitor	1 unit = 20-30 cc *Dose:* 1 unit/6 kg body weight initially, then 1 unit/3 kg every 6-12 hr *Storage:* 4°C for 2 yr; room temperature for variable periods
Human Albumin • Made from pooled normal human blood, plasma, or serum • 5% and 25% solution	Expand plasma volume; treat hypoalbuminemia and severe protein loss	*Dose:* 500-1,500 cc given IV with or without dilution (NS) at 1 cc/min, using a filter; administered more rapidly as treatment for shock: 100-200 cc of 25% solution as rapidly as tolerated.

The Patient Undergoing Angiography

Definition/Discussion

Angiography is the radiologic study of blood vessels through the injection of a radiopaque dye. An arteriogram is the visualization of arteries, usually in the head, neck, heart abdomen, or legs. A venogram is the visualization of veins, usually in the lungs or extremities.

Nursing Assessment

☐ **PERTINENT HISTORY**

Medical diagnosis, planned or emergency procedure, allergies to iodine (e.g., Betadine, shellfish)

☐ **PHYSICAL FINDINGS**

Peripheral circulation including presence, strength, location of pulses; warmth and color of skin; mobility and sensations in extremities; vital signs, skin temperature; level of consciousness; hydration status; patency of intravenous route for emergency drugs

☐ **PSYCHOSOCIAL CONCERNS/ DEVELOPMENTAL FACTORS**

Age; sex; occupation; expressions of anxiety regarding procedure/anticipated findings; usual roles and responsibilities; available support system; usual coping mechanisms; meaning of the procedure and possible abnormal findings; potential alteration in life-style

☐ **PATIENT AND FAMILY KNOWLEDGE**

Previous experience/level of knowledge concerning procedure and rationale; readiness and willingness to learn; method to be used; patient participation; when results will be known, usual postprocedure care, self-care needs upon discharge

Nursing Care

☐ **LONG-TERM GOAL**

The patient will undergo angiography free from preventable complications; the patient will understand the diagnostic findings and recommendations for future treatment.

NURSING DIAGNOSIS #1

Alteration in tissue perfusion related to decreased peripheral blood flow, obstruction, and/or hemorrhage

Rationale: *Atherosclerotic plaques can break loose during the procedure and migrate to distant vessels resulting in an obstruction of blood flow and ischemia of tissues distal to the obstruction. Hemorrhage/clot formation at the catheter insertion site may also obstruct flow. Early recognition of decreased tissue perfusion facilitates medical correction of problem before serious problems occur.*

☐ **GOAL**

The patient will have normal tissue perfusion after the procedure.

☐ **IMPLEMENTATION**

- Mark location of pulses with a felt-tip pen to serve as a baseline against which to measure postprocedure observations.
- Check vital signs and tissue perfusion every 15 minutes for 1 hour, then every 30 minutes for 4 hours, and every hour thereafter; compare findings with preprocedure assessment and report changes to physician promptly.
- Keep involved extremity extended to avoid

pressure and potential hemorrhage at insertion site.
- Report bleeding or hematoma formation at insertion site to physician.

☐ EVALUATION CRITERIA/DESIRED OUTCOMES

The Patient
- Has normal peripheral pulses, color, temperature, sensation, and movement in catheterized extremity after the procedure
- Is free from bleeding
- Has normal mentation, no chest pain, and stable vital signs after procedure

> **NURSING DIAGNOSIS #2**
>
> **Alteration in comfort** related to impaired mobility during and after the procedure
>
> ***Rationale:*** *The x-ray table used during the procedure is usually narrow and hard, and the patient may have to lie still for up to 3 hours. After the procedure, the patient must keep the involved extremity straight for several hours to prevent clot formation and/or hemorrhage.*

☐ GOAL

The patient will experience minimal discomfort during and after the procedure.

☐ IMPLEMENTATION

- During preprocedure teaching, explain reason for immobility and methods used to decrease discomfort.
- Have patient void immediately before the procedure to preclude discomfort of a full bladder during the procedure; however, do not limit fluids unless specifically ordered as adequate hydration is needed to promote excretion of the dye.
- Place needed items on tables, in drawers, and near bed within patient's reach to avoid moving involved extremity; secure call signal nearby and instruct patient on its use.
- Use 1 or 2 pillows under patient's head to vary position slightly; do not raise head or foot of bed; lock client controls to avoid accidental flexion of involved extremity.
- Medicate with analgesics as needed; evaluate effectiveness and document response.
- Utilize distraction (visitors, TV, conversation) or other pain-relief measures to remove focus of attention from discomfort.

☐ EVALUATION CRITERIA/DESIRED OUTCOMES

The Patient
- States discomfort is tolerable
- Relieves discomfort with minor position changes, analgesics, noninvasive pain relief measures
- Maintains desired immobility

> **NURSING DIAGNOSIS #3**
>
> a. **Potential for infection** related to invasive procedure
>
> b. **Potential for injury** related to reaction to dye
>
> ***Rationale:*** *Angiography involves a break in the skin and the insertion of a foreign object into the vascular system, thereby enabling the introduction of microorganisms that could result in infection. The patient may be sensitive to the dye and have a reaction varying from vertigo, nausea, skin rash, sneezing, or runny nose to severe reactions resulting in congestive heart failure, anaphylaxis, or loss of consciousness requiring emergency treatment, including CPR.*

☐ GOAL

The patient will be monitored closely for early signs of untoward reactions to the dye; will be protected from potential infection.

☐ IMPLEMENTATION

- Maintain asepsis when changing dressing after the procedure; observe wound for redness or discharge and report immediately; teach how to clean wound at home; obtain cultures of drainage as ordered.
- Administer prophylactic/therapeutic antibiotics on time to ensure appropriate blood levels; monitor for side effects.
- Monitor temperature every 2-4 hours and report elevation.
- Maintain hydration to avoid concentration of dye; keep IV patent and infusing at prescribed rate until patient is able to take adequate oral fluids; teach patient to drink at least 2 liters fluid/day for several days.

- Observe for and report any dye reactions so that treatment may be started immediately.

☐ EVALUATION CRITERIA/DESIRED OUTCOMES

The Patient

- Is free from rash, nausea/vomiting, cold symptoms, tachycardia, hypotension, pulmonary edema
- Maintains a temperature of 98°-99°F (37°-37.5°C) orally
- Has a clean wound with no redness, swelling, or discharge

NURSING DIAGNOSIS #4

a. **Fear** related to invasive procedure, potentially serious findings

b. **Ineffective individual coping** related to anxiety, fear, and/or a diagnosis of serious illness requiring major life-style changes, medical intervention

Rationale: *Many patients fear the procedure or what is partially known about it. Some are anxious about the procedure itself and its inherent discomfort/complications. Others fear the diagnosis may result in the need for further treatment. Some people do not have adequate support mechanisms or coping behaviors to deal with this anxiety and fear.*

☐ GOAL

The patient will express anxiety and fears related to procedure.

☐ IMPLEMENTATION

- Discuss meaning of procedure with patient; encourage expression of concerns and feelings ("Many people are concerned about . . . the feelings they will have when the catheter is inserted, what the doctor will find during the test." "How are you feeling about that?"); give realistic reassurance.
- Identify and encourage patient to use usual coping mechanisms (it is easier to use existing support systems in a stressful experience than it is to learn new behaviors).
- Report observations of excessive anxiety and fear; procedure may need to be delayed until fear and anxiety are reduced.

☐ EVALUATION CRITERIA/DESIRED OUTCOMES

The Patient

- Verbalizes anxieties and fears
- Utilizes available coping mechanisms and support systems to manage anxiety/fear

NURSING DIAGNOSIS #5

Knowledge deficit regarding procedure and self-care upon discharge

Rationale: *New procedures need to be explained to patient to promote full participation in the procedure and discharge care. The informed patient understands the reason for restrictions, is prepared for what to expect, is less frightened when normal sensations occur, and is more willing to cooperate in own care.*

☐ GOAL

The patient will understand and participate in the procedure and discharge care.

☐ IMPLEMENTATION

- Teach about and, if possible, orient to the angiography environment.
- Explain what is expected of the patient during the procedure (to lie still; the physician may ask patient to cough, deep breathe, or hold breath at certain times).
- Tell about sensations commonly experienced during the procedure (e.g., feelings of pressure as the catheter is inserted, sensations of heat or flushing when the dye is injected, feelings of nausea or palpitations).
- Teach to report any pain, shortness of breath, dizziness, or other unusual feelings immediately.
- Explain that the procedure may take up to 2-3 hours because of the time involved in preparing and manipulating the equipment.
- Tell the family/patient when to expect the test results and who will discuss it with them.
- Instruct about care after procedure (keep the involved extremity straight for the specified time, [about 6 hours]; the nurse will check vital signs and circulation frequently; report to nurse numbness, pain, bleeding, or other unusual sensations immediately).

- Instruct to drink extra fluids to help excrete the dye.
- Teach patient/family how to care for the insertion site at home (soap and water and dry Band-Aid) and what observations to make and report to physician (e.g., numbness, pain, drainage from insertion site); write down instructions, phone number to call for assistance, and when to see the physician for follow-up appointment.

☐ EVALUATION CRITERIA/DESIRED OUTCOMES

The Patient

- Describes the procedure and the reasons for it
- States what to expect during the procedure and own role in it
- Complies with activity restrictions immediately after procedure; lists what sensations to report
- Drinks at least 2 liters fluid daily
- Explains and demonstrates wound care before discharge
- States when to see physician again and how to call for answers to questions about self-care before the next regular appointment

The Patient Undergoing an Angioplasty

Definition/Discussion

Angioplasty is an alternative to coronary bypass surgery. Percutaneous transluminal coronary angioplasty (PTCA) is one of the methods used and involves the insertion of a balloon-tipped catheter through one of the conventional cardiac catheterization sites. The balloon is inflated inside a coronary artery to compress plaque against the artery walls and open the lumen of the artery. The procedure is sometimes combined with intracoronary streptokinase treatment. Another type of angioplasty may involve the use of a laser beam.

Angioplasty is usually done for patients with a proximal noncalcified blockage of less than 2 cm in fewer than 2 vessels.

Patients who develop complications during an angioplasty procedure may require coronary bypass surgery.

Nursing Assessment

☐ **PERTINENT HISTORY**

Previous similar episodes of chest pain including frequency and treatment; onset of current chest pain (time, symptoms, precipitating factors, treatment); history of bleeding problems; allergies; current medications; coronary disease risk factors

☐ **PHYSICAL FINDINGS**

Chest pain characteristics (location, radiation, intensity on a scale of 0-10), aggravating or relieving factors; associated symptoms (cough, shortness of breath, nausea and vomiting, palpitations); hemodynamic parameters and vital signs (blood pressure, apical/radial pulse, rhythm disturbances, respirations, temperature, pressure readings from arterial line and/or pulmonary artery catheter if in place); visible pulsations (jugular venous distention, peripheral pulses), warmth of extremities, capillary filling; heart and lung sounds on auscultation; laboratory data (cardiac enzymes, electrolytes, coagulation studies); 12-lead ECG (with and without chest pain) and continuous rhythm monitoring; current chest x-ray results

☐ **PSYCHOSOCIAL CONCERNS/ DEVELOPMENTAL FACTORS**

Coronary risk factors (age, sex, smoking, stress, weight, heredity); occupation; usual coping mechanisms; patient/family reaction to acute illness and planned procedure; roles and responsibilities; available support systems

☐ **PATIENT AND FAMILY KNOWLEDGE**

Level of knowledge; readiness and willingness to learn; possibility of failure and need for emergency coronary bypass surgery; length of procedure (2-3 hours) and patient participation during procedure; expectations of results

Nursing Care

☐ **LONG-TERM GOAL**

The patient will undergo successful angioplasty free from complications; the patient will return home to a pre-illness state of health.

NURSING DIAGNOSIS #1

Alteration in comfort: chest pain related to decreased oxygenation, inadequate perfusion, dysrhythmias

Rationale: *Coronary obstruction causes decreased flow of oxygenated blood to the myocardium; this results in anaerobic metabolism with lactic acid end products that are irritating*

to muscle and cause pain. Dysrhythmias may alter normal filling time of ventricles resulting in decreased cardiac output and decreased coronary blood flow. Dysrhythmias may be caused by myocardial ischemia or inadequate dye excretion during the procedure.

☐ GOAL

The patient will report chest pain promptly; will experience relief of chest pain within 5 minutes of nursing intervention.

☐ IMPLEMENTATION

- Assess the level of discomfort using a 0-10 point self-rating scale to obtain an objective measure of the pain.
- Teach to report chest pain (or other pain in neck, jaw, arm, or shoulder) when it first occurs; explain that delay in reporting may result in further heart damage; discourage the idea that the patient should be tough and wait until the pain is unbearable before notifying the nurse.
- Administer analgesics (morphine), vasodilators (nitroglycerine), and/or antianginal agents; evaluate and record effectiveness.
- Monitor heart rhythm and ECG changes (ST segment changes may indicate ischemia); perform 12-lead ECG during episodes of chest pain; administer antidysrhythmic drugs and monitor effectiveness.
- Assess for shortness of breath and anxiety associated with chest pain; administer oxygen by nasal cannula.
- Maintain bedrest before and for 24 hours after procedure to decrease myocardial oxygen demands.

☐ EVALUATION CRITERIA/DESIRED OUTCOMES

The Patient

- Reports chest pain (or other coronary pain) when it first occurs
- States pain is decreased/relieved with rest, the use of oxygen, or drugs

NURSING DIAGNOSIS #2

Potential for injury (bleeding) related to anticoagulant and thrombolytic therapies

Rationale: *Before, during, and immediately after angioplasty, the patient will be heparinized to decrease the chance of clot formation around the catheter and at the insertion site. Streptokinase may be given either by an IV or by an intracoronary route. These drugs have systemic effects that may produce slight or severe bleeding.*

☐ GOAL

The patient will be monitored for early indications of bleeding.

☐ IMPLEMENTATION

- Observe the catheter-insertion site (usually in femoral area) every 15-30 minutes for bleeding; treat mild to moderate bleeding with manual pressure and, if severe, a sandbag; notify physician who may continue heparinization if bleeding is not severe as reversal of anticoagulation may precipitate undesired clotting.
- Monitor vital signs every 15 minutes for the first 2 hours, every 30 minutes for following 2 hours, every hour for 4 hours, then every 4 hours.
- Assess mental status to monitor for intracerebral bleeding; check urine, stool, nasogastric drainage, and emesis for occult blood; observe sputum for blood; report any positive findings.
- Monitor coagulation studies (therapeutic response to heparin is a partial thromboplastin time (PTT) or an activated PTT (APTT) 2–2½ times the control for 3 days).
- Administer warfarin (Coumadin), aspirin, dipyridamole USP (Persantine) as ordered for long-term anticoagulant and antiplatelet therapy; monitor effectiveness (therapeutic response is prothrombin time [PT] of 2 times normal activity).

☐ EVALUATION CRITERIA/DESIRED OUTCOMES

The Patient

- Maintains usual mental status
- Has clear sputum, negative tests for occult blood
- Has coagulation studies at therapeutic levels without severe bleeding
- Receives prompt treatment for any bleeding

NURSING DIAGNOSIS #3

a. **Fear** related to uncertain success of angioplasty, loss of control
b. **Ineffective individual coping** related to anxiety, fear
c. **Anxiety** related to fear of unknown

Rationale: *Although most angioplasties are successful, the patient needs to understand that complications may develop necessitating emergency cardiac surgery. Loss of personal control is especially frightening to the patient who has type A personality characteristics (as these patients often do). This results in anxiety, fear, and altered coping responses.*

☐ GOAL

The patient will effectively cope with feelings of anxiety and fear before undergoing angioplasty.

☐ IMPLEMENTATION

- Provide a calm environment; include patient in care planning and decision making as much as possible.
- Provide adequate information to decrease fear of the unknown and to enable the patient to cope with realistic concerns.
- Encourage patient/family to share mutual concerns; answer all questions honestly.
- Instruct in alternative coping measures such as verbalization or use of social support systems.
- Administer sedation, if necessary; evaluate and record effectiveness.

☐ EVALUATION CRITERIA/DESIRED OUTCOMES

The Patient

- Expresses feelings about the upcoming procedure
- Identifies and uses adaptive coping mechanisms to decrease anxiety
- Verbalizes realistic concerns about the procedure

NURSING DIAGNOSIS #4

Alteration in cardiac output: decreased related to decreased tissue perfusion, complications of procedure Refer to *The Patient Undergoing Cardiac Catherization,* Nursing Diagnosis #1, page 51.

NURSING DIAGNOSIS #5

Alteration in tissue perfusion related to compromised circulation to catheterized extremity Refer to *The Patient Undergoing Cardiac Catherization,* Nursing Diagnosis #2, page 52.

NURSING DIAGNOSIS #6

Alteration in comfort related to immobility Refer to *The Patient Undergoing Cardiac Catherization,* Nursing Diagnosis #3, page 52.

NURSING DIAGNOSIS #7

Potential for infection related to invasive procedure Refer to *The Patient Undergoing Cardiac Catherization,* Nursing Diagnosis #4, page 53.

NURSING DIAGNOSIS #8

Knowledge deficit regarding procedure, postprocedure care, care after discharge

Rationale: *Inadequate knowledge may add to anxiety and interfere with the patient's ability to cooperate with nursing care. After discharge, the patient will need to administer own medications, have regular blood tests done, and receive continuing medical care.*

☐ GOAL

The patient will understand the purpose of angioplasty and expected results before the procedure; will cooperate with postprocedure restrictions; will understand own role in home care before discharge.

☐ IMPLEMENTATION

- Refer to *The Patient Undergoing Cardiac Catherization,* page 51.
- Tell patient that s/he may feel chest pain when the balloon is inflated, but that the pain will be relieved in 5-7 seconds when the balloon is deflated.
- Teach that the catheter as well as the arterial and pulmonary artery lines will remain in place (usually the groin) for several hours after the procedure.
- Reinforce the need for bedrest with head of the bed elevated less than 30° for 24 hours, or longer if there is bleeding.
- Reinforce physician's teaching that angioplasty may be unsuccessful or result in complications necessitating emergency cardiac surgery; give brief pre-op cardiac surgery instructions; refer to *The Patient Undergoing Cardiac Surgery: Preoperative Phase,* page 61.
- Encourage the patient/family to ask questions and express feelings.
- In preparation for discharge, explain indications, effects, and toxic effects of anticoagulant and antiplatelet therapy; instruct to notify physician of any signs of bleeding (e.g., tarry stools, flank pain, hematuria).
- Instruct not to substitute acetaminophen for aspirin (does do not have platelet-inhibiting effects).
- Instruct not to take over-the-counter drugs without physician's consent.
- Assist to identify coronary disease risk factors and to plan how to modify these to decrease chance of future coronary obstruction.
- Make referrals as appropriate for follow-up care, reinforcement of instructions, assessment of compliance, medical follow-up, dietary modification, or smoking cessation classes.

☐ EVALUATION CRITERIA/DESIRED OUTCOMES

The Patient

- Explains purpose of procedure correctly
- Lists possible complications of procedure and their treatment
- Explains own role and activity restrictions during and immediately after the procedure
- Lists discharge medications and precautions to be taken with anticoagulants
- Identifies coronary disease risk factors and states how to modify them
- Makes plans for medical follow-up

The Patient with an Aortic Aneurysm

Definition/Discussion

An aortic aneurysm is a localized dilated area of the thoracic or abdominal aorta. It can be *saccular* (not affecting entire circumference of vessel) or *fusiform* (involving entire circumference). In *dissecting-type* aneurysm blood is forced between layers of the vessel wall. Type A aneurysms involve the ascending aorta; type B identifies those in the descending aorta.

Treatment involves prompt surgical resection with replacement of affected section by a Dacron or Teflon graft. Surgery may be ruled out as a treatment option depending on site (descending aorta) or patient condition (over 80 years of age, concomitant unrelated terminal illness, or documented renal failure). Pain is the predominant symptom and varies with the type and speed of aneurysm development; patient may also be asymptomatic.

Nursing Assessment

☐ PERTINENT HISTORY

Family history of aneurysms or arteriosclerosis; hypertension, trauma, syphilis, or infection with necrosis of the media vessel layer

☐ PHYSICAL FINDINGS

Palpable, pulsating mass in the abdominal aorta region; pain in upper back or lumbar region that may radiate to the buttocks; hyper/hypotension, tachycardia/bradycardia; hemoptysis, bloody stools, nausea/vomiting

☐ PSYCHOSOCIAL CONCERNS/ DEVELOPMENTAL FACTORS

Age, sex (most common among middle-aged males); complications following surgery; physical, psychologic strengths; life-style (e.g., need to stop smoking, lose weight, eliminate maladaptive stress factors); fear of dying

☐ PATIENT AND FAMILY KNOWLEDGE

Understanding of condition, risks of surgery, level of knowledge, readiness and willingness to learn

Nursing Care

☐ LONG-TERM GOAL

The patient will be hemodynamically stable in preparation for surgical intervention; the patient will recover from surgery and return to usual roles in home, family, and community after a moderate convalescence. If inoperable because of critical condition, the patient will be sustained for as long as possible; the patient/family will be helped to cope with the crisis of loss.

NURSING DIAGNOSIS #1

a. **Anxiety** related to condition, impending surgery
b. **Knowledge deficit** regarding surgery, post-op course

Rationale: *The grave prognosis associated with aneurysm and the need for emergency surgery is likely to cause concern for the patient and family. Anxiety may be minimized with explanation/demonstration of procedures, treatments. Pre-op teaching is necessary to increase patient's active role in care and to promote compliance with treatment plan postoperatively.*

☐ GOAL

The patient/family will experience a decrease in anxiety; will express realistic expectations of post-op regimen; patient will be able to carry out post-op deep breathing, coughing, and exercise routines.

☐ IMPLEMENTATION

- Provide time to listen to feelings/concerns of patient/family; answer questions and try to calm fears; reassure that these feelings/concerns are valid.
- Consult with surgeon regarding expected post-op regimen; explain to patient what to expect (e.g., ventilator; central venous pressure, arterial pressure, or pulmonary catheter line(s); nasogastric tube).
- Explain pre-op procedures; provide additional explanations as needed; refer to *The Patient Undergoing Angiography,* page 20.
- Instruct about post-op routine, importance of coughing; demonstrate plantar flexion leg exercises and have patient return demonstration.
- Assure that adequate pain medication will be given.
- Assess previous coping strategies and assist patient/family to find effective strategies; initiate referrals to clergy or social worker as needed.

☐ EVALUATION CRITERIA/DESIRED OUTCOMES

The Patient/family

- Expresses decrease anxiety
- Describes immediate post-op regimen

The Patient

- Satisfactorily demonstrates coughing and exercises

NURSING DIAGNOSIS #2

Alteration in cardiac output: decreased related to effects of untreated aneurysm

Rationale: *An aortic aneurysm can lead to hemodynamic instability. When an aneurysm begins to leak, rapidly enlarge, or dissect, hypoperfusion of organs results. The patient may become hypertensive as the body attempts to compensate for the decreased blood supply. Immediate treatment with potent vasodilators to lower blood pressure should be initiated/monitored.*

☐ GOAL

The patient will maintain hemodynamic stability.

☐ IMPLEMENTATION

- Monitor and record vital signs and hemodynamic readings every 4 hours or as needed; check for bruits in femoral arteries; watch for widening pulse pressure; record peripheral pulse readings (dorsalis pedis) in both legs.
- Be alert for signs of peripheral vasoconstriction (e.g., cold, clammy skin or weak/absent peripheral pulses) and impaired renal tissue perfusion (e.g., decreased urinary output), which may be indicators of compensated decreased cardiac output; report significant findings to physician.
- If systolic blood pressure exceeds parameter established by physician, administer vasodilator prescribed; obtain systemic blood pressure reading every 5-15 minutes and titrate medication to achieve systolic pressure reading indicated by physician; monitor for effectiveness and toxicity.

☐ EVALUATION CRITERIA/DESIRED OUTCOMES

The Patient

- Demonstrates adequate/stable circulatory status

NURSING DIAGNOSIS #3

a. **Alteration in tissue perfusion: peripheral** related to low circulating blood volume, hypotension
b. **Fluid volume deficit** related to blood loss during aortic aneurysm repair

Rationale: *It is imperative to keep the patient adequately hydrated and to maintain normal cardiopulmonary status to ensure adequate tissue perfusion and decrease the likelihood of the graft occluding. Abnormally low blood pressure and/or decreased fluid volume may lead to decreased vascular perfusion.*

☐ GOAL

The patient will maintain normal vital signs; will demonstrate adequate tissue perfusion; will maintain adequate intake of fluid and electrolytes.

☐ IMPLEMENTATION

- Check dressings for blood or drainage at least every 4 hours; use abdominal binder to provide support and comfort for moving or coughing.
- Take vital signs frequently, report changes; monitor and record dorsalis pedis pulses at same times (use Doppler if pulses not palpable).
- Record warmth, color, sensation, and movement of extremities.
- Record intake and output carefully and accurately; report urinary output of 30 cc or less/ hour; adjust IV rate as ordered by physician or hospital protocol.
- Maintain patient in relatively flat position for about a week, avoiding extreme flexion that would increase abdominal pressure or impair leg circulation.
- Report post-op back pain (may indicate retroperitoneal hemorrhage or a thrombus developing at graft site).
- Report leg numbness or inability to move (may indicate transient local edema exerting pressure on femoral nerve or a developing arterial thrombus).
- Encourage and monitor leg exercises at least every 2-3 hours; remove and reapply elastic stockings at least every 8 hours.
- Give ice chips while NPO; after bowel sounds return and patient is allowed oral fluids, note amount and tolerance; progress to regular diet as ordered and tolerated.
- Give analgesics, sedatives, antibiotics, and other medications as ordered; monitor for effectiveness and observe for untoward reactions.

☐ EVALUATION CRITERIA/DESIRED OUTCOMES

The Patient

- Has balanced intake and output, stable electrolytes
- Maintains stable cardiopulmonary status, vital signs, and circulation

NURSING DIAGNOSIS #4

Fear related to severity of illness, inoperable condition, possible death

Rationale: *In the critically ill patient, the physiologic parameters are indicators of the overall success or failure of treatment regimens. Frequently, the condition is so severe that surgery cannot even be performed. The patient is powerless over own condition and faces the threat of dying. Fear of dying, whether surgery is performed or not, is an emotional response consciously recognized by the patient, and is related to the internal or external source of danger.*

☐ GOAL

The patient will identify/verbalize fears; will experience a reduction in the level of fear.

☐ IMPLEMENTATION

- Observe for behavioral manifestations of fear (e.g., refusal of treatment; increased vital signs; aggressive/critical attitude to staff; frequent use of call light; constant crying; somatic symptoms/complaints such as nausea, diarrhea; constant questioning).
- Assess patient's response to and perceptions regarding the diagnosis, treatments, equipment in a calm, unhurried manner.
- Provide time for patient to ventilate specific fears concerning future/dying.
- Reduce environmental stimulation (e.g., use dim lights, lower auditory stimuli, promote privacy).
- Allow family to participate in care as much as possible.
- Administer sedation/analgesics; evaluate effectiveness.
- Provide verbal/nonverbal support (e.g., hand holding while patient verbalizes feelings; sitting next to patient when the opportunity exists); if on ventilator, provide alternate means of communication (e.g., pad and paper, erasable slate, system of nods or taps to indicate yes or no).
- When patient feels upset, stay at bedside.
- Organize care to reduce sleep deprivation, increase rest periods.
- Encourage patient/family interaction (e.g.,

telephone calls to home, pictures of family in room, extending visitation rules).
- Assess religious preference and offer to contact clergy of choice; provide privacy to carry out religious practices.
- Implement referrals to social services, psychiatric liaison as needed.

☐ EVALUATION CRITERIA/DESIRED OUTCOMES

The Patient
- Identifies specific source(s) of fear
- Discusses fears with others
- Expresses reduction in level of fear
- Demonstrates relaxed posture, calm facial expression

NURSING DIAGNOSIS #5

Knowledge deficit regarding care of operative site, length of convalescence, diet, medications

Rationale: *If the patient is to return to normal roles in the home/job/community, s/he must have sufficient knowledge to be able to care for the incisional site and to adhere to the medical regimen. In addition, the patient may need strategies to adjust life-style (e.g., smoking cessation, low-salt diet, weight reduction, moderate exercise).*

☐ GOAL

The patient will verbalize risk factors that can increase blood pressure and decrease circulation; will satisfactorily demonstrate the ability to care for the operative site; will know indications, expected effects, names, dosage, and how to take prescribed medications; will verbalize the need for gradually increasing physical activity.

☐ IMPLEMENTATION

- Provide a written appointment, date, and time for follow-up visit to surgeon.
- Instruct on prescribed operative site care; plan to provide this instruction to permit time for patient/family to return demonstration; reinforce correct procedure and reinstruct as needed.
- Teach about prescribed diet (sodium-restricted to prevent hypertension); avoid constipating foods to decrease strain and pressure on graft site.
- Discuss ways of maintaining normal blood pressure by adapting to a more sedentary, less stressful life-style; initiate referral to psychologist if needed.
- Instruct about prescribed medications: explain any expected action, dosage, administration schedule, and side effects; advise to contact physician should side effects develop.

☐ EVALUATION CRITERIA/DESIRED OUTCOMES

The Patient
- Demonstrates correct care of the operative site
- Verbalizes accurate knowledge of diet, medications, activity, follow-up care
- Expresses a willingness to modify life-style in necessary ways

The Patient with Asthma

Definition/Discussion

Asthma is an intermittent, reversible, obstructive disorder of the respiratory tract. It is one of the three conditions (along with chronic bronchitis and pulmonary emphysema) collectively known as chronic obstructive pulmonary disease (COPD). Asthma, manifested by wheezing, dyspnea, and coughing, results when the individual experiences bronchial smooth muscle constriction, mucosal edema, and excess mucus production. Asthmatic episodes fall on a continuum from infrequent, mild events to severe, life-threatening crises (e.g., status asthmaticus).

Extrinsic (allergic) asthma is most frequently seen in patients with known allergies (e.g., hay fever, nasal allergies) or with a family history of allergy. The bronchospasm associated with extrinsic asthma is part of the immune response to the causative allergen. The onset of extrinsic asthma is usually during childhood or adolescence.

Intrinsic asthmatic episodes may be precipitated by infection, environmental changes, emotional stress, and ingestion of medications. Bronchospasm is associated with an imbalance of the individual's autonomic nervous system. Onset of intrinsic asthma is typically after age 35 and it develops into a chronic, fulminating condition. Patients with either intrinsic or extrinsic asthma may experience exercise-induced episodes.

Medical treatment aims at prevention and relief of symptoms during asthmatic episodes. Preventive measures prescribed may include avoidance of known bronchial irritants, desensitization to unavoidable irritants (e.g., house dust), and prophylactic use of medications by oral and inhalant routes. Medical treatments aimed at allaying symptoms during acute asthmatic episodes include the use of bronchodilators (e.g., theophylline, epinephrine), adrenocorticosteroids, and intermittent positive pressure breathing. When mucus plugs cannot be expelled by coughing or removed by suctioning, a bronchoscopy may be performed for lavage and aspiration. In severe crisis situations, mechanical ventilation may be required.

Nursing Assessment

☐ PERTINENT HISTORY

Duration of wheezing; precipitating events (e.g., upper respiratory infection, allergens, exercise, stress); medications used (prescribed regimen and specific medication/s last taken, including dose and time); prior experience with asthmatic episodes; allergies; smoking; high-risk occupation (involving inhalation of known respiratory irritants); physical environment (living in a geographic area with known air pollution); family history

☐ PHYSICAL FINDINGS

Tachypnea; increased breathing effort; dyspnea in chronic conditions; use of accessory muscles; breath sounds: rhonchi, rales, wheezing (with very little air flow, wheezing may be minimal or absent); chest x-rays: usually clear, with hyperinflation in persistent, long-standing conditions; arterial blood gases: normal or may indicate hypoxia with acidosis in acute crises; pulmonary function studies: forced expiratory volume (FEV), peak flow (PEFR), and vital capacity are abnormally low while total lung capacity (TLC) and residual volume (RV) are increased; tachycardia; ECG: prominent P waves with chronic asthma; increased eosinophil count; theophylline levels: toxicity or within therapeutic range

☐ PSYCHOSOCIAL CONCERNS/ DEVELOPMENTAL FACTORS

Age (present and at time of onset); coping mechanisms; support system; disease-related changes in habits (smoking) and/or life-style (occupation, activity level, or residence); anxiety regarding air hunger, hospitalization, treatment, diagnostic procedures; with chronic condition, increasing dependence upon others

☐ PATIENT AND FAMILY KNOWLEDGE

Disease process/treatment; precipitating factors; preventive measures; guidelines for self-care, medications, exercise regimen, and use of ventilatory aids; level of knowledge, readiness and willingness to learn

Nursing Care

☐ LONG-TERM GOAL

The patient will attain optimal health and maintain a normal life-style through control of asthmatic episodes. The patient in a severe asthmatic crisis will regain adequate respiratory function.

NURSING DIAGNOSIS #1

a. **Ineffective airway clearance** related to bronchospasm, mucosal edema, and ineffective cough
b. **Ineffective breathing pattern** (tachypnea) related to anxiety, "air hunger," fear of suffocating
c. **Impaired gas exchange** related to obstruction (mucus/inflammation) of trachea, bronchi, bronchioles, and hyperinflation of alveoli

Rationale: *Irritants/allergens/stressors create a change in the lower airway environment, triggering an immune and/or autonomic nervous response producing bronchoconstriction, mucosal wall edema, and increased mucus production. Hyperinflation of the lungs results in trapped air in the alveoli, decreasing the volume that can be forcefully expelled as a cough.*

In times of distress, the "air-hungry" patient may increase the rate but not the depth of respirations, using all energy just to breathe, making respiration a muscular rather than normal, involuntary act. With intrinsic asthma, the parasympathetic component of the autonomic nervous system dominates the sympathetic component, producing bronchoconstriction and bronchospasm rather than promoting bronchodilation as with healthy individuals.

Interference with alveolar ventilation may occur because of chronic obstruction of the air flow in and out of the lungs. Hyperinflation of the alveoli alters the ventilation/perfusion balance with resultant impaired gas exchange.

☐ GOAL

The patient will maintain an unobstructed airway; will be able to inspire and exhale air without wheezing or the use of accessory muscles; will demonstrate an effective respiratory rate with normal air exchange in the lungs.

☐ IMPLEMENTATION

- Monitor respiratory rate/effort, blood pressure, heart rate, skin color, mental status, and auscultate breath sounds every 15-30 minutes during severe episodes, then every 1-4 hours; watch for signs of acute respiratory insufficiency/failure (e.g., tachycardia with dysrhythmias, initial hypertension changing to hypotension, restlessness or agitation, impaired judgment, loss of consciousness, apnea); obtain pulmonary function studies as ordered.
- Call for assistance should respiratory failure occur; remain with patient, initiate resuscitative measures; prepare for possible endotracheal/tracheal intubation and mechanical ventilation; refer to *The Patient who is Ventilator-Dependent*, page 239.
- Ensure that ventilator is functioning properly
  - check alarm system
  - remove excess moisture from tubing
  - maintain closed system/ordered settings
  - monitor response by observation, auscultation, and obtaining/reviewing arterial blood gases as ordered
- Administer oxygen at ordered flow rate (usually 4-8 liters/minute, unless patient has chronic carbon dioxide retention; then, 2 liters/minute); use nasal prongs since mask tends to increase anxiety about suffocating; ensure proper humidification to decrease upper airway irritation and liquefy secretions.
- Assess need for suctioning (e.g., inability to expectorate, dyspnea, tachycardia, rhonchi,

diminished/distant breath sounds, restlessness/agitation) every 1-2 hours; gently suction as needed, monitor for signs of distress (e.g., bloody aspirant, bradycardia, bronchospasm); record amount and appearance of secretions; obtain sputum specimens as ordered.

- Disconnect catheter if bronchospasm occurs while suctioning (disconnected catheter serves as artificial airway); remove catheter after spasm has ended; remain with patient, calmly provide reassurance and explain what happened.
- Prepare patient, as ordered, for bronchoscopy to remove mucus plugs; provide concise explanations, reinforce what physician has told patient/family; correct misunderstood concepts; validate appropriate understanding; answer specific questions.
- Position for comfort and to decrease energy expenditure (e.g., high-Fowler's with additional pillows as needed; leaning on pillow on overbed table, in chair, or on side of bed); use hypoallergenic bed linens/pillow cases if available.
- Maintain patent IV line for administration of medications; monitor for desired response and untoward effects of drugs (e.g., increased heart rate/dysrhythmias with theophylline preparations).
- Provide intermittent positive pressure breathing (IPPB), percussion/vibration of lower lobes, and postural drainage as ordered; collaborate with respiratory therapist to reinforce regimen; administer pain medication PRN prior to procedures to enhance patient participation/comfort; monitor/record results.
- Plan time, after acute episode has subsided, for patient/family to express feelings about asthma attacks; listen attentively, acknowledge that many other patients have expressed similar feelings.

☐ EVALUATION CRITERIA/DESIRED OUTCOMES

The Patient

- Has normal respiratory rate without use of accessory muscles, breath sounds, blood gases, and pulmonary function studies
- Expectorates secretions
- Expresses decreased anxiety about suffocating

NURSING DIAGNOSIS #2

Fluid volume deficit related to tachypnea, dyspnea, decreased oral fluid intake

Rationale: *Insensible water loss from tachypnea and water loss from diaphoresis secondary to dyspnea will deplete total body water. During the acute episode, the patient will likely have a decreased oral intake because of fatigue, difficulty swallowing, or nausea secondary to prescribed medications (e.g., theophylline preparations).*

☐ GOAL

The patient will maintain adequate hydration.

☐ IMPLEMENTATION

- Ensure adequate fluid intake (combined oral/IV of at least 3,000 cc/day, unless contraindicated [e.g., patients with congestive heart failure]); administer prescribed IV fluids; encourage oral fluids as tolerated.
- Ascertain fluid preferences and offer frequently (clear, warm/tepid liquids will likely be best tolerated during acute episode, although some patients may prefer cold drinks and Popsicles; avoid milk since it tends to increase mucus secretions).
- Record intake; report increased tolerance of oral fluids to physician and collaborate regarding decreasing rate of IV fluids accordingly.
- Monitor urinary output/record weight as an indication of fluid balance (output should equal 2/3 to 3/4 of intake; weight should remain stable).
- Assess skin, mucous membranes, conjunctiva every 8 hours for signs of dehydration (e.g., brittle, dry skin with decreased turgor, dry, pale mucous membranes/conjuctiva); report significant findings to physician.
- Monitor serum electrolytes for detection of related imbalances; report abnormal levels to physician.

☐ EVALUATION CRITERIA/DESIRED OUTCOMES

The Patient

- Ingests 2,500-3,000 cc/fluid/day
- Has urinary output (800-2,500 cc/day) indica-

tive of fluid balance when compared with intake
- Maintains stable weight
- Displays moist mucous membranes/conjunctiva and good skin turgor
- Has serum electrolytes within normal limits

NURSING DIAGNOSIS #3

a. **Alteration in nutrition: less than body requirements** related to increased energy expenditure, decreased intake during acute asthmatic episode
b. **Potential for infection** related to compromised nutritional status, immunosuppression secondary to pharmacologic regimen (corticosteroids)

Rationale: *Oral intake during the initial phase of an acute asthmatic episode is likely to be negligible, especially if it is a severe episode. Even after the crisis has been resolved, fatigue after prolonged increased respiratory effort may prevent the patient from attaining adequate nutritional intake orally.*

If sufficient protein and calorie intake is not provided, the patient catabolizes muscles for fuel, contributing to atrophy of the respiratory muscles. Nutritional support may improve respiratory muscle functioning and increase energy levels, thus decreasing the effort required for breathing.

When nutritional status is impaired, the patient is at greater risk for infection than when adequate nutrition is provided. Moreover, patients receiving corticosteroids to decrease inflammation of the respiratory passages may be further at risk for infection because of the suppressive action on the immune system initiated by these drugs.

☐ GOAL

The patient will maintain adequate nutrition; will remain free from infection.

☐ IMPLEMENTATION

- Assess the patient's nutritional status: consider height, weight, body frame, ideal weight; condition of hair, skin, nails, and mouth; provide prescribed diet, recording oral intake/calorie count.
- Assess prehospitalization dietary regimen, noting food preferences; collaborate with dietician to plan acceptable diet.
- Encourage full consumption of prescribed diet; consider smaller, more frequent meals if easily fatigued; have family and friends bring in favorite foods; provide small high-protein, high-calorie supplements between meals; administer supplemental vitamins and minerals as ordered.
- Consult with physician about starting tube feedings if patient is unable to maintain oral intake (total parenteral nutrition may also be considered but it is not the usual choice since it increases the risk for infection).
- Monitor daily weight; report loss of 3 lb or more to physician.
- Monitor laboratory studies for indications of negative nitrogen balance (decreased serum proteins), immunosuppression (immunoglobulin deficiencies), and infection (positive cultures, increased WBC, presence of acute-phase proteins); report abnormal findings to physician.
- Monitor vital signs as ordered, watching for signs indicative of infection (e.g., elevated temperature, hypotension); report significant findings to physician.
- Observe/record amount and character of secretions; send purulent secretions for culture and monitor lab results.
- Caution visitors and staff with colds to wear mask or to not enter patient's room.
- Keep tissues handy at bedside; provide disposable container for soiled tissues; remove when filled or every 4-8 hours.
- Administer antibiotics on time to maintain blood levels; monitor for desired and untoward effects.

☐ EVALUATION CRITERIA/DESIRED OUTCOMES

The Patient

- Ingests an oral intake sufficient to provide required nutritients
- Maintains a stable weight
- Remains free from infection

NURSING DIAGNOSIS #4

Activity intolerance related to dyspnea and fatigue

Rationale: *During an acute asthmatic episode the patient may be unable to perform tasks re-*

quiring even minimal energy expenditure without exertional dyspnea. Exercise may have been a precipitating factor of the asthmatic episode. Physical activity should be gradually increased after resolution of the acute crisis. Strategies that promote self-awareness of fatigue and recognition of early signs of exertional dyspnea may be effective in preventing future acute episodes.

☐ GOAL

The patient will be able to perform activities of daily living free from dyspnea or fatigue.

☐ IMPLEMENTATION

- Determine usual patterns of activity and fatigue; attempt to schedule required activities at times when the patient usually has more tolerance.
- Plan care to conserve patient's limited amount of energy, providing rest periods before and after planned activities/treatments.
- Keep supplies within easy reach of patient.
- Assist in discovering point of fatigue so that patient does not exceed it; if current episode was exercise induced, allow patient to ventilate feelings/concerns about the specific situation and/or the disease process in general.
- Encourage attempts to decrease or stop smoking; explain the compounding effect of this additional irritant; if close family members smoke, encourage them to curtail smoking in patient's presence.
- Discuss prescribed exercise regimen and physical conditioning program with physician and exercise physiologist; encourage patient participation in plan; explain purpose of regimen/program (to increase exercise tolerance by gradually increasing activity while promoting optimal pulmonary functioning).

☐ EVALUATION CRITERIA/DESIRED OUTCOMES

The Patient

- Demonstrates decreased dyspnea on exertion
- Has increased ability to perform daily activities with less fatigue
- Has pulmonary function studies within normal limits

NURSING DIAGNOSIS #5

a. **Ineffective individual coping** related to recurrent asthmatic episodes and required life-style changes
b. **Disturbance in self-concept: role performance** related to increased dependency caused by effects of chronic illness
c. **Ineffective family coping** related to role performance change of patient

Rationale: *When asthma becomes a chronic condition, it may disrupt the normal lifestyle/roles of the patient and family. With frequent acute episodes and related activity intolerance, the individual may find that s/he is more dependent upon others than previously. Depending upon the precise role the individual has in the family and his/her self-concept, this may be distressing to the patient, family, or both. Financial expenditures related to treatment or time lost from work may upset the family's financial stability. Healthy members of the family may feel that too much attention is being given to the patient.*

☐ GOAL

The patient/family will adapt to illness-related role and life-style changes with minimal alteration in family functioning.

☐ IMPLEMENTATION

- Plan care to permit time to sit with patient or family members at least 15 minutes each day to elicit feelings/concerns regarding this hospitalization and the changes having a family member with asthma has brought about; recognize/accept negative feelings, indicating that others have expressed similar complaints.
- Review baseline assessment for previously effective coping mechanisms; explore with patient/family the possibilities for employing similar strategies at this time; when possible, offer alternatives, encouraging patient/family to choose solutions.
- Recognize the financial and emotional strains on the patient/family; initiate referral to social service if assistance required.
- Identify available community informational and supportive resources.

☐ EVALUATION CRITERIA/DESIRED OUTCOMES

The Patient/family

- Identify impact of patient's asthma on individual role/family life
- Develop strategies for making required changes
- State they are receiving adequate family support
- Identify appropriate community resources for continued assistance in coping as needed

> **NURSING DIAGNOSIS #6**
>
> **Knowledge deficit** regarding treatment regimen
>
> ***Rationale:*** *Knowledge of factors that precipitate asthmatic episodes and reasons for the treatment regimen will enable patient to have greater control over subsequent acute episodes, use health care assistance more appropriately, and maintain a more functional lifestyle.*

☐ GOAL

The patient will have sufficient information about precipitating factors, medications, and inhalers to promote control of asthma.

☐ IMPLEMENTATION

- Instruct to prevent acute asthmatic episodes by avoiding exposure to respiratory irritants (e.g., smoking, air pollution, pollens, allergens, extreme variations in temperature or humidity, excessive physical exercise).
- Discuss the signs of an impending acute episode (e.g., cough, wheezing, fever, nausea/vomiting, increased anxiety/tension); suggest measures to minimize distress (e.g., position changes, rest, medications, fluids, stress-reduction techniques).
- Teach to protect self from respiratory infections by avoiding exposure to persons with known infection, avoiding crowds and poorly ventilated spaces, being immunized against influenza (if not allergic), taking prescribed prophylactic antimicrobials, practicing good oral hygiene, and promptly reporting any sign of respiratory infection (e.g., chest pain; change in color, character, or amount of sputum; increased difficulty breathing or talking; sore throat, fever, or chills).
- Teach about the use of prescribed medications
  - provide list of medication names, actions, side effects, dosages, and schedules
  - remind the patient, if steroids are prescribed, that they may mask the signs of infection by suppressing the inflammation response
  - identify signs of toxicity and inform patient/family to contact physician if signs occur; explain that untoward effects may be eliminated by changing doses or medications
  - avoid self-medication with over-the-counter preparations that may suppress coughing and dry secretions.
- Discuss methods to remove secretions easily: maintaining an adequate fluid intake (8-10 glasses of fluid/day), using humidification to loosen and mobilize secretions, and following postural drainage and breathing exercises as prescribed.
- Review respiratory therapy aids to be used after discharge or reinforce respiratory therapist instructions; ensure the patient has a written list of instructions; have the patient practice assembling and disassembling equipment; review prescribed times for treatments and indications for use.
- Encourage maintenance of body tone by regular exercise as tolerated; instruct to use medications (e.g., cromolyn sodium) prior to exercise; refer to community service agencies or private exercise physiologist for specific programs if available.

☐ EVALUATION CRITERIA/DESIRED OUTCOMES

The Patient/family

- Identifies situations or agents that precipitate an asthmatic attack and strategies for avoiding precipitating factors
- Recognizes the signs of an impending attack and states measures to minimize distress
- Identifies factors that precipitate activity intolerance and strategies to prevent acute asthmatic episodes
- Knows prescribed medications, desired actions, schedule for administration, side effects
- States measures to prevent exposure to infection and reasons to contact physician

The Patient with an Automatic Implantable Cardioverter-Defibrillator

Definition/Discussion

The automatic implantable cardioverter-defibrillator (AICD) is an implantable device to prevent the occurrence of sudden cardiac death. The AICD continuously monitors the patient's heart rate and rhythm, detects rapid ventricular dysrhythmias above 150 beats/minute within seconds, and delivers a shock to the heart to restore normal sinus rhythm. The AICD's sensing system identifies ventricular tachycardia or fibrillation by detecting the amount of time the ECG signal does not spend at baseline. These 2 rhythms spend very little time at baseline, whereas the ECG configuration of normal sinus rhythm spends a great deal of time at the isoelectric line.

Nursing Assessment

☐ PERTINENT HISTORY

Life-threatening dysrhythmias, especially during electrophysiologic studies; failure of conventional drug therapy for dysrhythmias; idiopathic cardiac dysrhythmias; dilated cardiomyopathy; refractory coronary artery disease, both ischemic and nonischemic for which cardiac surgery is not a viable option; medical and surgical history.

☐ PHYSICAL FINDINGS

Vital signs, especially blood pressure, heart rate and rhythm; ECG, 24-hour Holter monitor; *with dysrhythmia*: level of consciousness (LOC), palpitations, syncope, vertigo; *with surgical procedure*: site of incision including condition of wounds and dressing, patency of IV, rate and character of respirations, breath sounds, oxygen therapy utilized, pain, hematoma at generator site, localized edema.

☐ PSYCHOSOCIAL CONCERNS/ DEVELOPMENTAL FACTORS

Age, sex, type of work, educational and developmental level, present and past coping patterns, interpersonal relationships, available support systems, body image, patient/family anxieties about procedure/anticipated prognosis and ability of AICD to function correctly, previous experience with illness and hospitalization.

☐ PATIENT AND FAMILY KNOWLEDGE

Level of knowledge and understanding of present condition, readiness and willingness to learn, expectations of post-op site, understanding of therapy especially when AICD is activated, expectations for discharge and home care, ability to follow through on discharge instructions, need for continued follow-up care.

Nursing Care

☐ LONG-TERM GOAL

The patient will successfully undergo insertion of the automatic, internal cardioverter-defibrillator; the patient will understand discharge instructions and the need for routine follow-up.

NURSING DIAGNOSIS #1

a. **Alteration in cardiac output: decreased** related to dysrhythmias, compromised myocardial function
b. **Alteration in tissue perfusion: cardiac, cerebral** related to dysrhythmias, compromised myocardial function

Rationale: *Dysrhythmias, especially lethal ventricular dysrhythmias, will result in decreased filling time and, with a compromised myocardium, ineffective pumping action. Over the course of time, decreased cardiac output results in reduced organ and tissue perfusion due to an extended period of hypoperfusion that occurs with ventricular tachycardia or fibrillation. Decreased blood flow to the brain also causes alteration in consciousness and thought process. Underlying cardiomyopathy and advanced coronary artery disease further reduce the effectiveness of the heart as a pump. These conditions are usually present in patients who require an AICD. Patients who require an AICD usually have a long history of alteration in cardiac output/tissue perfusion.*

☐ GOAL

The patient will have improved cardiac output and tissue perfusion.

☐ IMPLEMENTATION

- Note and document the on/off status of the AICD and number of seconds required to start the sequence of events that lead to discharge by the AICD; obtain an ECG strip to document actual discharge by the AICD.
- Monitor vital signs, especially blood pressure and pulse, every 1 to 2 hours and progress to every 4 hours; if applicable, monitor hemodynamic parameters, including cardiac output, at least every 4 hours.
- Monitor ECG for ventricular dysrhythmias, especially premature ventricular contractions (PVC) or bursts of ventricular tachycardia.
- Observe and assess patient's mentation during periods of dysrhythmias.
- Have on hand IV antidysrhythmic medications (e.g., lidocaine, procainamide hydrochloride [Pronestyl], bretylium tosylate [Bretylol]).
- Be prepared to institute cardioversion or defibrillation
  - defibrillate only if ventricular fibrillation occurs (cardioversion is the preferred countershock treatment)
  - do not place paddles over the AICD
  - set voltage at 50-100 watt seconds and increase if the patient is not successfully cardioverted
- Institute cardiopulmonary resuscitation (CPR) if countershock is unsuccessful or if the AICD malfunctions and dysrhythmias persist.

☐ EVALUATION CRITERIA/DESIRED OUTCOMES

The Patient

- Has warm, dry skin with normal peripheral pulses, color, and capillary filling
- Maintains cardiac output of 4-7 liters/minute and a cardiac index of 2.5-4 liters/m^2
- Has normal mentation
- Is free from cardiac dysrhythmias

NURSING DIAGNOSIS #2

a. **Powerlessness** related to inadequate knowledge of the need, function, and placement of the AICD
b. **Anxiety** related to impending surgery, misinformation, concern over AICD, unknown causes
c. **Fear** related to impending surgery, concern over AICD, unknown causes

Rationale: *Fear, anxiety, and powerlessness are quite common considering the patient's diagnosis and prognosis if AICD is not successful. Patient fears are usually compounded by previous hospitalizations in which dysrhythmia therapy was either unsuccessful or patient had numerous episodes requiring countershock.*

☐ GOAL

The patient will experience decreased fear and anxiety during hospitalization; will express sense of control over some aspects of treatment.

IMPLEMENTATION

- Encourage patient/family to verbalize fear and anxieties once information has been reviewed.
- Provide reassurance to the patient/family during the course of the hospitalization, with daily update of the patient's progress and activities.
- Provide frequent one-to-one interactions as necessary to decrease patient's apprehension (this can be done while giving direct patient care, when the family is visiting, or when nurse has assessed that patient is experiencing fear and/or anxiety).
- Allow patient choices when possible; permit increasing independence.

EVALUATION CRITERIA/DESIRED OUTCOMES

The Patient

- Identifies sources of fear/anxiety
- Discusses fears with nurses/family
- Makes rational choices regarding treatments
- Has realistic concerns concerning implantation of AICD

NURSING DIAGNOSIS #3

a. Impaired gas exchange related to surgical incision site, ineffective cough, pain, immobility, inadequate lung expansion

b. **Ineffective breathing pattern** related to surgical incision site, ineffective cough, pain, immobility inadequate lung expansion

Rationale: *If a thoracotomy is utilized, the patient will be prone to developing respiratory complications such as pneumonia and pneumothorax. In the post-op phase, the patient is reluctant to cough and deep breathe for fear of rupturing the suture line or because of pain. Immobility results in pooling of secretions in dependent areas of the lung, inadequate lung expansion predisposes the patient to developing atelectesis and/or pneumonia.*

GOAL

The patient will maintain adequate oxygenation; will have improved gas exchange.

IMPLEMENTATION

- Assess need for pain medication by asking patient to rate pain on a 0-10 scale.
- Provide moderate analgesic for pain; administer 1 hour prior to respiratory treatments to make the patient more comfortable.
- Assess vital signs, especially if respiratory depressant is administered.
- Auscultate breath sounds at least every 4 hours.
- Establish turning schedule; assist to ambulate 3 times a day during the first 1-2 post-op days or until s/he can ambulate by self.
- Encourage deep breathing and effective coughing at least every 2 hours; splint area with a pillow, tell patient to take 3 breaths and cough.
- Encourage use of incentive spirometer; hve patient perform the exercise at least every 2 hours.
- Increase IV or oral fluids to liquify secretions; weigh patient each morning to ensure that patient with compromised cardiac status is not overhydrated.
- Maintain precise intake and output; check for sacral and pedal edema at least every 8 hours.
- Auscultate breath sounds every 2 to 4 hours.

EVALUATION CRITERIA/DESIRED OUTCOMES

The Patient

- Coughs and deep breathes effectively
- Has clear breath sounds bilaterally
- Has blood gases within an acceptable range for the patient
- Is free from respiratory complications

NURSING DIAGNOSIS #4

Potential for infection related to invasive procedure, surgical incision

Rationale: *AICD implantation involves interruption of skin integrity, thereby making the patient susceptible to postimplant infectious process. Site of infection could be systemic or local. In addition, all patients have some type of invasive line, including peripheral IVs or pulmonary artery catheters. Long-standing cardiac disease patients may be weak and debilitated, significantly delaying wound healing.*

GOAL

The patient will be free from infection.

IMPLEMENTATION

- Monitor incision site for redness, swelling, warmth, hematoma, or fluid accumulation at least every 8 hours.
- Clean incision with hydrogen peroxide using aseptic technique on a daily basis.
- Observe for bleeding onto the dressing site for the first 24 hours.
- Leave incision open to air after the first 24 hours to promote wound healing.
- Monitor vital signs, especially temperature, every 4 hours.
- Monitor WBC and differential count.
- Administer prophylactic IV antibiotics as ordered; monitor for side effects.
- Monitor BUN and creatinine as necessary.

EVALUATION CRITERIA/DESIRED OUTCOMES

The Patient

- Maintains normal temperature
- Has evidence of good wound healing with clean dry incision line
- Has no hematoma or fluid accumulation at generator site

NURSING DIAGNOSIS #5

Alteration in comfort: pain related to surgical incision, invasive line, shock from AICD, AICD wire becoming displaced or broken

Rationale: *The patient will experience post-op pain depending on the surgical site and the patient's own pain threshold. A lateral thoracotomy or median sternotomy is frequently performed and the resulting pain is similar to that after cardiac surgery. If the subxyphoid or subcostal approach is utilized, the patient should experience less discomfort. When the AICD fires, the shock produces a physical jolt that is similar to countershock; it is also described by patients as a sharp blow to the chest. A displaced or broken wire causes pain where the wire is malfunctioning. This pain is similar to chest pain and radiates from the subclavian area to the abdomen.*

GOAL

The patient will maintain an adequate level of comfort.

IMPLEMENTATION

- Assess level of discomfort and determine origin of pain (e.g., incisional, AICD firing, wire malfunction); use a 0-10 self-rating scale to obtain an objective measure.
- Record location, duration, intensity, and precipitating and relieving factors.
- Administer analgesics as ordered; evaluate for effect after 30 minutes.
- Instruct patient that the shock from AICD will be felt and to anticipate a discomfort that is similar to a sharp blow to the chest.
- Determine if pain is noncardiac; prepare patient for x-ray and possible surgery for replacement of misplaced wire.

EVALUATION CRITERIA/DESIRED OUTCOMES

The Patient

- Has minimal discomfort
- Verbalizes where the pain originates
- Differentiates discomfort from AICD from other possible sources of discomfort

NURSING DIAGNOSIS #6

Knowledge deficit regarding implantation procedure, post-op care, discharge instructions, and routine follow-up care

Rationale: *Patients frequently report a variety of treatment modalities utilized before the decision to have an AICD is recommended. The treatments usually include either frequent countershock, multiple hospitalizations, multiple attempts at testing various dysrhythmic drugs. The AICD is a relatively new treatment and the patient/family will need realistic reassurance regarding the actual procedure and what to expect after implantation. Patients need explicit discharge instructions regarding what to do when the AICD fires and how to anticipate complications (e.g., battery failure, AICD malfunction). Routine follow-up is essential for this patient population.*

GOAL

The patient will understand the purpose of the AICD implantation procedure and what to expect in the post-op phase; will verbalize discharge activity instructions and participate in routine follow-up care.

IMPLEMENTATION

- Provide patient/family with booklet on AICD provided by manufacturer; ensure that patient understands written material; if unable to comprehend the material, provide additional clear, simple information.
- Orient about what to expect the day of the implantation.
- Explain post-op care especially if sternotomy or thoracotomy approach is utilized; review coughing and deep breathing, use of incentive spirometer, need for pain medication.
- Review the sensations the patient should experience when AICD fires.
- Provide patient/family with written discharge instructions on what to do when the AICD fires
  - have patient lie down
  - initiate CPR if AICD fails after 4 fires or after 30 seconds and unconsciousness occurs
  - if patient is alone, s/he should call ambulance at the first sign of palpitations.
- Stress need for battery check every month for the first year, then every 2 months, and generator check every 3 months after the first year.
- Explain the need for family to learn CPR; provide with a list of resources to obtain instruction.
- Provide with written self-care instructions
  - patient can exercise, swim, jog, have sexual relations
  - patient cannot drive since threat of dysrhythmias and loss of consciousness still exist
  - patient can swim or bathe without fear of electrocution

EVALUATION CRITERIA/DESIRED OUTCOMES

The Patient

- Verbalizes knowledge of implantation procedure
- Describes post-op care accurately in own words
- Complies with discharge instructions
- Keeps follow-up appointments

The Patient with Burns

Definition/Discussion

Burns are injuries to tissues caused by thermal (e.g., flame, liquid), chemical, electrical, and/or radioactive agents. The outcome of burn injury is the denaturation of protein, resulting in cell injury or death. The care of the patient following burn injury oftentimes requires a lengthy physiologic, emotional, and functional rehabilitation.

Nursing Assessment

☐ **PERTINENT HISTORY**

Mechanism of burn injury, past medical history, allergies, medications taken, loss of function of actual body part, dietary habits

☐ **PHYSICAL FINDINGS**

Vital signs, level of consciousness; depth of burn (layers involved); extent of burn (percentage of total body surface area involved); presence of factors indicative of smoke inhalation (e.g., stridor, carbonaceous sputum, blackened tongue, dry cracked lips, singed nasal hairs, erythema of pharynx); cherry-red lips; urinary output; circumferential burns; arterial blood gases; serum electrolytes; fluid status; bowel sounds, presence of infection, constipation, diarrhea, level of pain, activity tolerance, sleep patterns.

☐ **PSYCHOSOCIAL CONCERNS/ DEVELOPMENTAL FACTORS**

Age, sex, patient/family interaction, ethnicity, cultural background, financial status, usual coping mechanisms, changes in role or responsibility, uncooperativeness, sleeplessness, pain, acceptance/adaptation to altered body image, anxiety, fear, grief, feelings of powerlessness, isolation caused by susceptibility to infection, noncompliance with health care treatments

☐ **PATIENT AND FAMILY KNOWLEDGE**

Perception of health status, disease condition, noncompliance with treatment; educational level, readiness and willingness to learn

Nursing Care

☐ **LONG-TERM GOAL**

The patient will recover from the burn without loss of function of any body part; the patient will recover maximum potential use of the involved body part(s).

NURSING DIAGNOSIS #1

a. **Impaired gas exchange** related to heat exposure, inhalation injury, edema of laryngeal structures
b. **Ineffective breathing pattern** related to heat exposure, inhalation injury, edema of laryngeal structures
c. **Ineffective airway clearance** related to retained secretions, imposed position

Rationale: *Byproducts of combustion cause pneumonitis, resulting in destruction of respiratory cell protein and loss of cilia. Heat exposure results in an increased capillary leak in the respiratory structures causing edema of the respiratory passages. Inability to expectorate retained secretions as a result of a decreased cough reflex may lead to an altered respiratory status.*

☐ **GOAL**

The patient will maintain an adequate airway.

IMPLEMENTATION

- Maintain patent airway with high-flow oxygen (100%) unless contraindicated.
- Monitor respiratory rate and characteristics of respiration at least every hour and as necessary.
- Monitor for level of consciousness changes every hour to determine cerebral oxygenation.
- Observe for communication difficulties that may indicate increasing edema of laryngeal structures.
- Monitor for dyspnea, stridor, or hoarseness.
- Auscultate breath sounds every 2 hours to detect abnormal sounds.
- Measure tidal volume and vital capacity to assess for changes indicating decreasing respiratory ability.
- Suction gently as needed using aseptic technique to maintain patent airway.
- Assist with bronchoscopy to determine extent of respiratory injury.
- Monitor arterial blood gas values for acid-base abnormalities and decreased oxygen saturation.
- Monitor carboxyhemogloblin level to determine carbon monoxide poisoning.
- Monitor eschar formation on chest or neck that could compromise respiratory status.
- Administer drugs to support immune response (e.g., GamImmune).
- Administer intermittent positive pressure breathing treatments to prevent alveolar collapse.
- Provide chest physical therapy to maintain patent airway.
- Turn, cough, and deep breathe patient every 2 hours to mobilize secretions.
- Be ready for intubation with an endotracheal tube or tracheostomy; refer to *The Patient with a Tracheostomy*, page 236; have emergency tray nearby.

EVALUATION CRITERIA/DESIRED OUTCOMES

The Patient

- Is free from laryngeal edema, stridor, or hoarseness
- Maintains arterial blood gases within normal limits
- Has no adventitious breath sounds
- Exhibits lucid level of consciousness

NURSING DIAGNOSIS #2

a. **Alteration in cardiac output: decreased** related to evaporative fluid loss, hemorrhage, inadequate fluid resuscitation
b. **Fluid volume excess** related to iatrogenic fluid overload
c. **Fluid volume deficit** related to inadequate fluid resuscitation, evaporative fluid loss, hemorrhage
d. **Alteration in tissue perfusion: cardiopulmonary/renal** related to fluid loss, edema, thrombosis, stasis, hypovolemia
e. **Alteration in patterns of urinary elimination** related to inadequate fluid resuscitation, fluid loss, hemoconcentration

Rationale: *Capillary destruction in burn injury initiates an initial plasma-to-interstitial-fluid shift causing hypovolemia, which may also result from inadequate fluid replacement. In the absence of adequate fluid replacement, hemolysis of red blood cells and release of myoglobin from damaged muscles leads to decreased renal perfusion. Following the initial plasma-to-interstitial-fluid shift, fluid then begins to leak back into the plasma from the interstitium, causing hypervolemia if fluid resuscitation is not carefully monitored.*

GOAL

The patient will maintain adequate blood volume and fluid and electrolyte balance; will excrete adequate urinary output.

IMPLEMENTATION

- Record weight of patient as soon as possible after admission.
- Monitor vital signs at least every hour and as needed; observe for trends.
- Record accurate fluid intake (e.g., oral, IV) and output (e.g., urine, nasogastric [NG] suction) every hour.
- Start IV with large-bore needle (#14 or #16).
- Insert Foley catheter utilizing aseptic technique.
- Titrate fluid replacement based on urine output, central venous pressure (CVP), level of

consciousness, or other parameters used in your institution.
- Administer crystalloid and/or colloid fluid per hospital protocol.
- Observe hemodynamic parameters for changes in stability caused by fluid overload or hypovolemia.
- Assess for signs and symptoms of inadequate fluid replacement/impending shock (e.g., restlessness, disorientation, excessive thirst, increased pulse, decreased blood pressure, decreased urine output, CVP less than 5 cm water).
- Assess for signs and symptoms of excessive fluid replacement/pulmonary congestion/pulmonary edema (e.g., dyspnea, venous engorgement, moist rales, increased blood pressure, CVP greater than 15 cm water).
- Assess ECG for dysrhythmias that may result from electrical burn injury or hemodynamic instability.
- Monitor laboratory results and report those that directly reflect a fluid and electrolyte imbalance (most frequent laboratory requests include electrolytes, hemoglobin, hematocrit, glucose, serum proteins, serum potassium, serum sodium, BUN, creatinine, and urinalysis).
- Administer potassium-restricted foods/fluids if patient is hyperkalemic; refer to Table 1, *Common Fluid and Electrolyte Imbalances,* page 14.
- Measure circumference of burned areas to determine if edema is increasing.
- Prepare for escharotomy and/or fasciotomy if circumferential edema or constriction of burn eschar compromises circulation.
- Elevate, if possible, all burned areas to allow for venous return.
- Monitor distal peripheral pulses utilizing a Doppler if necessary; notify physician immediately and prepare for fasciotomy if pulses are unobtainable.
- Observe urine for hematuria or brownish red color indicative of intravascular hemolysis related to thrombosis/hemomyoglobinuria.

☐ EVALUATION CRITERIA/DESIRED OUTCOMES

The Patient

- Has body weight change of less than 1 lb
- Maintains CVP between 5 and 15 cm water
- Is hemodynamically stable
- Maintains electrolytes within normal levels
- Excretes at least 0.5-2.0 cc/kg/hour

NURSING DIAGNOSIS #3

a. **Alteration in comfort: pain** related to tissue edema and destruction, eschar debridement, other treatments
b. **Ineffective thermoregulation** related to loss of protective layer of skin
c. **Hypothermia** related to loss of protective layer of skin

Rationale: *Pain receptors left intact will respond to pressure caused by edema or manipulation during treatments resulting in pain. Patients rarely experience total burn anesthesia since deep partial thickness or superficial partial thickness burns are usually peripheral to full thickness injuries. The skin functions to conserve body heat. Destruction of skin disrupts that ability thus promoting rapid cooling of the body.*

☐ GOAL

The patient will maintain an adequate level of comfort.

☐ IMPLEMENTATION

- Determine level of discomfort considering depth and extent of injury, areas of involvement, age, other pathology present, and previous treatment.
- Assess the level of discomfort using a 0-10 point self-rating scale to obtain an objective measure of the pain.
- Maintain an accurate record of amount, time, and type of medication utilized (too much medication, too soon, can cause respiratory difficulties); chart effect.
- Administer sedation/pain medication IV to increase adequate absorption; give 30 minutes-1 hour prior to treatments, debridement procedure, and application of topical agents to ensure patient comfort and adequate relaxation.
- Administer pain medication cautiously, judiciously, and conservatively, ensuring that patient is given adequate relief but is not overmedicated.
- Provide diversional activity to distract patient from the pain experience.
- Maintain environmental temperature at approximately 76°-82°F to ensure warmth and

comfort of patient. Monitor patient temperature every hour.
- Refer to *The Patient Experiencing Pain,* page 180.

☐ EVALUATION CRITERIA/DESIRED OUTCOMES

The Patient
- Verbalizes decreased pain
- Participates in care
- Maintains normothermia

NURSING DIAGNOSIS #4

a. **Impairment of skin integrity** related to loss of protective layer, poor wound healing, decreased nutritional replacement, decreased tissue perfusion
b. **Potential for infection** related to open wounds, poor wound healing, inadequate healing of skin grafts.
c. **Impaired tissue integrity** related to open wounds, poor wound or skin graft healing

Rationale: *Decreased tissue perfusion causes aggregation of cellular debris in the microcirculation, thus preventing adequate blood supply for healing. Decreased nutritional intake, especially of proteins, increases the risk of poor wound healing because insufficient nutrients are provided for tissue repair. Loss of the first line of defense against infection and formation of eschar provides an excellent culture medium for growth of infectious bacteria on the original burn wound or donor skin and recipient sites. In addition, the patient with a burn has a compromised immune response. Multiple exogenous factors contribute to the risk of infection (e.g., Foley catheter, IV, CVP) as well as nonadherence to aseptic practices by staff and visitors.*

☐ GOAL

The patient will be free from wound infection.

☐ IMPLEMENTATION

- Determine the type of isolation techniques to be used; wear gowns, gloves, and masks to help keep the bacterial count to a minimum.
- Maintain an aseptic environment using sterile equipment and supplies.
- Observe for signs and symptoms of infection (e.g., malodorous wound drainage, elevated leukocyte count, elevated temperature).
- Use strict sterile technique when changing dressings.
- Administer antibiotics and observe response.
- Prepare for hydrotherapy treatments and eschar debridement (tangential excision, enzymatic debridement). Explain importance. Encourage participation.
- Apply topical antimicrobials and bacteriostatic agents.
- Prepare for grafting procedures, maintaining asepsis of donor and recipient sites.
- Obtain cultures from wounds, preventing contamination from skin flora.
- Prevent skin surfaces from touching to prevent autocontamination.
- Assess the necessity to continue isolation techniques; monitor laboratory data.
- Shave or clip body hair that may harbor bacteria.
- Provide special site care for face, eyes, ears, or perineum.
- Observe for signs and symptoms of infection (e.g., malodorous wound drainage, elevated leukocyte count, elevated temperature).
- Observe for signs and symptoms of septicemia (e.g., positive blood cultures, hemodynamic changes).
- Discourage visits from family or friends with infections.
- Administer tetanus immunization prophylactically.
- Use strict sterile technique when changing a dressing.
- Administer antibiotics, medications to support immune response, and observe patient response.
- Apply topical antimicrobials and bacteriostatic agents; evaluate and document effectiveness.
- Prepare for tangential excision, enzymatic debridement by explaining procedures, providing pre-op care.
- Prepare for grafting procedures maintaining asepsis of donor and recipient sites; utilize wet soaks to injured tissue; observe viability of donor and recipient sites during dressing changes; identify patient concerns and questions regarding the procedure.
- Know about various skin grafts that may be used including

- *homograft* (allograft): skin taken from another living person or from a cadaver; this type of graft is usually temporary but with the advent of newer immunosuppressant drugs such as cyclosporin A, the graft may be more permanent
- *heterograft* (xenograft): a temporary graft taken from an animal, usually porcine, or made of synthetic material
- *autograft:* skin taken from the patient's own viable tissue.

- Provide post-op skin graft care; elevate grafted extremity or part; avoid excessive pressure on area from tight dressings; do not use tape on skin; observe for excessive bleeding at sites; monitor lifting up of graft resulting from edema, which decreases viability of graft; observe for decreased viability of recipient site evidenced by darkening of graft edges (violaceous borders) or purulent drainage.

☐ EVALUATION CRITERIA/DESIRED OUTCOMES

The Patient

- Has negative wound and blood cultures
- Exhibits evidence of autograft acceptance
- Maintains temperature within normal limits
- Is free from drainage or odor from wound
- Exhibits no edema or decreased viability of recipient skin graft site

NURSING DIAGNOSIS #5

a. **Alteration in nutrition: less than body requirements** related to increased caloric requirement, decreased caloric intake, inadequate intake of nutrients, paralytic ileus

b. **Alteration in bowel elimination: constipation/diarrhea** related to inadequate intake of nutrients, nasogastric (NG) tube feedings, paralytic ileus

c. **Alteration in oral mucous membranes** related to inadequate oral intake or oral hygiene

Rationale: *Patients with burns become hypermetabolic, requiring increased caloric intake to maintain nutritional state. Gastric hemorrhage caused by Curling's ulcer and paralytic ileus are results of the gastric dilatation that occurs during the stress response to the burn injury. Hypertonic tube feedings may cause diarrhea, while inadequate fluid intake may cause constipation and disruption in the oral mucous membranes.*

☐ GOAL

The patient will maintain adequate nutrition; will demonstrate adequate gastrointestinal motility.

☐ IMPLEMENTATION

- Insert NG tube; attach to low intermittent suction.
- Administer hyperalimentation; refer to *The Patient Receiving Total Parenteral Nutrition,* page 229.
- Administer tube feedings.
- Monitor pH of gastric aspirate for a decrease indicating hyperacidity.
- Administer antacids through the NG tube, clamping tube following administration.
- Administer high-calorie, high-protein tube feedings or oral diet when tolerated; establish small, frequent feeding interspersed with high-calorie, high-protein snacks; work with patient/family regarding food likes and dislikes; refer to dietician as necessary.
- Provide an environment conducive to eating (e.g., remove soiled dressings, bedpans, and other distractors; eliminate offensive odors).
- Assess ongoing nutritional status; observe oral mucous membranes; assess skin turgor.
- Provide oral hygiene every 4 hours.
- Provide adequate rest to ensure that patient is not too tired to eat.
- Weigh patient daily.
- Maintain accurate intake and output records.
- Auscultate bowel sounds every 4 hours.
- Assess ongoing nutritional status.
- Monitor bowel evacuation for constipation or diarrhea.

☐ EVALUATION CRITERIA/DESIRED OUTCOMES

The Patient

- Consumes 75% of ordered diet
- Maintains weight at least at preburn level
- Is free from paralytic ileus
- Has gastric aspirate negative for occult blood
- Exhibits pink, moist oral mucosa without lesions

NURSING DIAGNOSIS #6

a. **Ineffective individual coping** related to body-image changes
b. **Alteration in family process** related to severity of injury, possible death of self or family member, helplessness
c. **Fear** related to physiologic and emotional disruption, painful procedures
d. **Grieving** related to actual/perceived loss of body part
e. **Anxiety** related to unknown outcome of burn therapy, anticipation of pain, unfamiliar and painful procedures
f. **Ineffective family coping** related to body image changes of patient
g. **Spiritual distress** related to seriousness of situation
h. **Powerlessness** related to inability to change situation
i. **Social isolation** related to perceived appearance
j. **Noncompliance** with treatment protocols related to perceived hopelessness

Rationale: *The burn patient/family is unprepared for the traumatic nature of the devasting injury and is maybe unable to manage both the internal and external stressors because of compromised resources. Responses to loss following a burn injury usually include fear of physical discomfort, disfigurement, mutilation, or death. In addition, patients will demonstrate concerns regarding abandonment, surgical procedures, and lengthy convalescence. These fears and concerns may be real or unfounded. Resolution in either event may take from several weeks to months or years depending on the severity of burn, course of treatment, and individual response to treatment.*

☐ GOAL

The patient/family will verbalize feelings about changes in own body; will cope with the extent and number of losses; the patient/family will adapt to changed life-style.

☐ IMPLEMENTATION

- Give as much information as patient/family want to help decrease fear and anxiety.
- Encourage to talk about current situation and feelings; provide empathic listening.
- Encourage participation and cooperation in care.
- Continue to help to express feelings about current status, fears; listen actively; incorporate other health care personnel as appropriate.
- Reinforce use of adaptive defenses while patient/family moves through grieving stages; refer to *The Patient Experiencing Grief and Loss,* page 272.
- Plan experiences for the patient to control, manipulate, and succeed in to decrease feelings of powerlessness (e.g., allow to make some decisions regarding own care, schedule).
- Refer patient for cosmetic counseling as appropriate since an enhanced physical appearance may improve patient's body image.
- Assess importance and impact of appearance changes; discuss with patient/family.
- Provide careful explanation of procedures to dispel fears.
- Organize care to prevent undue pain and anxiety.
- Inform patient/family of any signs of progress.
- Project calm, unhurried attitude while performing procedures.
- Demonstrate respect for patient/family.
- Allow for privacy when visitors are with patient.
- Provide for financial and spiritual counseling as desired.
- Refer to *The Patient Experiencing Grief and Loss,* page 272, and *The Patient Experiencing a Body-Image Disturbance,* page 253.

☐ EVALUATION CRITERIA/DESIRED OUTCOMES

The Patient/family

- Experiences anxiety at no more than a minimum level
- States realistic perception of burn injury
- Expresses fears, grief, anxieties, feelings about self
- Utilizes family for support
- Uses situational support for adaptation
- Refer to clergy for support

NURSING DIAGNOSIS #7

a. **Potential for injury** related to contractures and immobility
b. **Self-care deficit: total** related to immobility, reduced range of motion
c. **Diversional activity defit** related to impaired mobility, decreased self-care ability
d. **Activity intolerance** related to impaired range of motion (ROM)

Rationale: *The burn patient is at increased risk for contracture formation as a result of immobilization of a body part. Immobilization of a burn wound encourages formation of hypertrophic scarring, a powerful tightening of skin and underlying structures. The patient is at risk for the development of other complications resulting from immobility, including decubitus ulcer formation, bone demineralization, and sensory alterations. Decreased sensory stimulation, sensory monotony, and sensory deprivation may alter the patient's perception of the environment.*

☐ GOAL

The patient will be free from complications associated with immobility.

☐ IMPLEMENTATION

- Provide for proper positioning and immobilization of burn wound/graft site using splints, traction, etc.; consult with physical or occupational therapist to plan adaptive devices for patient use; encourage patient/family participation in planning.
- Provide active and passive ROM exercises at least daily; utilize hydrotherapy as necessary.
- Turn at least every 2 hours to prevent formation of pressure areas.
- Provide diversional therapy; encourage visits from family and friends; place a clock and calendar within patient's field of vision; reorient to surroundings as necessary; refer to *The Patient Experiencing Sensory Alteration,* page 275.

☐ EVALUATION CRITERIA/DESIRED OUTCOMES

The Patient

- Performs ROM exercises of all joints at least daily
- Participates in activities of daily living to extent possible
- Participates with staff to develop activity/rest schedule

NURSING DIAGNOSIS #8

Knowledge deficit regarding burn injury

Rationale: *Following an acute burn injury, measures to maintain life will be the priority in patient care. Most interventions utilized during this phase are not part of routine health maintenance procedures and therefore will be new to the patient. Inadequate preparation may lead to patient/family misconceptions of current and future health status.*

☐ GOAL

The patient will demonstrate adequate knowledge of all procedures and their rationale.

☐ IMPLEMENTATION

- Assess patient's/family's level of understanding of treatment.
- Explain all procedures prior to beginning new and ongoing procedures.
- Encourage verbalization and questions by patient/family; correct misconceptions.
- Discuss impact of returning to home/work/family after a prolonged hospitalization; identify specific physical and emotional needs necessary to function at home.
- Monitor patient's/family's continuing level of understanding of treatment and home care; teach as necessary.
- Encourage to ask questions.
- Explain and demonstrate new procedures that need to be done after discharge; have patient/family return demonstration.
- Assist to plan for economic, creative, and social needs upon return to home environment.
- Instruct on medication effects, side effects, dosage, and reportable symptoms of medication overdosage; give written instructions.
- Discuss patient's future with regard to the rehabilitation phase of burn injury.

EVALUATION CRITERIA/DESIRED OUTCOMES

The Patient

- Verbalizes knowledge of procedures and their rationale
- Cooperates with health team in all phases of care
- Identifies effects, side effects, dosage, and reportable symptoms of prescribed medications
- Plans homebound economic, social, and creative activities
- Outlines specific goals for rehabilitation

The Patient Undergoing Cardiac Catheterization

Definition/Discussion

Cardiac catheterization is a procedure in which a catheter is placed in the heart chambers and arteries to determine the functioning and condition of the heart and arteries.

Nursing Assessment

☐ PERTINENT HISTORY

History of cardiovascular symptoms; family history of cardiovascular disease; patient/family history of related diseases/risk factors; allergies (especially to iodine, Betadine, or shellfish); current medications

☐ PHYSICAL FINDINGS

Vital signs, especially blood pressure, heart rate and rhythm, pulse deficits; ECG pattern; peripheral perfusion; urine output; level of consciousness; syncope; fluid balance; respiratory status; chest pain, shortness of breath; intermittent claudication

☐ PSYCHOSOCIAL CONCERNS/ DEVELOPMENTAL FACTORS

Age, sex, type of work; smoking habits; drinking habits; use of recreational drugs; hobbies/ ways to relax; relationships with others; eating patterns; educational level; sexual activity; usual coping mechanisms; available support systems; patient/family anxieties about procedure/anticipated diagnosis/treatment

☐ PATIENT AND FAMILY KNOWLEDGE

Knowledge of cardiac anatomy and of procedure to be done including preparation for procedure, technique to be used, patient's participation in procedure, and postprocedure care; level of knowledge; readiness and willingness to learn

Nursing Care

☐ LONG-TERM GOAL

The patient will experience a successful cardiac catheterization with minimal anxiety, free from preventable complications.

NURSING DIAGNOSIS #1

Alteration in cardiac output: decreased related to decreased tissue perfusion, complications of procedure (i.e., hemorrhage, cardiac perforation, excessive diuresis, myocardial infarction).

Rationale: *During the catheterization, the underlying valvular, coronary, or myocardial disease may result in less blood volume to the ventricle for ejection, excessive blood volume causing congestion, or poor pumping action of the ventricle. All of these result in decreased cardiac output and decreased blood flow to tissues. In addition, complications such as hemorrhage and excessive diuresis cause decreased venous return, decreased left ventricular filling, and decreased cardiac output. The most severe complications, myocardial infarction and cardiac perforation, result in decreased functioning of the myocardium and poor pumping action of the heart.*

☐ GOAL

The patient will have adequate cardiac output and tissue perfusion.

☐ IMPLEMENTATION

- Monitor vital signs and periperal pulses after procedure every 30 minute for 3 hours to detect changes from patient's baseline; decreased blood pressure, increased pulse rate, decreased peripheral pulse volume may indicate low cardiac output.
- Monitor level of consciousness and report confusion or disorientation to physician immediately.
- Record accurate intake and output; if patient has Foley catheter in place, measure output every hour to detect fluid imbalance from rapid osmotic diuresis due to dye, or low output due to decreased blood flow to kidneys.
- Auscultate lungs and inspect neck for jugular venous distension (JVD) every hour.
- Assess and treat angina promptly; report to physician any chest pain unrelieved by 3 doses of nitroglycerin.
- Assess perfusion to extremities (e.g., color, temperature, capillary filling, sensation, peripheral pulses).
- Assess catheter insertion site for bleeding or hematoma formation.
- Administer cardiotonic and afterload-reducing drugs as ordered to stimulate the myocardium, to strengthen contractility, and increase cardiac output.
- Elevate legs to promote venous return.

☐ EVALUATION CRITERIA/DESIRED OUTCOMES

The Patient

- Has normal blood pressure, heart rate, heart rhythm, clear mentation
- Maintains urine output of at least 30 cc/hour
- Has warm extremities with normal color and peripheral pulses
- Is free from signs of venous engorgement
- Is relieved of anginal pain

NURSING DIAGNOSIS #2

Alteration in tissue perfusion related to compromised circulation in catheterized extremity

Rationale: *Trauma at the site of the catheterization can cause obstruction to arterial flow by a hematoma or thrombus. The extremity will become cool and pale or mottled and will have compromised tissue metabolism if this occurs. If venous obstruction occurs, extremity may become edematous and slightly cyanotic until collateral veins take over.*

☐ GOAL

The patient will have normal circulation to catheterized extremity.

☐ IMPLEMENTATION

- Assess color, warmth, sensation, capillary filling, and peripheral pulses of extremity distal to catheterization site before the procedure (to provide a baseline for comparisons) and with each assessment of vital signs following the procedure; report deviations from normal.
- Apply heat to opposite extremity (with physician's order) to provide reflex vasodilation of affected extremity if arterial flow is decreased; do not apply heat to affected extremity (it will increase oxygen needs of tissues that are already compromised).
- Elevate affected extremity to increase venous return if venous flow is decreased.
- Monitor for bleeding or hematoma formation at catheterization site with each vital sign check.
- Keep affected extremity straight for 3-6 hours or as ordered to prevent bleeding and mechanical obstruction to flow.

☐ EVALUATION CRITERIA/DESIRED OUTCOMES

The Patient

- Has normal pulse, color, temperature, movement and sensation, and capillary filling in affected extremity
- Is free from bleeding or hematoma, peripheral edema

NURSING DIAGNOSIS #3

a. **Alteration in comfort** related to bedrest, immobility, restricted movement
b. **Impaired physical mobility** related to forced immobility of catheterized extremity
c. **Noncompliance** with activity orders related to misunderstanding of need for immobility

Rationale: *The patient is not permitted to move the catheterized extremity for several hours after the procedure to prevent bleeding or mechanical obstruction to blood flow. This forced immobility on a patient who feels well and wishes to move about can be uncomfortable and stressful, thereby increasing the risk of nonadherence to medical regimen.*

☐ GOAL

The patient will be as comfortable as possible while maintaining activity restrictions.

☐ IMPLEMENTATION

- Explain reasons for activity restrictions and anticipated duration of restrictions.
- Assist patient with armboard, soft restraints, or pillow rolls around leg if unable to maintain extremity in straight position; explain interventions as a way to encourage cooperate rather than to punish.
- Reposition in bed and give back rubs to promote comfort; keep personal articles within easy reach.
- Keep call bell within reach and explain how to use it.

☐ EVALUATION CRITERIA/DESIRED OUTCOMES

The Patient

- Maintains catheterized extremity in straight position for as long as ordered
- Verbalizes comfortable position within necessary limitations
- Calls for assistance as needed

NURSING DIAGNOSIS #4

Potential for infection at catheterization site, intracardiac structures related to invasive procedure

Rationale: *Catheterization involves breaking the skin barrier and inserting a foreign object through arteries and veins into the heart. Any microorganisms that may be inadvertently introduced are in a rich culture medium (blood) and may proliferate, causing infection.*

☐ GOAL

The patient will undergo catheterization free from evidence of infection.

☐ IMPLEMENTATION

Preprocedure

- Cleanse catheterization site as prescribed to minimize number of microorganisms present on skin.

Postprocedure

- Use sterile technique when changing dressings to prevent introduction of microorganisms.
- Monitor temperature every 1-2 hours for first 4-6 hours after catheterization and then every 4 hours; report elevations above 100°F (37.8°C) orally.
- Obtain blood cultures per protocol for temperature elevations to help identify causative organism and antibiotics needed.
- Observe insertion site for edema, redness, heat, or discharge.
- Monitor chest sounds for new heart murmurs and friction rubs (may indicate endocarditis); notify physician immediately.
- If infection occurs or is suspected, monitor white blood cells and administer antibiotics as ordered.

☐ EVALUATION CRITERIA/DESIRED OUTCOMES

The Patient

- Is free from redness, heat, edema, discharge at catheterization site
- Maintains temperature 100°F (37.8°C) orally, a normal white blood cell count
- Has normal (for patient) heart sounds

NURSING DIAGNOSIS #5

a. **Ineffective individual/family coping** related to serious nature of procedure, possible diagnoses, treatment
b. **Anticipatory grieving** related to loss of body function, role, occupation
c. **Alteration in family process** related to role change
d. **Disturbance in self-concept** related to change in perception of self as healthy person

Rationale: *Heart disease carries with it both physical and emotional implications. The pa-*

tient's physical condition may result in an inability to continue working and a role change in family affairs. The patient may see self as a sick person or as healthy healthy and deny physical limitations, resulting in a nontherapeutic response to illness. The diagnosis of heart disease may suggest severe disability or death to some. The varied possible responses to the actual/potential diagnosis of heart disease may result in one or more of the above diagnoses.

☐ GOAL

The patient will realistically discuss catheterization and feelings about potential diagnosis of heart disease.

☐ IMPLEMENTATION

- Explain catheterization procedure clearly (see Nursing Diagnosis #6).
- Encourage patient/family to discuss fears and concerns.
- Explain that fear and grieving are common.
- Help patient identify usual coping mechanisms and support use of them.
- Assist to describe self-perceptions and identify and capitalize on strengths.

☐ EVALUATION CRITERIA/DESIRED OUTCOMES

The Patient

- Verbalizes concerns about catheterization and potential diagnosis
- Identifies potential effects of illness on family dynamics and finances
- Identifies and employs usual coping mechanisms

NURSING DIAGNOSIS #6

Knowledge deficit regarding procedure, postprocedure care

Rationale: *Inadequate knowledge about what is to happen may create excessive anxiety that can interfere with the patient's ability to cooperate with the health team during and after the procedure.*

☐ GOAL

The patient will describe the cardiac catheterization procedure, the reason for having it done, what will be experienced during the procedure, and how to participate in procedure and postprocedure care.

☐ IMPLEMENTATION

- Assess patient's/family's knowledge regarding the procedure; ask what the physician has told them about the purpose of the procedure and what will be done.
- Teach about the procedure in terms patient/family can understand
  - basic anatomy of the heart, purpose of catheterization
  - preprocedure care including diet, shaving of intended site (antecubital area or groins), IV line in arm for medications, medication before procedure to help patient relax, need to empty bladder before procedure, length of the procedure (1-4 hours).
  - what the catheterization lab looks like
  - what will happen during procedure, including safety measures
  - what will happen after the procedure
- Use pictures, drawings, booklets, films or other audiovisual aids to help clarify and reinforce instructions.
- Ensure the patient understands the procedure and potential complications before signing the consent.
- Give instructions for discharge care; an informed patient will be able to take better care of self and report problems early so they can be treated effectively; instructions include
  - how to clean site, recognize infection, change the dressing
  - to notify physician of signs of infection, pain, numbness or tingling in extremity, chest pains, shortness of breath; give patient physician's phone number
  - to return to physician for suture removal (usually 5 days)
- Discuss results of catheterization (after physician has discussed them) and assess patient's understanding of recommended treatment
  - what medications to take
  - to drink extra fluids to continue excreting the dye for about 2 days
- Write down discharge instructions that may otherwise be forgotten or misunderstood so patient can refer to them at home.

☐ EVALUATION CRITERIA/DESIRED OUTCOMES

The Patient

- States purpose of cardiac catheterization
- Explains cardiac catheterization procedure, including preprocedure care and participation during and after the procedure
- Lists symptoms to report to physician during and after procedure
- Demonstrates/describes how to care for insertion site at home, what symptoms to notify physician for, when to see physician again, and what medications to take
- Discusses results of study and implications for care; asks questions freely

The Patient Undergoing Cardiac Surgery: Postoperative Phase

Definition/Discussion

The postoperative phase of cardiac surgery begins when the patient leaves the operating room. It includes postanesthesia recovery, intensive care, home care, and rehabilitation.

Nursing Assessment

☐ PERTINENT HISTORY

Type of surgery done, complications during surgery, course of operation

☐ PHYSICAL FINDINGS

Arterial blood pressure, heart rate and rhythm, ECG, peripheral pulses, skin temperature and color, capillary filling, neck vein distension, edema, pulmonary artery pressure, pulmonary capillary wedge pressure, right atrial or central venous pressures, rate and character of respirations, breath sounds, oxygen therapy utilized, use of accessory muscles, arterial blood gases, chest tube function, level of consciousness, reflexes, sensation, movement, hourly urine output and specific gravity, skin turgor, mucous membranes, electrolytes, condition of wounds and dressings, temperature, pain, IVs

☐ PSYCHOSOCIAL CONCERNS/ DEVELOPMENTAL FACTORS

Patient behavior including confusion, combativeness, quiescence, tearfulness, anger, anxiety; hallucinations (visual or auditory), nightmares

☐ PATIENT AND FAMILY KNOWLEDGE

Awareness of environment, condition, and treatment; ability to comprehend and follow instructions; expectations of post-op appearance; understanding of therapy; expectations for home care and ability to follow through with health team prescriptions, readiness and willingness to learn

Nursing Care

☐ LONG-TERM GOAL

The patient will recover free from preventable complications and return to usual roles in home and job while adhering to the prescribed medical regimen.

NURSING DIAGNOSIS #1

a. **Alteration in cardiac output: decreased** related to blood loss, fluid deficit, compromised myocardial function, dysrhythmias
b. **Alteration in tissue perfusion: cardiac, renal, cerebral** related to blood loss, fluid excess or deficit, compromised myocardial function, dysrhythmias
c. **Fluid volume deficit** related to blood loss, compromised myocardial function
d. **Fluid volume excess** related to iatrogenic fluid overload, fluid shifts

Rationale: *Decreased blood return to the heart following severe blood loss or fluid deficit will* *result in decreased left ventricular filling, increased heart rate, decreased stroke volume, and therefore decreased cardiac output. Dysrhythmias also cause a decreased output by the same mechanism of decreased filling time. Decreased cardiac output may result in reduced organ and tissue perfusion. Low blood flow to the kidneys could precipitate acute renal failure. Decreased blood flow to the brain causes an alteration in level of consciousness and thought processes.*

☐ GOAL

The patient will have normal cardiac output for body size (i.e., cardiac index); will have adequate tissue perfusion.

☐ IMPLEMENTATION

- Monitor hemodynamic parameters including cardiac output; refer to *The Patient Requiring Hemodynamic Monitoring*, page 117.
- Assess hourly urine output and specific gravity to monitor renal arterial blood flow.
- Monitor fluid balance to detect excess or deficit before cardiac output is affected; refer to Table 1, *Common Fluid and Electrolyte Imbalances*, page 14.
- Monitor blood loss through the chest tube at least every hour; report blood loss of more than 100 cc/hour for 2 consecutive hours or more than 150 cc in 1 hour; replace blood loss as ordered.
- Observe for signs of hypovolemia including decreasing blood pressure, increasing heart rate, decreasing CVP, pulmonary artery pressure, and pulmonary capillary wedge pressure.
- Monitor blood pressure especially for hypertension (could cause a bypass graft to break resulting in hemorrhage and decreased myocardial perfusion), hypotension (resulting from hemorrhage, cardiac tamponade, pain, or dysrhythmias), and narrowed pulse pressure (caused by cardiac tamponade).
- Monitor heart rate and rhythm via ECG for tachydysrhythmias, bradydysrhythmias, and ectopic beats.
- Prepare to institute the following treatments if necessary: fluid/blood replacement, inotropic agents to increase myocardial contractility, afterload reducing agents or treatments to decrease systemic pressure, diuretic therapy if patient is in fluid overload, antidysrhythmic medications, or return to surgery for hemostasis or pericardiocentesis.
- Utilize Glasgow Coma Scale to monitor ongoing level of consciousness regularly.

☐ EVALUATION CRITERIA/DESIRED OUTCOMES

The Patient

- Has warm, dry skin with normal peripheral pulses, color, and capillary filling
- Has urine output of at least 25-30 cc/hour
- Maintains/regains pre-op level of consciousness
- Maintains a cardiac output of 4-7 liters/minute (cardiac index 2.5-4 liter/m^2)
- Has hemodynamic parameters within normal limits
- Is free from cardiac dysrhythmias

NURSING DIAGNOSIS #2

a. **Ineffective breathing pattern** related to anesthetic, analgesic sedation, pain, restrictive bandages, poor body position, inadequate lung expansion

b. **Impaired gas exchange** related to retained secretions, ineffective cough effort, obstruction of pulmonary blood flow

c. **Alteration in tissue perfusion: cardiopulmonary** related to anesthetic agents, analgesic sedation, ineffective cough effort, obstruction to pulmonary blood flow

Rationale: *Anesthesia and analgesia depress the cough reflex. Anesthesia also makes normal pulmonary secretions thick and tenacious. The post-op patient with chest pain is unwilling to breathe deeply or cough to mobilize those secretions. Restrictive bandages, chest tubes, and a supine position may also deter a patient from coughing. The retained secretions build up in the airways and settle along the alveolar capillary membrane blocking the normal exchange of oxygen and carbon dioxide between the lung and the blood. Occasionally, an obstruction to pulmonary blood flow can prevent blood from making contact with the alveolus.*

☐ GOAL

The patient will maintain optimal oxygenation.

☐ IMPLEMENTATION

- Provide adequate dosages of pain medication to relieve pain without oversedating; evaluate and record effectiveness.
- Turn patient from side to side and position on opposite sides every 2 hours to mobilize secretions and permit full expansion of upper lung.
- Position with head elevated to allow diaphragm to drop, creating more room for lung expansion.
- Instruct to take a series of 3 progressively larger breaths and then cough; cough is most effective at maximal inhalation because the force of exhaled air is behind the mucus.
- Help patient splint the incision with a pillow while coughing to decrease pain.
- Teach how to use assistive devices (e.g., intermittent positive pressure breathing, incentive spirometer) when ordered; emphasize slow, deep inhalation rather than forced exhalation.
- Assist with/perform percussion and postural drainage as needed.
- Suction using aseptic technique if patient is unable to cough out secretions.
- Encourage to drink liquids within the restrictions imposed by cardiac status.
- Maintain closed chest drainage to promote lung expansion (refer to *The Patient with a Pneumothorax,* page 197).
- Auscultate chest every hour in the immediate post-op period to assess lung expansion and remove secretions; if patient is intubated, there is a possibility that endotracheal tube may slip into right mainstem bronchus resulting in absence of breath sounds on left.
- Refer to *The Patient with Pneumonia,* page 194, *The Patient with Pulmonary Edema,* page 201, *The Patient Undergoing a Thoracotomy,* page 226, and *The Patient with a Tracheostomy,* page 236, for additional considerations as needed.

☐ EVALUATION CRITERIA/DESIRED OUTCOMES

The Patient

- Has clear breath sounds bilaterally
- Participates in breathing exercises, coughs effectively
- Has arterial blood gas results within an acceptable range

NURSING DIAGNOSIS #3

a. **Impaired communication: verbal** related to post-op intubation, neurologic deficit

b. **Alteration in thought process** related to inadequate cerebral oxygenation, sensory alteration, stress response

Rationale: *Most cardiac surgery patients remain intubated for several hours postoperatively until they are able to breathe unassisted. Some may be intubated longer following respiratory complications. The endotracheal tube passes between the vocal cords preventing speech. The patient's hands are frequently restrained to prevent injury caused by pulling on tubes, thereby decreasing the ability to gesture. The patient who has a decreased cerebral perfusion or a cerebral vascular accident postoperatively may be aphasic and have difficulty understanding others and/or expressing self (refer to* The Patient with a Cerebral Vascular Accident, page 71).

☐ GOAL

The patient will be able to communicate needs postoperatively.

☐ IMPLEMENTATION

- Reinforce to the patient/family reason for inability to talk while intubated; the patient who understands that this is both a temporary disability and a normal post-op problem will be able to accept it better, thus decreasing anxiety.
- Ask yes/no questions to which the patient can nod head; know and anticipate common patient concerns including the urge to void with an indwelling Foley; the desire to see family/friends; the need for pain relief, airway suctioning, or reassurance that everything is all right; the desire to have hands unrestrained; explain each answer.
- Allow patient to write or gesture; be alert to patient's possible attempt to extubate self, which could result in severe respiratory distress and death.
- Have patient point to letters on a spelling board to communicate messages; this is sometimes better than writing because coordination may be poor and writing illegible.

- Attempt to lip read the patient who is nasally intubated.
- Be honest with the patient if unable to understand and offer to try again later; refer to *The Patient Experiencing Sensory Alteration,* page 275.

☐ EVALUATION CRITERIA/DESIRED OUTCOMES

The Patient

- Uses at least one successful method of communication
- Indicates that message/request is understood
- Indicates understanding of instructions from staff

NURSING DIAGNOSIS #4

Potential for infection related to invasive procedure, decreased body resistance

Rationale: *Many cardiac surgery patients are weak and poorly nourished preoperatively. Serum proteins may be low, interfering with ability to heal normally. Some patients have taken steroids that suppress their immune system and lower their resistance to infection. All cardiac surgery patients have some type of invasive lines, including central and peripheral IVs, pulmonary artery catheters, arterial lines, chest tubes, Foley catheters, nasogastric (NG) tubes, and endotracheal or tracheostomy tubes. Infection can be prevented with scrupulous attention to aseptic technique.*

☐ GOAL

The patient will be free from infection.

☐ IMPLEMENTATION

- Maintain closed drainage systems for chest tubes and Foley catheters (refer to *The Patient with a Pneumothorax,* page 197).
- Handle IV and arterial lines with strict aseptic technique.
- Use strict aseptic technique when suctioning a patient; note characteristics of secretions obtained.
- Handle NG tubes with clean technique; inspect nares for pressure sores from the tube; lubricate the nares every shift with water-soluble lubricant; report any skin breakdown.
- Change dressings and cleanse incisions daily; note appearance of wounds and incisions including wound edges and presence of redness, swelling, drainage, or odor; chart observations, compare with previous assessment; chart and report abnormalities.
- Monitor patient's temperature every 2-4 hours; report immediately elevations above 101°F (38.3°C) rectally; prepare to assist with blood cultures or to obtain cultures of sputum, urine, or wound drainage.
- Administer antibiotics; check culture and sensitivity reports to be sure microorganism is sensitive to antibiotic being used; evaluate and record effectiveness and side effects; monitor appropriate laboratory data for toxic effects.
- Monitor serum proteins; encourage high-protein foods or administer parenteral nutrition, tube feedings, serum albumin, or plasmanate as needed.

☐ EVALUATION CRITERIA/DESIRED OUTCOMES

The Patient

- Maintains normal temperature
- Has evidence of good wound healing from from redness, drainiage
- Produces only clear or white tracheal aspirate
- Drains clear urine without sediment or pus

NURSING DIAGNOSIS #5

The following diagnoses occur frequently in the post-op cardiac surgery patient.

a. **Alteration in comfort: pain** related to surgical incision, invasive tubes, prolonged bedrest; refer to *The Patient Experiencing Pain,* page 458.
b. **Impairment of skin integrity** related to poor tissue perfusion, edema, immobility
c. **Fear/anxiety** related to unknown causes, decreased cerebral perfusion; refer to *The Patient Experiencing Anxiety,)* page 250

☐ GOAL

The patient/family will demonstrate sufficient understanding of the clinical situation to cooperate with nursing care; will understand home care needs and a rehabilitation plan.

☐ IMPLEMENTATION

- Explain each procedure before doing it, even if it has been explained before; keep explanation brief.
- Reinforce pre-op instructions.
- Emphasize normal nursing care; explain abnormal situations briefly; include family in instructions.
- Encourage physical closeness of family.
- Begin to teach information about medications, activity, incision care, and diet therapy
- Instruct in fluid restrictions if any, importance of taking daily weight in same clothes at same time of day; if continued weight gain, notify physician.
- Advise to avoid smoking or smoke-filled rooms and to avoid crowds and people with infections; limit visitors.

☐ EVALUATION CRITERIA/ DESIRED OUTCOMES

The Patient/family

- Asks for explanations of procedures and care
- Understands explanations and can explain them in own words, where appropriate
- Cooperates with nursing care
- States how the patient will increase activity, and how signs of activity intolerance will be handled
- Explains reason for daily weight taking
- States how to limit visitors until strength returns
- Describes program for follow-up care

NURSING DIAGNOSIS #6

a. **Knowledge deficit** regarding immediate post-op care, home care, rehabilitation

b. **Disturbance in self-concept** related to altered perception of self (refer to *The Patient Experiencing a Body-Image Disturbance*, page 253)

c. **Ineffective individual/family coping** related to recovery from serious illness (refer to *The Patient Requiring Crisis Intervention*, page 256)

d. **Grieving** related to perceived or actual loss of body function, role, occupation (refer to *The Patient Experiencing Grief and Loss*, page 272)

e. **Alteration in family process** related to role change (refer to *The Patient Requiring Crisis Intervention*, page 256)

Rationale: *Patients/families in a stressful situation may not understand what has been taught because they are unable to concentrate on information given. Although the post-op care is routine for the nurse, the multiple tubes and machines are frightening for the patient/family. Lack of understanding may result in a misinterpretation of the situation, needless additional stress, and failure to cooperate with nursing care. There are important things the patient/family also needs to know about rehabilitation. A moderate amount of anxiety may increase their concern about health care and make them eager learners. Too much anxiety will render them unable to focus their attention well enough to learn.*

The Patient Undergoing Cardiac Surgery: Preoperative Phase

Definition/Discussion

Cardiac surgery is the surgical correction of congenital or acquired abnormalities of the heart. It may include repair of valvular lesions, closure of atrial or ventricular septal defects, excision of ventricular aneurysms, or bypassing of obstructed coronary arteries. During the preoperative phase the patient is stabilized and prepared emotionally and physically for surgery.

Nursing Assessment

☐ **PERTINENT HISTORY**

Medical and surgical history; coronary disease, valvular lesion, septal defect, or ventricular aneurysm; duration of problem; effect or limits of problem on everyday activities; coronary risk factors; current prescribed medications or treatments; cardiac catheterization, echocardiogram, CBC, electrolytes, cardiac enzymes, coagulation studies, chest x-ray

☐ **PHYSICAL FINDINGS**

Refer to nursing care plans appropriate to diagnosed cardiac problem (e.g., myocardial infarction, hypertension, congestive heart failure); refer to *The Patient Undergoing Cardiac Catheterization,* page 51.

☐ **PSYCHOSOCIAL CONCERNS/ DEVELOPMENTAL FACTORS**

Age, sex, occupation, usual coping mechanisms, available support systems, roles and responsibilities

☐ **PATIENT AND FAMILY KNOWLEDGE**

Concept of health problem and planned treatment, understanding of post-op care, possible complications, fears about surgery, level of knowledge, readiness and willingness to learn

Nursing Care

☐ **LONG-TERM GOAL**

The patient will express adequate knowledge of the existing pathologic condition, technique of correction, and pre- and post-op care; the patient will be in a stabilized physiologic and psychologic state prior to surgery; the patient will exhibit only moderate anxiety regarding surgery.

NURSING DIAGNOSIS #1

a. **Fear** related to impending surgery, possible surgical outcome, misinformation, unknown causes
b. **Anxiety** related to unknown causes, misinformation

Rationale: *The unknown, as well as exaggerated or inaccurate reports from others, can result in pre-op fear or anxiety, which is correlated with an increase in post-op delirium and morbidity. Some anxiety is normal; the patient who is not anxious at all all may not understand what is happening.*

☐ GOAL

The patient will experience no more than moderate anxiety regarding impending surgery.

☐ IMPLEMENTATION

- Monitor how patient feels about impending surgery; suggest that most people are anxious and talking about it may be helpful.
- Ask if patient has had friends or relatives who have shared their own heart surgery experiences; finding out what the patient knows and expects helps identify misconceptions as well as realistic fears.
- Give information appropriate to surgery (see Nursing Diagnosis #4).
- Assist to use usual coping mechanisms to decrease stress if adaptive; instruct in alternative coping measures such as relaxation, guided imagery as needed.
- Encourage verbalization of fears and anxieties; allow time to share feelings.
- Evaluate and chart ongoing level of anxiety and coping behavior; report excessive anxiety, suggest appropriate referrals.
- Refer to *The Patient Experiencing Anxiety,* page 250.

☐ EVALUATION CRITERIA/DESIRED OUTCOMES

The Patient

- Identifies sources of anxiety
- Discusses fears with nurses/family
- Identifies at least one method to decrease stress and uses it preoperatively
- Has realistic pre-op fears about surgery

NURSING DIAGNOSIS #2

Sleep pattern disturbance related to anxiety, unfamiliar environment

Rationale: *The patient may find it difficult to relax in the hospital environment and wake up frequently during the night. Anxiety and worry about the surgery may prevent the patient from sleeping. A patient who is not rested is at a greater risk for post-op problems.*

☐ GOAL

The patient will sleep through the night.

☐ IMPLEMENTATION

- Ask patient for details of usual sleeping pattern, including use of sleep aids (e.g., warm milk, hot bath, eyeshades, night light).
- Offer a backrub, straighten bed, provide patient's usual sleep aids when possible.
- Deal with anxiety (see Nursing Diagnosis #1) during the day hours to permit relaxation at night.
- Administer sedatives or hypnotics when needed; evaluate and record effectiveness; put up side rails to protect patient who may be disoriented because of medications.

☐ EVALUATION CRITERIA/DESIRED OUTCOMES

The Patient

- Maintains usual sleeping patterns
- Feels rested on awakening

NURSING DIAGNOSIS #3

Spiritual distress related to fear of death, disability

Rationale: *Diseases of the heart involve fears of death or disability because the heart is vital for life. Some people view illness as punishment for sin. Many who may or may not regularly practice their religion feel a need to consult a spiritual advisor before this major surgery and to find spiritual comfort through organized religion or identified religious leaders.*

☐ GOAL

The patient will experience spiritual comfort and peace of mind preoperatively.

☐ IMPLEMENTATION

- Ask if patient practices any particular religion; inform of available services of hospital priest, chaplain, or rabbi; offer to call patient's own spiritual advisor.
- Ask for any requests for spiritual care postoperatively (may wish to have spiritual minister visit postoperatively or assist family members).
- Offer to pray with the patient if need is expressed; although you may not share the pa-

tient's religious beliefs, this gesture may provide spiritual comfort.

- If patient wishes, discuss plans for care in case of irreversible coma or death; some fear prolongation of suffering more than death itself and wish to leave a living will; others wish to follow specified religious practices in the event of death.

☐ EVALUATION CRITERIA/DESIRED OUTCOMES

The Patient

- Accepts or declines spiritual services
- Identifies desires for post-op spiritual care

NURSING DIAGNOSIS #4

Knowledge deficit regarding cardiac surgery

Rationale: *Cardiac surgery is considered more serious than most other types of surgery in terms of its physiologic and psychologic implications. It also requires active patient participation to effect a normal post-op recovery. In order for the patient to participate in the postop course, correct and accurate information is needed.*

☐ GOAL

The patient will understand the impending surgery; will take an active role in post-op care.

☐ IMPLEMENTATION

- Provide information as wanted and needed but do not overburden since this may only increase anxiety.
- Give general, practical information concerning visiting hours, length of stay in ICU, availability of chaplain, etc.
- Orient to pre-op routines and procedures, laboratory studies, x-ray, ECG, and skin shave.
- Orient to ICU environment, staff, procedures to be carried out, equipment utilized and types of sounds normally heard in the ICU.
- Explain use of the intermittent positive pressure breathing (IPPB) apparatus, incentive spirometer, extremity exercises, and the proper techniques of coughing and deep breathing.
- Explain that because of anxiety, medications, major surgery, the lack of uninterrupted sleep, etc., it is normal to have unusual dreams or nightmares, feel depressed, exhausted, or irritable, and that these will pass.
- Assure that a nurse will be nearby at all times in the ICU and that staff members will be monitoring progress closely.

☐ EVALUATION CRITERIA/DESIRED OUTCOMES

The Patient

- Explains the surgical procedure accurately on a basic level
- Demonstrates coughing and deep breathing techniques, use of IPPB/incentive spirometer, leg exercises
- Asks questions or makes comments to clarify concepts explained
- States health team's expectations during the post-op period
- Verbalizes a willingness to report hallucinations, depression

The Patient with Cardiogenic Shock

Definition/Discussion

Cardiogenic shock is the acute state of decreased cardiac output and decreased tissue perfusion caused by left ventricular pump failure (e.g., after myocardial infarction), ineffective pumping (e.g., dysrhythmias), flow obstruction (e.g., cardiac tamponade, valvular disease, pulmonary embolus, thoracic aortic aneurysm), or complications of open-heart surgery. The effect of this decreased ability to maintain pulmonary and systemic circulation is self-perpetuating since the coronary vessels are inadequately perfused as well, causing further damage to the injured heart muscle.

Medical treatment aims to preserve coronary perfusion while decreasing the cardiac workload and increasing cardiac output. Mechanical ventilation may be required to promote adequate oxygenation while decreasing required energy expenditures. Specific fluid volumes to be infused are dependent upon pulmonary and renal functioning.

Pulmonary capillary wedge pressure (PCWP) reflects the functioning of the left ventricle and gives an indication of pulmonary congestion. It is used as the main indicator of fluid status for patients with cardiogenic shock. Diuretics and fluid restriction will likely be ordered for the patient with an elevated PCWP (above 18 mm Hg); fluid replacement will be provided for the patient with a decreased PCWP (below 15 mm Hg) and urinary output of less than 20-30 ml/hour.

Drugs with inotropic and vasoconstrictive effects are used to increase blood flow to the heart and vital organs. Peripheral vasodilators may be required as well. Commonly prescribed drugs are dopamine, epinephrine, and norepinephrine. Dobutamine, isoproterenol, nitropusside, and phentolamine may be used as well. All these drugs are titrated according to the patient's condition and therefore require constant nursing vigilance when being administered. If improvement does not occur, an intra-aortic balloon pump (IABP) may be inserted to reduce left ventricular filling pressure and improve output and flow. If the balloon pump is also not effective, the patient may be prepared for cardiac catheterization and possible open-heart surgery to correct the cause of the cardiovascular failure.

Nursing Assessment

☐ PERTINENT HISTORY

Severe congestive heart failure, cor pulmonale, myocardial pericarditis, acute myocardial infarction

☐ PHYSICAL FINDINGS

Cerebral hypoxia (confusion, restlessness, apathy); tachycardia; peripheral vasoconstriction (skin cold, profuse sweating, pallor); decreased or absent peripheral pulses; decreased urinary output (less than 20 cc/hour); decreased blood pressure (systolic below 80 mm Hg or more than 30 mm Hg below patient's "normal" systolic pressure), with narrowing of pulse pressure; increased respirations with short, shallow respiratory efforts; rales upon auscultation; arterial blood gases reflecting respiratory alkalosis (early) or metabolic acidosis (late), hemodynamic readings: increased PCWP, decreased cardiac output, increased peripheral vascular resistance

☐ PSYCHOSOCIAL CONCERNS/ DEVELOPMENTAL FACTORS

Heightened anxiety and fear increasing stress; possible change in life-style; changes in role performance

PATIENT AND FAMILY KNOWLEDGE

Disease process and potential outcome, community support systems, readiness and willingness to learn

Nursing Care

LONG-TERM GOAL

The patient will regain optimum perfusion of vital organs with gradual withdrawal of supportive measures through correction of underlying causes and improvement of cardiovascular action.

NURSING DIAGNOSIS #1

Alteration in cardiac output: decreased related to ineffective cardiac pumping mechanism

Rationale: *Cardiogenic shock consists of sustained systemic arterial hypotension with increased perfusion of the lungs, kidneys, brain, and extremities. Symptoms reflect compensatory mechanisms as the body attempts to maintain adequate blood pressure by redistributing blood volume in the presence of decreasing cardiac output. While the nurse cannot independently initiate the measures to correct the condition causing the decreased cardiac output of a patient in cardiogenic shock, s/he is responsible for collaborating with the physician to continually monitor the patient's status, assess possible complications, titrate medications, and evaluate patient responses to medical therapy.*

GOAL

The patient will have adequate cardiac output with perfusion to all body tissues.

IMPLEMENTATION

- Place patient in a supine position with head of bed slightly elevated to decrease cardiac workload (Trendelenburg's position is contraindicated because it increases diaphragmatic pressure).
- Maintain strict bedrest; inspect skin and provide prophylactic measures every 2 hours (when activity is contraindicated, preventive nursing care becomes high priority); use alternating pressure mattress or consult physician regarding order for egg-crate mattress.
- Monitor blood pressure and pulse every 5-15 minutes; watch for decreased systolic pressure, narrowing pulse pressure, increased pulse; assess quality and rhythm of pulse; report changes from baseline/physician established parameters.
- Maintain patent IV line; record intake; adjust IV flow rate and titrate prescribed medications (e.g., dopamine, dobutamine, isoproterenol, diuretics, vasodilators) according to physician-established parameters; monitor for desired/untoward effects.
- Monitor cardiac rhythm continuously; record a rhythm strip every 4 hours, more often if irregular; administer antidysrhythmic drugs; record and report response.
- Assess for signs of potassium imbalance while monitoring vital signs (e.g., decreased muscle tone/flaccidity/cramping, malaise, nausea, diarrhea, mental confusion, irritability); check laboratory studies for increased/decreased potassium levels.
- Assess effectiveness of counterpulsation via IABP; refer to *The Patient Requiring Intra-Aortic Balloon Pumping*, page 128.
  - expect to find decreased PCWP and increased cardiac output
  - assess for signs/symptoms indicating improved peripheral, renal, and cerebral perfusion
  - check leg perfusion especially carefully as balloon may cause decreased vascular perfusion of leg used for insertion
  - adjust rate of augmentation of cardiac output according to physician-established parameters
- Measure urinary output/specific gravity hourly; expect concentrated or normal urinary specific gravity; report output less than 20 cc/hour for 2 consecutive hours.

EVALUATION CRITERIA/DESIRED OUTCOMES

The Patient

- Has stable blood measurement similar to preshock state
- Has normal cardiac rhythm and peripheral pulses
- Has hemodynamic pressures and cardiac output within normal limits
- Has urinary output greater than 30 cc/hour

- Is mentally alert or maintains preshock level of consciousness

NURSING DIAGNOSIS #2

Impaired gas exchange related to decreased cardiac output

Rationale: *When cardiac output is decreased, the ventilation/perfusion ratio is altered. Initially, increased respiratory and heart rates may compensate for the decreased stroke volume, but these compensatory mechanisms increase the cardiac workload. High-flow oxygen therapy (50% concentration via mask) is part of the initial medical treatment for cardiogenic shock. If arterial blood gases indicate decreased oxygen and increased carbon dioxide partial pressures, mechanical ventilation may be ordered.*

☐ GOAL

The patient will experience improved gas exchange in the lungs with resultant adequate oxygenation of all body tissues.

☐ IMPLEMENTATION

- Assess respiratory rate, depth, effort, and rhythm; auscultate lungs for pulmonary congestion/atelectasis and inspect skin for pallor/cyanosis every hour.
- Note changes in respiratory pattern (increased respiratory rate is expected; Cheyne-Stokes respirations may occur in late stages).
- Administer oxygen via mask at prescribed flow rate; ensure proper humidification; remove mask every 2 hours to clean/ inspect skin underneath.
- Monitor arterial blood gases; prepare patient for endotracheal intubation and mechanical ventilation if oxygen therapy is not effective.
- Suction as needed to maintain patent airway; turn from side to side and percuss basilar areas prior to suctioning when patient condition permits (check with physician regarding gradually increasing activity). Refer to *The Patient Who is Ventilator-Dependent*, page 239.

☐ EVALUATION CRITERIA/DESIRED OUTCOMES

The Patient

- Has a normal respiratory rate and pattern
- Has normal arterial blood gases, clear breath sounds
- Is free from pallor, cyanosis

NURSING DIAGNOSIS #3

Anxiety related to guarded prognosis, ICU environment

Rationale: *When a patient is admitted to a coronary care unit and the physician has examined the patient and explained the treatment plan, the patient/family are likely to be aware of the gravity of the situation. Initially, they may not fully understand the condition and may express feelings of helplessness and fear that the patient will die. It is essential to control patient anxiety to reduce physiologic reactions (e.g., increased pulse, respirations) that increase the cardiac workload and contribute to the gravity of the situation. Measures aimed at promoting relief from anxiety for family members may be just as important as allaying the patient's anxiety as one person's anxiety may increase another's.*

☐ GOAL

The patient/family will express fears/concerns regarding the patient's status; will relate a reduction in anxiety.

☐ IMPLEMENTATION

- Explain the coronary care setting/monitoring equipment; indicate how the nurses are able to continuously monitor the patient's status; if the patient requires a ventilator, establish a means of communicating (e.g., gestures, taps, pen/pencil, erasable slate).
- Allow patient/family to express feelings and ask questions; reinforce what physician has said; clarify explanations as necessary; indicate acceptance of expressed feelings by validating that others have had similar concerns.
- Describe procedures and give a rationale prior to carrying them out; give brief, clear explanations; share physical signs of improvement (e.g., improved vital signs, hemo-

dynamic readings, blood gases) with patient/family.
- Minimize auditory/visual stimuli to decrease environmental stress as much as possible; use gentle touch and supportive words, especially with family members.
- Allow family to spend as much time as possible with patient; when it is necessary to ask family to leave bedside, tell them when they can return.
- Assess family for signs of fatigue; encourage them to rest/eat regularly; provide them with the unit telephone number and reassure them that they may call at any time and that the nurses will carefully watch the patient and call concerning condition changes.
- Contact religious representative if patient/family so desires.
- Initiate referral for crisis intervention to assist family and offer emotional support if needed.

☐ EVALUATION CRITERIA/DESIRED OUTCOMES

The Patient

- Establishes a means of communicating concerns
- Has needs met

The Patient/family

- Express/demonstrate no more than a moderate level of anxiety

NURSING DIAGNOSIS #4

Knowledge deficit regarding guidelines for follow-up care

Rationale: *While the patient may not require instruction specific for care after recovering from cardiogenic shock, s/he will need teaching regarding the posthospitalization regimen for the precipitating condition.*

See The Patient with a Myocardial Infarction, *page 151,* The Patient with a Pulmonary Embolus, *page 205,* The Patient Undergoing Cardiac Surgery: Postoperative Phase, *page 56, for pertinent nursing diagnoses, goals, implementations, and evaluation criteria/desired outcomes.*

The Patient with a Cerebral Aneurysm

Definition/Discussion

A cerebral aneurysm is the dilated (outpouched) area of an intracranial arterial wall that is weakened and susceptible to leakage or rupture. A five-grade system is used to categorize levels of severity based on symptomatology.

- *Grade 1:* alert, no neurologic deficit, minimal headache, and minimal nuchal (neck) rigidity
- *Grade 2:* mild to severe headache and nuchal rigidity, neurologic deficit relatd to cranial nerve III palsy (drooping eyelid, diplopia, unilateral pupil dilation or visual loss due to compression of optic chiasm)
- *Grade 3:* drowsy, confused, mild neurologic deficit
- *Grade 4:* stupor, mild to severe hemiparesis
- *Grade 5:* deep coma, decerebrate posture, moribund appearance

Signs and symptoms vary according to the patient and amount of bleeding (subarachnoid hemorrhage), unruptured intracranial aneurysms are often asymptomatic.

Treatment may include measures to stabilize the patient or sustain vital functions, emergency intracranial surgery to control the bleeding or evacuate a hematoma, or medical management to prevent rupture until the aneurysm can be operated on.

Nursing Assessment

☐ **PERTINENT HISTORY**

Medical and surgical history, age; sudden, severe headaches; nausea, vomiting; seizures; neurologic deficits; hypertension; visual disturbances; stiff neck; activity at time of symptoms

☐ **PHYSICAL FINDINGS**

Vital signs, altered level of consciousness, increased intracranial pressure, xanthochromic (yellow-tinged) or grossly bloody cerebral spinal fluid (CSF) with increased protein or cell count, results of CT scan or cerebral angiograms

☐ **PSYCHOSOCIAL CONCERNS/ DEVELOPMENTAL FACTORS**

Age, sex, occupation, life-style, support systems, usual coping strategies, roles and responsibilities

☐ **PATIENT AND FAMILY KNOWLEDGE**

Level of knowledge; definition and etiology of aneurysm; planned treatment (e.g., surgery); readiness and willingness to learn, rehabilitation

Nursing Care

☐ **LONG-TERM GOAL**

The patient will recover from aneurysm free from disability or complications and return to usual role and activities. If the aneurysm is inoperable, the patient and family will demonstrate adequate knowledge and skills to manage care.

NURSING DIAGNOSIS #1

Alteration in tissue perfusion: cerebral related to bleeding/rebleeding, vasospasm

Rationale: *Bleeding or rebleeding and vasospasm cause an increase in intracranial pressure (ICP). A ruptured or leaking aneurysm causes bleeding into the subarachnoid space. Elevations in blood pressure can cause rebleeding, which usually occurs 7-14 days after the initial bleed as lysis of the clot begins. Vasospasm occurs most frequently 4-12 days post-subarachnoid bleed and peaks around the 5th or 7th day. Postoperatively, there is an* *increased incidence of vasospasm with symptoms usually becoming evident on the 4th to 11th post-op day.*

☐ GOAL

The patient will demonstrate adequate cerebral perfusion.

☐ IMPLEMENTATION

- See *The Patient with Increased Intracranial Pressure,* page 122, *The Patient with a Head Injury,* page 105, and *The Patient Undergoing Intracranial Surgery,* page 132, for all pertinent nursing care.
- Institute aneurysm precautions (e.g., private, darkened room; limited visitors; bedrest; no television) to prevent increased blood pressure and rebleed.
- Administer antihypertensives and/or antifibrinolytic agents to prevent bleeding; monitor for hypotension if patient is receiving antihypertensives; deep vein thrombosis, phlebitis, pulmonary embolus, diarrhea, tinnitis if receiving antifibrinolytics.
- Monitor for side effects of vasospasm therapy (kanamycin and reserpine: diarrhea, hypotension; isuprel and aminophylline: tachycardia and cardiac dysrhythmias; calcium channel blockers: hypotension, dysrhythmias).

☐ EVALUATION CRITERIA/DESIRED OUTCOMES

The Patient

- Has blood pressure within specified parameters
- Has unchanged neurologic status
- Complies with activity restrictions

NURSING DIAGNOSIS #2

Alteration in comfort (headache, nausea/vomiting) related to increased ICP

Rationale: *Blood in the subarachnoid space from a leaking or ruptured aneurysm results in a rise in CSF pressure, meningeal irritation, and cerebral edema causing a headache and/or nausea and vomiting.*

☐ GOAL

The patient will be comfortable.

☐ IMPLEMENTATION

- Assess patient's level of discomfort using a 0-10 point self-rating scale to obtain an objective measure of the pain.
- Administer analgesics and/or antiemetics and evaluate effectiveness.
- Provide alternative comfort measures such as guided imagery, relaxation
- Insert a nasogastric tube and attach to suction for gastrointestinal upset as needed.
- Reduce or eliminate activities that would increase blood pressure, ICP and aggravate headache (see aneurysm precautions, Nursing Diagnosis #1).
- Refer to *The Patient Experiencing Pain,* page 180.

☐ EVALUATION CRITERIA/DESIRED OUTCOMES

The Patient

- Verbalizes decreased pain
- Retains fluids and food
- Rests quietly

NURSING DIAGNOSIS #3

a. **Anxiety** related to fear of unknown, uncertain future
b. **Fear** related to surgical intervention
c. **Disturbance in self-concept: body image, role performance** related to loss of function
d. **Ineffective individual/family coping** related to actual or potential loss of well-being and function

Rationale: *The patient may or may not present with actual neurologic deficits such as hemiparesis, hemiplegia, dysarthria, or aphasia but there is the potential risk for such alterations postoperatively. Added to these concerns about the patient's physical status is the lengthy hospitalization required for diagnostic tests and preparation prior to surgical intervention, as well as the post-op course.*

☐ GOAL

The patient/family will effectively adapt to actual or potential altered abilities; will exhibit only moderate amount of anxiety.

IMPLEMENTATION

- Explain reason for lengthy hospitalization (e.g., bleeding prevents early surgical intervention, risk of rebleed).
- Explain rationale for tests/procedures, frequent neurologic assessments, treatments.
- Encourage verbalization of feelings and concerns.
- Reinforce capabilities, progress.
- Refer patient/family to other professional resources as necessary.

EVALUATION CRITERIA/DESIRED OUTCOMES

The Patient/family

- Verbalizes feelings related to fears
- Identifies potential and actual stressors
- Demonstrates effective coping strategies

NURSING DIAGNOSIS #4

Knowledge deficit regarding disease process, treatment, prognosis, rehabilitation

Rationale: *Individuals with aneurysms are often not aware of their condition until the aneurysm ruptures, necessitating unexpected hospitalization and often emergency surgery. The treatment plan, activity restrictions, and rehabilitation plan will need to be explained when the crisis has passed or upon diagnosis.*

GOAL

The patient/family will demonstrate adequate knowledge regarding the plan of treatment.

IMPLEMENTATION

- Explain all tests and procedures as time allows.
- Encourage verbalization and questions if possible.
- Discuss patient's future as honestly as possible.
- Plan for rehabilitation as necessary; refer to *The Patient with a Cerebral Vascular Accident*, page 71.

EVALUATION CRITERIA/DESIRED OUTCOMES

The Patient

- Complies with restricted activity
- Verbalizes understanding of illness, therapy, prognosis
- Participates in selected rehabilitation activities

The Patient with a Cerebral Vascular Accident

Definition/Discussion

A cerebral vascular accident (CVA), also known as a stroke, is an interruption in the intracerebral circulation related to a vascular insufficiency, thrombosis, embolism, or hemorrhage.

Nursing Assessment

☐ PERTINENT HISTORY

Medical history including hypertension, diabetes mellitus, cardiovascular disease, transient ischemic attacks (TIA) or reversible ischemic neurologic deficit (RIND); cigarette smoking; oral contraceptive use; motor/sensory disturbances; visual disturbances

☐ PHYSICAL FINDINGS

Level of consciousness (LOC), mental status; motor and sensory deficits; aphasia; vision; cranial nerve function; vital signs; blood studies (clotting profile, CBC, triglycerides, cholesterol, glucose); CT scan; angiogram; ECG; EEG; weight/obesity

☐ PSYCHOSOCIAL CONCERNS/ DEVELOPMENTAL FACTORS

Age, sex, available support systems, life-style, usual coping strategies, occupation, usual roles and responsibilities, emotional reaction to illness

☐ PATIENT AND FAMILY KNOWLEDGE

Cause of stroke, risk factors, prognosis/expected outcome, level of knowledge, readiness and willingness to learn

Nursing Care

☐ LONG-TERM GOAL

The patient will maintain body function and be free from preventable complications.

> NURSING DIAGNOSIS #1
>
> **Alteration in tissue perfusion: cerebral** related to inadequate cerebral blood supply, increased intracranial pressure (ICP), decreased cerebral oxygenation
>
> ***Rationale:*** *An alteration in cerebral blood flow as a result of vascular insufficiency, thrombosis, embolism, or hemorrhage compromises the delicate intracranial balance of brain tissue, blood volume, and cerebrospinal fluid. An inadequate blood supply and reduced oxygen to brain tissue results in necrosis or infarction.*

☐ GOAL

The patient will demonstrate adequate cerebral perfusion.

☐ IMPLEMENTATION

- Assess patient's neurologic status including LOC/mental status, pupils and eye movements, motor and sensory function, verbal response every 1-4 hours to detect changes indicative of altered cerebral function.
- Monitor vital signs every 1-4 hours.
- Administer antihypertensive medication and monitor effect.
- Maintain a patent airway and adequate ventilation.
- Promote venous outflow from the brain by

elevating the head of the bed and aligning head/neck.
- Utilize restraints only when absolutely necessary because agitation will increase ICP.
- Organize care to allow for optimal rest periods.
- Administer medications to prevent further blood clots (e.g., heparin, Coumadin, aspirin, Persantine).
- Administer diuretics to reduce fluid volume; monitor intake and output.
- Administer steroids to prevent cerebral edema.
- Monitor for toxic and side effects related to therapeutic drug interventions.
- Monitor pertinent laboratory tests (e.g., PTT, PT, electrolytes) to determine therapeutic drug blood levels or electrolyte imbalances that may alter patient's sensorium.
- Notify physician of neurologic and other significant hemodynamic changes immediately.
- Refer to *The Patient with Increased Intracranial Pressure,* page 122, for specific measures to treat increased ICP.
- Assist with diagnostic procedures (CT scan, angiography) as needed.

☐ EVALUATION CRITERIA/DESIRED OUTCOMES

The Patient

- Demonstrates unchanged or improved neurologic status
- Maintains blood pressure within specified parameters

NURSING DIAGNOSIS #2

a. **Ineffective breathing pattern** related to obstructed airway, increased ICP, alteration in LOC

b. **Ineffective airway clearance** related to obstructed airway, poor cough reflex, alteration in LOC

Rationale: *A patient with a decreased LOC resulting from impaired cerebral circulation may be unable to maintain a patent airway. The patient with a CVA may experience an obstructed airway from the tongue, mucus plugs, pulmonary congestion from aspiration, a poor cough reflex, or the effects of immobility.*

☐ GOAL

The patient will maintain a patent airway with adequate pulmonary ventilation; will expectorate accumulated bronchial secretions; will be free from hypoxia and pulmonary congestion.

☐ IMPLEMENTATION

- Assess patient's ability to maintain an open airway.
- Maintain a patent airway: place patient in semi-Fowler's position, suction airway, and employ airway adjuncts (e.g., oral airway, endotracheal tube with or without mechanical ventilation).
- Monitor respiratory rate, rhythm, and depth every 1-4 hours.
- Auscultate breath sounds every 4 hours to determine adequate aeration and to detect adventitious sounds.
- Encourage coughing and deep breathing every 2-4 hours to mobilize secretions.
- Assess amount, color, consistency of pulmonary secretions; obtain culture and sensitivity of secretions to determine need for additional treatments.
- Monitor arterial blood gas values for abnormalities and decreased oxygen saturation.
- Administer oxygen.
- Assess for signs of hypoxia and hypercapnia (restlessness, cyanosis, increased respiratory rate and heart rate, symptoms of increased ICP).
- Administer bronchodilators, pulmonary expectorants.
- Monitor intake and output.
- Notify physician of significant findings.

☐ EVALUATION CRITERIA/DESIRED OUTCOMES

The Patient

- Has adequate bilateral lung aeration with minimal or absent adventitious sounds
- Maintains regular respiratory rate of 12-24 breaths/minute
- Maintains blood gases within normal limits
- Is free from clinical signs of hypoxia

NURSING DIAGNOSIS #3

Impaired physical mobility related to decreased LOC, paresis/plegia

Rationale: *Mobility may be limited because of a decreased LOC or as a result or loss of motor/sensory function.*

☐ GOAL

The patient will maintain muscle strength; will be free from complications of immobility.

☐ IMPLEMENTATION

- Assess patient's motor function, sensation, and reflexes in all extremities to determine abilities and limitations.
- Maintain therapeutic body alignment with head, shoulders, and hips level on a firm mattress with bed board.
- Brace feet against footboard, in line with legs, heels off the mattress and protected from pressure to prevent footdrop and skin breakdown.
- Utilize trochanter rolls to prevent external or internal hip rotation, pain and discomfort.
- Support arms and hands in functional positions: elbows slightly flexed, wrists extended, a hard handroll or rubber ball to keep fingers in "grasp" position and to control spasm; hand elevated to prevent dependent edema.
- Reposition patient every 2 hours.
- Perform passive range of motion every 2-4 hours if not contraindicated to prevent contractures and atrophy.
- Utilize trapeze bar over bed to assist patient with mobility and encourage independence.
- Assist with ambulation as needed, maintaining patient safety.
- Coordinate efforts with physical and occupational therapists.

☐ EVALUATION CRITERIA/DESIRED OUTCOMES

The Patient

- Is repositioned, up in chair, or ambulated on a regular basis
- Is free from pressure sores, muscle atrophy, contractures

NURSING DIAGNOSIS #4

a. **Alteration in nutrition: less than body requirements** related to dysphagia, difficulty with chewing, loss of appetite

b. **Impaired swallowing** related to loss of motor function

Rationale: *Diminished blood flow to the areas of the brain responsible for the motor and sensory functions of chewing, swallowing, and arm/hand movement can result in nutritional problems. In addition, depression and immobility may contribute to loss of appetite.*

☐ GOAL

The patient will maintain optimal nutritional status, fluid intake, and electrolyte balance.

☐ IMPLEMENTATION

- Assess patient's gag reflex, ability to swallow, presence of facial paralysis, motor and sensory function of upper extremities, evidence of perceptual deficits to determine functional eating ability.
- Monitor intake and output and dietary intake to determine deficits.
- Monitor electrolytes (poor oral intake and fluid deficit can cause sodium, potassium, and chloride imbalances).
- Administer IV fluids.
- Administer nasogastric feedings and water.
- Administer hyperalimentation therapy (refer to *The Patient Receiving Total Parenteral Nutrition,* page 229).
- Assist with oral feedings when indicated starting with thickened/full liquids, which are more easily managed than clear liquids.
- Assess patient's food likes and dislikes to motivate adequate intake.
- Advance diet as tolerated (full liquid→soft or pureed→regular).
- Consult dietician as necessary.
- Coordinate efforts related to swallowing and ability to feed self with speech and occupational therapists.
- Provide oral hygiene before/after each oral feeding.
- Monitor patient's weight.

EVALUATION CRITERIA/DESIRED OUTCOMES

The Patient

- Maintains weight within 10% of admission weight
- Tolerates parenteral nutrition or tube feedings with minimal residual, no diarrhea, balanced electrolytes
- Swallows soft food without aspiration

NURSING DIAGNOSIS #5

Impairment of skin integrity related to altered sensation, immobility, incontinence, altered nutritional status

Rationale: *The patient who has had a stroke may be unable to feel pressure/pain and move self, all of which puts the patient at risk for skin breakdown. Keeping the skin clean and dry is essential.*

GOAL

The patient will maintain skin integrity, tone, turgor, and circulation.

IMPLEMENTATION

- Assess patient's skin for intactness, color changes, turgor, temperature, and presence of edema every 4 hours and as necessary.
- Keep skin clean and dry.
- Promote circulation with frequent changes of position, massages, suitable room ventilation and loose, absorbent bedclothes.
- Utilize pressure prevention aids (e.g., cushions, devices, pads).

EVALUATION CRITERIA/DESIRED OUTCOMES

The Patient

- Has intact skin
- Is free from erythema over bone prominences

NURSING DIAGNOSIS #6

Alteration in patterns of urinary elimination: functional incontinence related to sensory/motor impairment, immobility, impaired communication

Rationale: *A CVA can cause actual damage to motor and sensory nerve innervation of the bladder. Other factors contributing to urinary elmination problems include the inability to communicate the need to void and the inability to ambulate to the bathroom or commode.*

GOAL

The patient will remain continent of urine; will be protected from complications of incontinence.

IMPLEMENTATION

- Observe for incontinence, note type and pattern.
- Assess whether patient is aware of need to void or able to communicate need (observe for nonverbal clues such as restlessness).
- Offer bedpan/urinal frequently.
- Establish regular voiding schedule.
- Stimulate voiding utilizing privacy, running water, comfortable position, Credé's maneuver as needed.
- Palpate bladder for distention as needed.
- Perform catheter care twice daily if Foley catheter in use (perineal washing, application of bacteriostatic ointment to urinary meatus, tape catheter to prevent traction); utilize Foley catheter only if necessary since invasive measures increase the possibility of infection.
- Assess character/appearance of urine to determine concentration and possible urinary tract infection; obtain urine specimens as indicated.

EVALUATION CRITERIA/DESIRED OUTCOMES

The Patient

- Is continent
- Communicates need to void
- Remains clean and dry
- Is free from evidence of urinary tract infection

NURSING DIAGNOSIS #7

Alteration in bowel elimination: constipation, diarrhea, incontinence related to fluid and dietary intake, loss of voluntary control, impaired communication, peristaltic changes, intolerance to tube feedings, immobility

Rationale: *Inability to communicate the need to defecate, to ambulate to the bathroom or commode, or to obtain food and fluid by oneself results in a variety of bowel elimination problems. Neurologic damage to the bowel, or the inability to swallow and chew necessitating tube feedings can compound the problem. Impaired mobility can slow peristalsis causing constipation.*

☐ GOAL

The patient will evacuate bowel on a regular basis.

☐ IMPLEMENTATION

- Assess whether patient is aware of or able to communicate need to defecate.
- Assess patient's previous bowel habits.
- Assist with mobilization and increased activity as needed to stimulate peristalsis.
- Administer stool softeners, bulk-forming laxatives, suppositories, enemas.
- Assess patient's nutritional status and encourage high-fiber foods and roughage.
- Offer extra fluids if able to tolerate.
- Observe for incontinence at lease every shift.
- Assess and record character and frequency of bowel movements.
- Stimulate evacuation by providing privacy and comfortable position.

☐ EVALUATION CRITERIA/DESIRED OUTCOMES

The Patient

- Has soft, formed bowel movements on a regular basis
- Communicates the need to defecate

NURSING DIAGNOSIS #8

Impaired communication: verbal related to expressive/receptive aphasia, dysarthria, altered thought processes

Rationale: *Impaired circulation and resultant brain damage can affect the individual's ability to communicate resulting in the inability to express or correctly express oneself despite intact muscular control, the inability to understand written/verbal messages, the inability to express oneself verbally due to problems with the muscles used in speech, or incorrect or inappropriate verbal expression as a result of changes in mentation.*

☐ GOAL

The patient will establish/reestablish an effective means of communication.

☐ IMPLEMENTATION

- Assess patient's ability to communicate (express self, understand others, remain oriented).
- Maintain eye contact with patient when communicating.
- Address patient in a slow and unhurried manner.
- Utilize simple one-step word commands with gestures or pictures if necessary.
- Ask questions that can be answered with "yes" or "no" or gestures.
- Inform patient of staff's understanding of and empathy with communication problem.
- Respond to patient's nonverbal behavior.
- Consult with speech therapist for added help.

☐ EVALUATION CRITERIA/DESIRED OUTCOMES

The Patient

- Establishes an effective method of communication with verbal and nonverbal cues
- Is free from signs of frustration regarding communication of needs

NURSING DIAGNOSIS #9

a. **Sensory-perceptual alteration: visual, tactile, kinesthetic** related to visual defects, impaired sensation
b. **Unilateral neglect** related to disturbed perceptual abilities
c. **Potential for injury** related to impaired self-protective mechanisms

Rationale: *Damage to brain structures from impaired cerebral circulation can result in hemianopsia, diplopia, loss of touch or proprioception, pain, or decreased/absent temperature sensation. Unilateral neglect indicates the person may be inattentive to or unaware of the body parts affected by the sensory loss.*

☐ GOAL

The patient will adapt to visual deficits, compensate for sensory disturbances, and be free from injury caused by diminished or absent sensation.

☐ IMPLEMENTATION

- Assess patient's visual and sensory function to determine deficit.
- Position objects, call light, food tray within reach on unaffected side.
- Approach patient from the unaffected side and encourage family to do so.
- Cover affected eye with an eye patch or shield if diplopia is present.
- Assist in gauging distance of objects.
- Assist with activities of daily living and mobility as needed.
- Monitor temperature of food, bathwater to prevent accidental injury; teach patient/family to do the same.

☐ EVALUATION CRITERIA/DESIRED OUTCOMES

The Patient

- Is free from injury
- Verbalizes need for safety precautions necessitated by individual sensory deficits
- Adapts to sensory impairments

NURSING DIAGNOSIS #10

a. **Grieving** related to actual/perceived loss of function
b. **Ineffective individual coping** related to loss of well-being
c. **Disturbance in self-concept: body image, self-esteem, role performance, personal identity** related to loss of body functions, physical changes, role changes, dependence

Rationale: *Alterations in motor and sensory function, such as hemiplegia, as well as altered patterns of communication (aphasia) make the person dependent on others for even the most basic needs. Hospitalization and the CVA-induced disabilities disrupt the individual's life-style including roles in family, community/society, and career.*

☐ GOAL

The patient will effectively adapt to an altered appearance, disabilities, and roles.

☐ IMPLEMENTATION

- Explore with patient/family fears of dying, loss of independence, loss of control of body functions, crippling and permanent disability, and loss of speech.
- Encourage verbalization and expression of feelings (anger, depression, frustration, anxiety, helplessness, hopelessness).
- Determine impact of altered health status on patient and family on an ongoing basis.
- Refer to *The Patient Experiencing Grief and Loss,* page 272, and *The Patient Experiencing a Body-Image Disturbance,* page 253.
- Consult social services, counseling, clergy, as needed.
- Remind patient/family that progress is slow but possible; reinforce all positive gains (improvements in condition, patient accomplishments).

☐ EVALUATION CRITERIA/DESIRED OUTCOMES

The Patient

- Is able to view self in mirror
- Participates in care to the extent possible
- Demonstrates increased independence
- Verbalizes concerns, fears

NURSING DIAGNOSIS #11

Knowledge deficit regarding disease process/treatment, prognosis

Rationale: *The unexpected nature of a CVA as well as its seriousness and complexity make the patient/family need for information very acute. Communication problems may interfere with effective teaching.*

☐ GOAL

The patient/family will demonstrate adequate knowledge of cerebrovascular disease and the prognosis.

☐ IMPLEMENTATION

- Explain all treatments and procedures
- Encourage questions and answer as honestly as possible.
- Utilize resources (e.g., written materials, movies) to aid in teaching.

☐ EVALUATION CRITERIA/DESIRED OUTCOMES

The Patient/family

- Describes in own words what disease process is
- Acknowledges/understands care needs
- Participates in care appropriately and safely

The Patient With Chronic Renal Failure

Definition/Discussion

Chronic renal failure (CRF) is a progressive, irreversible deterioration of renal function leading to end-stage renal disease, which usually results in fatal uremia unless interventions of dialysis or kidney transplant are performed. The stages of CRF are

- *diminished renal reserve:* reduced renal function without the accumulation of metabolic wastes in the blood
- *renal insufficiency:* metabolic wastes begin to accumulate in the blood resulting in elevated BUN, serum creatinine, uric acid, and phosphorus levels
- *uremia:* excess amounts of nitrogenous wastes accumulate in the blood since the kidneys can no longer maintain homeostasis

Onset of CRF is usually slow with mild, intermittent symptoms.

Nursing Assessment

☐ PERTINENT HISTORY

Known renal disease, primary or secondary to trauma; surgery; metabolic disorders, especially diabetes mellitus and liver failure; family history of renal disease

☐ PHYSICAL FINDINGS

Refer to *The Patient with Acute Renal Failure,* page 10; in addition, bronzing of skin; dry, brittle hair; uremic frost (whitish crystals on skin from waste products being excreted through perspiration); osteodystrophy, joint pain; amenorrhea, impotence, decreased libido; metabolic acidosis; hepatitis B, non-A and non-B (from multiple blood transfusions)

☐ PSYCHOSOCIAL CONCERNS/ DEVELOPMENTAL FACTORS

Compliance with the treatment protocol; support system; depression, powerlessness, social isolation, grieving, motivation

☐ PATIENT AND FAMILY KNOWLEDGE

Options for treatment, participation in decision making, level of knowledge, readiness and willingness to learn

Nursing Care

☐ LONG-TERM GOAL

The patient will maintain predialysis status as long as possible, living within restrictions imposed by the disease; the patient will be able to deal with the possibility of long-term dialysis or renal transplant if feasible.

NURSING DIAGNOSES #1 to #3

Refer to Nursing Diagnoses #1, #2, and #3 in *The Patient with Acute Renal Failure*, page 10.

NURSING DIAGNOSIS #4

a. **Grieving** related to loss of renal function, required life-style changes, poor prognosis
b. **Fear** related to anticipated death
c. **Ineffective individual/family coping** related to diagnosis, life-style changes, necessary decision making

Rationale: *It is normal for a patient with a chronic, disabling diagnosis to experience the stages of the grieving process (i.e., denial, anger, depression, bargaining, and acceptance) as s/he mourns the loss of a normal bodily function, and changes in body image and normal life-style. Fear of dying is also a normal reaction to CRF. The many complications of CRF are life threatening and it is realistic to expect that the disease process will shorten the patient's life span.*

☐ GOAL

The patient will accept and adjust to body and role changes brought about by restrictions imposed by CRF; will express, and staff will accept without judgment, any and all feelings, including negative ones and those dealing with death.

☐ IMPLEMENTATION

- Plan nursing care to allow for some time each day to discuss with the patient specific aspects of the disease process, prescribed therapy, and treatment options; ask the patient to describe what this information means and how s/he feels about the current situation and the projected future; allow expression of any feelings, limiting only those that are destructive.
- Structure interventions according to the patient's/family's stage in the grieving process; refer to *The Patient Experiencing Grief and Loss*, page 272.
- Arrange for the patient to confer with the nephrology nurse specialist, transplant coordinator, or dialysis nurse for detailed information about options being considered.
- Discuss goals and ability to meet the desired goals; focus on short-term rather than long-term expectations.
- Support adaptive coping mechanisms; assist patient in finding alternatives if present strategies are not effective (e.g., asking for explanations when new regimen is presented rather than indicating agreement to a treatment not completely understood).
- If the patient is not adapting (e.g., expresses hopelessness, refuses to adhere to prescribed regimen), crisis intervention may be necessary; refer to *The Patient Requiring Crisis Intervention*, page 256, or initiate referral to appropriate counselor.
- Assist to realize that self-worth is not solely related to productivity (i.e., maintaining expected occupational role); discuss changes in usual role functioning and family relationships (often a problem if the spouse has to go to work); include spouse and other family members in discussion; inform patient/family of support groups available in the community; initiate referrals for family therapy as necessary; confer with social services department to initiate referrals for financial assistance.
- Recognize the patient's right for autonomy; know that a patient's right to refuse treatment to prolong life is supported in the American Hospital Association's "Patient's Bill of Rights," which states that patient has the right to do so after having been informed of the consequences; continue emotional support to patient/family if this decision is made.

☐ EVALUATION CRITERIA/DESIRED OUTCOMES

The Patient/family

- Expresses statements reflecting understanding and acceptance of the chronic course of renal failure
- Describes implications of life-style changes
- Verbalizes feelings about death

NURSING DIAGNOSIS #5

Alteration in comfort: pain related to osteodystrophy

Rationale: *Inability of the kidneys to maintain electrolyte balance may result in disturbance of the calcium-phosphorus ratio; when the calcium-phosphorus product (i.e., serum calcium multiplied by serum phosphorus) exceeds 40, calcium phosphate crystals precipitate into soft tissue, and blood vessels.*

☐ GOAL

The patient will be free from joint pain, or if present, will express relief from pain; will maintain normal serum calcium and phosphorus levels.

☐ IMPLEMENTATION

- Administer medications to regulate calcium/phosphorus balance.
- Monitor serum calcium and phosphorus levels; report elevated calcium-phosphorus product.
- Initiate comfort measures when joint pain is present.
- Medicate for relief of pain as needed: avoid analgesics that are detoxified by the kidneys; monitor effects.

☐ EVALUATION CRITERIA/DESIRED OUTCOMES

The Patient

- Maintains/regains normal serum calcium and phosphorus levels
- Experiences absence or relief of joint pain

NURSING DIAGNOSIS #6

Alteration in comfort (pruritus) related to uremic frost

Rationale: *In end-stage renal disease the kidneys are unable to excrete metabolic wastes so alternate routes of excretion are used by the body in an effort to compensate for the failure of this vital function. The patient's perspiration will contain end products of metabolism, leaving an irritating whitish powder on the skin called uremic frost.*

☐ GOAL

The patient will be free from pruritus.

☐ IMPLEMENTATION

- Bathe patient at least daily and as needed, using minimal soap, to remove accumulated wastes; apply lubricating lotion (without additives) to prevent dryness.
- If bedridden, turn at least every 2 hours, massaging back and coccyx; use sheepskin protection for bony prominences and other standard decubitus prevention measures.
- If uremic frost develops, use a solution of 2 tablespoons vinegar to 1 pint warm water to dissolve deposited crystals; rinse with warm water.
- Explain that dialysis removes the metabolic wastes and thus decreases the likelihood of uremic frost developing.

☐ EVALUATION CRITERIA/DESIRED OUTCOMES

The Patient

- Reports decrease in or absence of pruritus
- Is free from uremic frost

NURSING DIAGNOSIS #7

Potential for injury related to motor, cognitive, and sensory deficits secondary to uremic encephalopathy

Rationale: *Elevated serum ammonia levels are toxic to central nervous system tissues. In end-stage renal disease, decreased cognitive functioning may be evidenced. Problems with control of skeletal muscles may result in impaired physical mobility. Additionally, sensory perception may be impaired, especially in elderly patients or those whose renal disease is secondary to diabetes or arteriosclerotic lesions.*

☐ GOAL

The patient will be protected from physical injury; will be oriented to time, place, and person.

☐ IMPLEMENTATION

- Monitor blood pH, BUN, serum creatinine, and ammonia.
- Assess neurologic status at least every 8 hours; observe for apathy, decrease in recent memory, tremors, peripheral numbness or loss of muscle strength, asterixis, convulsions, or decreased levels of consciousness.
- If physical mobility is limited because of unsteady gait or decreased sensory perception, carefully inspect the patient's room for environmental hazards; discuss safety precautions with staff and patient/family; orient patient to unfamiliar surroundings, being sure to leave personal items and call button within reach prior to leaving room; assist with ambulation as tolerated; if patient requires a cane, walker, or wheelchair, ask that s/he call for assistance before getting out of bed or chair.
- Orient to time, place, and person as neces-

sary; encourage conversation to maintain mental alertness and active participation in activities of daily living.

☐ EVALUATION CRITERIA/DESIRED OUTCOMES

The Patient

- Is oriented to time, place, and person with no change in neurologic status
- Maintains physical safety

NURSING DIAGNOSIS #8

Altered sexuality pattern related to impotence, decreased libido

Rationale: *The exact mechanism causing sexual dysfunction associated with CRF is unknown but is thought to be related to uremic neuropathy as well as to general feelings of malaise, weakness, and fatigue. Not all patients experience sexual dysfunction.*

☐ GOAL

The patient will express understanding of sexual dysfunction in CRF; will be able to identify alternate means for sustaining a satisfying sexual relationship.

☐ IMPLEMENTATION

- If patient does not initiate the discussion, establish a trusting relationship before introducing the topic of sexual dysfunction.
- Ensure privacy/confidentiality; approach patient with an open, nonjudgmental attitude; permit patient to set the pace.
- Encourage patient to verbalize thoughts and feelings; ask about usual patterns of sexual expression; include partner if patient so desires; explain the importance of sharing concerns with the partner.
- Provide accurate information; discuss alternate methods for attaining a satisfying sexual relationship; initiate referral to qualified counselor as necessary.

☐ EVALUATION CRITERIA/DESIRED OUTCOMES

The Patient

- Acknowledges relationship between sexual dysfunction and CRF
- Indicates plans to use alternate methods for sharing satisfying sexual relationship

NURSING DIAGNOSIS #9

Knowledge deficit regarding posthospitalization treatment regimen

Rationale: *An understanding of the disease process of CRF, including effects on each body system, potential complications, and lifestyle changes required can increase compliance with treatment. This knowledge is essential to support the highest quality of life within the constraints of the individual's condition.*

☐ GOAL

The patient/family will understand the progression of CRF, expected symptomatology, avoidable complications, prescribed diet, fluid restrictions, medications (including toxic effects to be reported to physician), and treatment of choice for end-stage renal disease.

☐ IMPLEMENTATION

- Establish a teaching plan according to specific learning needs of patient/family.
- Include explanation of normal kidney function and explain the extent of renal functioning present; explain how laboratory studies reflect ongoing renal status; identify signs and symptoms that might indicate changes in fluid and electrolyte balance and instruct patient to contact physician should they develop.
- Instruct patient/family about the importance of daily weighing as an indication of fluid retention; confer with physician as to amount of weight gain or loss to be reported.
- Review the signs and symptoms of infection and bleeding, stressing the importance of immediately informing the physician of their occurence.
- Provide a list of prescribed medications; establish a daily schedule of administration with the patient/family, planning for specific medications to be given on an empty stomach or with milk or meals; if antibiotics are ordered, explain why constant blood levels are desirable; ensure that toxic effects to be reported to physician are clearly understood.
- Discuss prescribed dietary regimen to pa-

tient/family, explaining why protein, sodium, potassium, and fluid are restricted; request dietician to work with patient/family member who prepares meals to plan menus consistent with patient preferences as much as possible; provide a written menu plan, including lists of foods to be avoided and included; stress the importance of reading labels, especially for sodium and potassium content.

- Encourage patient/family to express feelings about current condition, prognosis, and treatment; discuss treatment options projected for end-stage renal disease; establish a plan for providing continuing emotional support via individual, family, or group sessions in the community.

☐ EVALUATION CRITERIA/DESIRED OUTCOMES

The Patient/family

- Describes disease course and acceptance of this diagnosis
- Lists significant signs and symptoms, including toxic effects of prescribed medications, to be reported to physician
- Verbally commits to comply with prescribed diet and fluid restrictions and to make arrangements for follow-up laboratory studies on an outpatient basis

The Patient with Cirrhosis

Definition/Discussion

Cirrhosis is a chronic, progressive disease in which scar tissue replaces liver tissue causing degeneration, decreased functioning, and increased resistance to portal blood flow. The most common types of hepatic cirrhosis are

- *Laënnec's portal cirrhosis:* scar tissue develops in the portal area
- *postnecrotic cirrhosis:* follows acute infections

Laënnec's cirrhosis occurs more frequently than postnecrotic cirrhosis.

Nursing Assessment

☐ PERTINENT HISTORY

Medical and surgical history; history of viral hepatitis; drug use (especially IV); medications taken; alcoholism; liver/infectious disease; exposure to chemicals, anesthetic agents; congestive heart failure; rheumatic heart disease; bleeding tendencies; esophageal varices

☐ PHYSICAL FINDINGS

Enlarged liver and/or abdominal tenderness; signs of poor nutritional status including tissue wasting, weakness, fatigue, or anorexia; edema; ascites; jaundice; dark urine; increased serum bilirubin, SGOT, SGPT, LDH; decreased serum albumin; spider telangiectasia; asterixis; palmar erythema; altered mental status; splenomegaly; esophageal varices; hemorrhoids; caput medusae; elevated temperature

☐ PSYCHOSOCIAL CONCERNS/ DEVELOPMENTAL FACTORS

Age (more frequent over age 50), sex (more common in males), occupation, roles and responsibilities, use of alcohol as coping mechanism, available support system

☐ PATIENT AND FAMILY KNOWLEDGE

Treatment modalities to maintain liver function and retard progression of the disease, level of knowledge, readiness and willingness to learn

Nursing Care

☐ LONG-TERM GOAL

The patient will maintain optimum level of functioning within the limitations of prescribed medical regimen in order to reduce the progress of liver damage.

NURSING DIAGNOSIS #1

Fluid volume deficit related to fluid and sodium retention, potassium excretion, ascites

Rationale: *Liver damage prevents proper detoxification of aldosterone, causing water and sodium retention and potassium excretion. In addition, albumin synthesis is altered and portal hypertension may be present resulting in ascites. The resulting sodium and water retention may cause a deficit in circulating fluid volume.*

☐ GOAL

The patient will adhere to prescribed diet in an effort to prevent further liver damage.

☐ IMPLEMENTATION

- Anticipate tube feedings to provide nutrition if patient is too nauseated or if bleeding complications occur.

- Teach that adequate nutrition is often as important as medications to retard progress of the disease.
- Provide a diet high in protein and calories as tolerated to aid in regeneration of liver cells; explain rationale to patient; make meals as attractive and interesting as possible; include family during meals if this is therapeutic for patient.
- Provide frequent small meals with protein supplements to decrease anorexia and nausea; consider patient preferences in choosing foods.
- Restrict sodium if ascites and edema are present, suggest use of salt substitute; teach patient to use other flavorings (e.g., lemon juice, oregano).
- Encourage bedrest and rest periods during the day to conserve energy and decrease metabolic demands if appropriate.
- Avoid roughage in diet if hemorrhoidal bleeding is present.
- Encourage vitamin supplements with iron, folic acid, and thiamine to help reduce dietary deficiencies.

☐ EVALUATION CRITERIA/DESIRED OUTCOMES

The Patient

- Adheres to prescribed diet
- Ingests all food on tray at each meal
- Actively participates in choosing foods

NURSING DIAGNOSIS #2

Ineffective breathing pattern related to positioning, impaired mobility, ascites

Rationale: *Fluid accumulation in the abdominal area causes pressure on the diaphragm resulting in decreased lung expansion, which may cause hypoxemia.*

☐ GOAL

The patient will maintain fluid volume and electrolyte levels within normal limits.

☐ IMPLEMENTATION

- Record intake and output accurately; weigh patient every day to assess fluid status.
- Determine daily amount of allowed fluids; provide oral fluids within dietary restrictions, personal likes/dislikes.
- Know normal laboratory values; if patient wants to know these values share this information, pointing out signs of positive change as they occur; refer to Table 1, *Common Fluid and Electrolyte Imbalances*, page 14.
- Observe amount and location of edema; chart daily and as changes occur.
- Monitor presence and depth of jaundice of skin and sclera; monitor color, odor, and character of feces; observe color of urine to monitor increasing liver damage.
- Measure abdominal girth every day to assess ascites; mark placement of tape on abdomen for consistent measurement.
- Administer diuretics to promote diuresis of accumulated fluid.

☐ EVALUATION CRITERIA/DESIRED OUTCOMES

The Patient

- Has balanced intake and output, electrolytes within normal limits
- Has decreased abdominal girth
- Experiences fluid weight loss of at least 1-2 lb/day until within normal limits

NURSING DIAGNOSIS #3

a. **Impairment of skin integrity** related to edema, ascites, pruritus
b. **Potential for infection** related to scratching, impaired skin integrity

Rationale: *Liver damage causes an obstruction of bile flow resulting in an accumulation of bile salts in the skin, causing pruritus. Edema of the extremities and abdominal ascites cause tautness of the skin, added weight on the tissues, and a decrease in peripheral circulation, predisposing skin to breakdown and infection.*

☐ GOAL

The patient will maintain intact skin; will be free from skin breakdown, decubitus ulcer, or infections; will experience relief of pruritus and skin discomfort.

☐ IMPLEMENTATION

- Know that patients with cirrhosis are prone to skin breakdown because of poor nutri-

tional state, edema, muscle wasting, and immobility.
- Turn patient every 2 hours and keep off back as much as possible.
- Consider using an air mattress, sheepskin, egg-crate mattress.
- Provide range-of-motion exercises as necessary; consult with physician and physical therapist regarding appropriate exercises.
- Keep room cool; administer antipruritic medication and lotions in an effort to control pruritus.
- Provide gentle rubbing, patting, or stroking of skin; apply powder, talc, or cornstarch; avoid soap; keep skin dry to prevent breakdown.
- Keep patient's fingernails short or apply gloves to patient to prevent abrasions from scratching.

☐ EVALUATION CRITERIA/DESIRED OUTCOMES

The Patient

- Is free from skin breakdown, decubitus, or infection
- Verbalizes relief from pruritus

NURSING DIAGNOSIS #4

Alteration in thought processes related to increased serum ammonia

Rationale: *Rising levels of ammonia result from the breakdown of protein and the breakdown of red blood cells from gastrointestinal bleeding or hemorrhage. The severely damaged liver is unable to detoxify the ammonia. Altered mental status ranging from drowsiness to hepatic coma is directly related to the increasing levels of ammonia.*

☐ GOAL

The patient will maintain adequate oxygenation.

☐ IMPLEMENTATION

- Explain to patient/family that shortness of breath often occurs with ascites; observe for changes in breathing, cyanosis.
- Place patient in semi- to high-Fowler's position as tolerated; support back and arms to allow for maximum lung expansion.
- Keep items within easy reach of patient.
- Turn patient every 2 hours; encourage deep breathing and position changes to maximize aeration of lungs.
- Encourage regular use of incentive spirometer to maximize lung expansion.
- Auscultate lungs each shift and as necessary for adventitious sounds and decreased breath sounds.
- Monitor arterial blood gases for respiratory dysfunction.
- Monitor vital signs, especially respiratory rate and temperature, for impending pulmonary infection.
- Encourage patient to use supplemental oxygen if ordered to prevent hypoxemia.
- Assist with paracentesis to decrease ascites and relieve pressure on diaphragm.

☐ EVALUATION CRITERIA/DESIRED OUTCOMES

The Patient

- Breathes regularly and comfortably
- Has arterial blood gases within normal limits
- Has lungs clear to auscultation and percussion

NURSING DIAGNOSIS #5

Alteration in nutrition: less than body requirements related to anorexia, nausea, vomiting, indigestion, inadequate intake

Rationale: *A long history of poor nutrition and a history of chronic alcohol abuse can predispose an individual to cirrhosis. Individuals who ingest large quantities of alcohol generally do so without maintaining an adequate intake of nutrients. Subsequent liver damage results in poor metabolism of the nutrients that are ingested. Anorexia, nausea and vomiting, and indigestion caused by the altered metabolism further increase the risk of altered nutrition.*

☐ GOAL

The patient will be free from mental status deterioration.

☐ IMPLEMENTATION

- Observe for early signs of hepatic encephalopathy including euphoria, inappropriate behavior, fatigue, irritability, restlessness, loss of judgment.

- Observe and chart mental status each shift.
- Observe for signs of impending hepatic coma including nausea and vomiting, low-grade fever, diarrhea, abdominal ache or pain; chart and report findings.
- Monitor ammonia and postassium levels and arterial blood gases.
- Restrict protein in diet to prevent increased ammonia production.
- Give narcotics, sedatives, and tranquilizers cautiously (may mask signs of hepatic coma).
- Prevent constipation; give stool softeners, maintain adequate hydration to decrease formation of ammonia in the intestines.
- Anticipate lactulose, magnesium sulfate, neomycin, or kanamycin enemas or oral antibiotics to decrease intestinal ammonia levels.

☐ EVALUATION CRITERIA/DESIRED OUTCOMES

The Patient

- Has serum ammonia levels within normal limits
- Remains awake, alert, and oriented

NURSING DIAGNOSIS #6

a. **Knowledge deficit** regarding disease process, complications, treatment
b. **Disturbance in self-concept: self-esteem, role performance, personal identity** related to alcoholism, serious illness
c. **Ineffective individual coping** related to alcoholism, serious illness, knowledge deficit
d. **Anxiety** related to fear of the unknown
e. **Ineffective individual/family coping** related to disease process, lifestyle changes
f. **Alteration in family process** related to lifestyle changes
g. **Powerlessness** related to treatment modalities
h. **Self-care deficit: total** related to imposed restrictions

Rationale: *Cirrhosis is a chronic, long-term, progressive illness with life-threatening complications that make recovery difficult. Many patients present with a long history of alcohol abuse; they identify alcohol as a major coping mechanism, but continued alcohol ingestion will cause further liver deterioration. Behavior and life-style changes are imperative for recovery and rehabilitation. Knowledge of the disease and its relationship to alcohol ingestion may encourage the patient to utilize more effective coping mechanisms, increase selfesteem, and allow resumption of former or more adaptive roles.*

☐ GOAL

The patient will verbalize knowledge of the disease process, complications, and treatment; will have an increased self-concept; will demonstrate adaptive coping mechanisms.

☐ IMPLEMENTATION

- Teach relationship of alcohol to progression of disease; stress importance of completely eliminating alcohol from diet.
- Refer to community resources for aid in eliminating alcohol (e.g., Alcoholics Anonymous, social worker, other alcohol rehabilitation facilities).
- Stress importance of adhering to prescribed diet.
- Teach about susceptibility to infections and preventive measures.
- Explore postdischarge sources of support to aid in adjusting to behavior and life-style changes.
- Include family in discharge teaching to provide support for treatments and life-style modifications.
- Explore alternative coping mechanisms and recreational or diversional activities to assist with adjustment after discharge.
- Teach patient/family signs and symptoms of reportable complications such as increased abdominal girth, weight gain, edema, fever, blood in stools or urine, vomiting, confusion, tremors, or change in personality/behavior.
- Encourage patient to ventilate feelings to help decrease anxiety related to life-style changes, decreased self-esteem, or problems with role adjustment.
- Instruct in importance of adequate rest to preserve liver function.

☐ EVALUATION CRITERIA/DESIRED OUTCOMES

The Patient

- Describes disease process, complications, and treatment in own words
- Participates actively in self-care
- Verbalizes an increase in self-esteem
- Demonstrates adaptive coping mechanisms
- Abstains from alcohol
- Describes an appropriate dietary regimen

The Patient with Congestive Heart Failure

Definition/Discussion

Congestive heart failure (CHF) results when the heart, because of impaired cardiac function or increased work load, cannot maintain an adequate blood supply to the lungs and/or other parts of the body. Congestive heart failure occurs when fluid accumulates in the body's tissues because of this inability to circulate blood.

CHF may be classified according to the side of the heart that is affected. During the acute phase only one side may be involved but impairment of the other is usually inevitable as the condition progresses. With *right-sided failure,* fluid accumulates in the systemic venous system, causing an increase in right atrial and peripheral venous pressures with resultant peripheral edema and congestion of the abdominal organs. Because of the decreased venous return to the right heart, the supply of unoxygenated blood pumped into the lungs is decreased.

In *left-sided failure,* fluid accumulates in the pulmonary circulatory system because the outflow of oxygenated blood into the systemic arterial system from the left ventrical is decreased. The pooling in the lungs causes an alteration of the ventilation/perfusion ratio resulting in impaired gas exchange and increased breathing effort. Severe left-sided failure may result in acute pulmonary edema (see *The Patient with Pulmonary Edema,* page 201).

During the acute phase of CHF, symptoms may reflect right-sided failure, left-sided failure, or both. Medical treatment aims toward correcting the cause, improving cardiac function, and maintaining fluid balance. Surgery (e.g., valve replacement, repair of ventricular defect) may be required to correct the underlying cause.

Nursing Assessment

☐ PERTINENT HISTORY

Damage to heart muscle or valves; congenital heart defect; disturbance in rate, rhythm, or conduction; pericarditis; hypertension; thyrotoxicosis; anemia; excessive infusion of IV fluids

☐ PHYSICAL FINDINGS

General: tachypnea, tachycardia, weak/thready pulse, narrowing pulse pressure, chest pain, pallor/cyanosis, diaphoresis, cool skin, altered mental status, dizziness, syncope, decreased urinary output
Right-sided failure: fatigue, dependent edema, jugular vein distension, hepatomegaly, splenomegaly, ascites, anorexia, elevated right atrial and central venous pressures
Left-sided failure: dyspnea on exertion, orthopnea, cough; blood-tinged, frothy sputum; elevated pulmonary capillary wedge pressure

☐ PSYCHOSOCIAL CONCERNS/ DEVELOPMENTAL FACTORS

Reactions to stress, fear of dying

☐ PATIENT AND FAMILY KNOWLEDGE

Causative factors; need for low-stress environment, protection from anxiety-provoking situations; procedures, treatments; level of knowledge, readiness and willingness to learn

Nursing Care

☐ LONG-TERM GOAL

The patient will recover from the acute episode and will adjust roles in home, work, and community to adhere to prescribed medical regimen.

NURSING DIAGNOSIS #1

a. **Alteration in cardiac output: decreased** related to inefficient heart action

b. **Alteration in tissue perfusion: peripheral** related to decreased cardiac output

Rationale: *CHF occurs when the heart is unable to perform normally as a pump, producing a cardiac output insufficient to meet the body's needs at rest or during activity. Nursing measures aimed at decreasing the cardiac workload will increase the efficiency of the heart as a pump, thus improving circulation throughout the body.*

☐ GOAL

The patient will maintain a cardiac output adequate to circulate blood to the body's tissues.

☐ IMPLEMENTATION

- Maintain complete bedrest to reduce cardiac workload (1 day of complete rest conserves about 25,000 heart contractions).
- Place patient in a semirecumbent position with pillows under arms and behind back longitudinally; provide footboard.
- Avoid unnecessary movement; give mouth care and partial bath only; change position, inspect skin, and massage pressure points every 2 hours.
- Limit visitors to immediate family for short intervals (5-10 minutes) every 1-2 hours when awake; if patient is fearful/anxious, extend time if visitors have a calming effect on patient.
- Monitor cardiac rhythm continuously, record a rhythm strip every 4 hours or more if irregular; administer antidysrhythmic agents, assess for expected response and untoward effects.
- Assess cardiac functioning (e.g., blood pressure, pulse, hemodynamic readings) every 1-2 hours or as ordered (cardiac output may be measured every 4-8 hours with other readings done more frequently); watch for signs of further impairment (e.g., decreased blood pressure with narrowing pulse pressure; increased pulse, central venous/right atrial pressure, or pulmonary capillary wedge pressure).
- Observe quality of peripheral pulses (e.g., full, bounding weak, regular/irregular) and skin appearance (e.g., temperature, color, moistness, turgor) every 4 hours.
- Administer inotropic agents, vasodilators, and alpha-adrenergic agents as ordered, monitoring for effectiveness and toxicity; assess response to digitalis preparations very carefully as electrolyte imbalances associated with fluid volume excess may potentiate the effects of digitalis and result in toxicity with what would normally be therapeutic doses.
- Give sedatives/hypnotics as ordered; assess respiratory status for shallow, irregular rate prior to administering known respiratory depressants; monitor patient response.

☐ EVALUATION CRITERIA/DESIRED OUTCOMES

The Patient

- Has improved, stable vital signs and hemodynamic readings
- Has strong peripheral phases
- Displays warm, dry skin with good turgor
- Is free from or controls dysrhythmias

NURSING DIAGNOSIS #2

a. **Impaired gas exchange** related to effects of altered pulmonary circulation

b. **Ineffective breathing pattern** related to pain, anxiety, and impaired circulation

Rationale: *Both right-sided and left-sided heart failure are likely to cause alterations in ventilation/perfusion. With right-sided failure, a decreased volume of unoxygenated blood is pumped into the lungs. In left-sided failure, blood backs up in the lungs because the left ventricle is unable to efficiently pump oxygenated blood to the body's tissues. In either* *case, the result is hypoxia, causing pain (in the chest and limbs most frequently) and feelings of breathlessness.*

One of the body's normal compensatory mechanisms for hypoxia is to increase oxygen intake. Unfortunately, the increased respiratory rate increases the cardiac workload further, intensifying rather than decreasing the hypoxic state.

☐ GOAL

The patient will maintain respiratory functioning adequate to oxygenate all body tissues.

☐ IMPLEMENTATION

- Administer oxygen as prescribed (usually 4-6 liters/minute unless contraindicated because of chronic hypoxia, then 2 liters/minute); use nasal prongs rather than mask, as mask tends to further increase anxiety.
- Medicate for pain promptly; monitor for expected relief; assess for untoward effects of medication and institute measures to modify.
- Assess respiratory status (rate, depth, character, breath sounds, productiveness of cough) every 1-2 hours; watch for orthopnea, increased rate, decreased depth, rales, frothy sputum (refer to *The Patient with Pulmonary Edema*, page 201).
- Prepare for intubation and assisted ventilation if indicated (refer to *The Patient with Asthma*, page 32).
- Monitor arterial blood gases for hypoxemia, decreased oxygen saturation, respiratory alkalosis.
- Position for comfort and ease of breathing; use semi-Fowler's or position described in Nursing Diagnosis #1; plan care to allow for rest periods before and after treatments/visitors.
- Watch for alterations in mental status (e.g., decreased level of consciousness, restlessness, agitation) suggestive of cerebral hypoxia.
- Explain procedures/treatments briefly; provide sufficient information to decrease anxiety but avoid overwhelming the patient/family during the acute phase.

☐ EVALUATION CRITERIA/DESIRED OUTCOMES

The Patient

- Has normal respiratory rate, depth, effort, and breath sounds
- Is free from dyspnea at rest
- Has normal arterial blood gases
- Maintains/regains mental alertness
- Relates decreased pain, anxiety

NURSING DIAGNOSIS #3

Alteration in fluid volume: excess related to effects of right-sided heart failure and/or decreased renal perfusion pressure with left-sided heart failure

Rationale: *When the right ventricle is unable to effectively pump blood into the pulmonary circulatory system, blood backs up into the right atrium and venous systemic circulatory system. If the left ventricle pumps an insufficient blood volume through the aorta to the body's tissues, compensatory mechanisms (e.g., decreased renal perfusion pressures) are enacted. With blood flow to the kidneys decreased, the glomerular filtration rate decreases as well, resulting in retention of sodium and water in an attempt to increase intravascular volume to compensate for the decreased cardiac output. Decreased excretion of sodium causes retention of potassium as well, with the possible risk of fatal dysrhythmias.*

☐ GOAL

The patient will maintain/regain fluid and electrolyte balance.

☐ IMPLEMENTATION

- Weigh patient on admission and daily, at same time, on same scale, and with same clothing; report daily gains or losses of more than 3 lb.
- Inspect extremities, sacrum, and periorbital areas for edema and assess for jugular vein distention every 4-8 hours.
- Monitor central venous pressure/hemodynamic readings as ordered; adjust IV intake according to physician's order.
- Restrict fluids and sodium as ordered; record intake carefully, including all IV medications and water taken with medications.
- Have patient rinse mouth well after using mouthwashes and toothpaste as many of these contain large amounts of sodium.
- Give preliminary explanations of the role of

sodium in the formation of edema; provide sodium-restricted diet as ordered, recording intake; confer with dietician regarding patient food preferences.
- Record urinary output and specific gravity every 1-8 hours; report changes in specific gravity and output of less than 20-30 cc/hour for 2 consecutive hours.
- Administer diuretics as ordered; monitor urinary output hourly; watch for signs of related electrolyte imbalances (e.g., hyponatremia, hypokalemia); refer to Table 1, *Common Fluid and Electrolyte Imbalances*, page 14.

☐ EVALUATION CRITERIA/DESIRED OUTCOMES

The Patient
- Has a daily fluid intake equal to or less than urinary output
- Shows a weight loss when compared to baseline
- Displays decreased peripheral, sacral, or periorbital edema
- Has normal serum electrolytes, BUN, and creatinine

NURSING DIAGNOSIS #4

Potential for infection related to invasive catheters (IVs, hemodynamic monitoring, Foley)

Rationale: *The acutely ill patient with CHF may require multiple invasive catheters to treat the cause, allay symptoms, and monitor progress of CHF-related problems. Each invasive line poses a risk for infection.*

☐ GOAL

The patient will remain free from infection.

☐ IMPLEMENTATION

- Inspect all catheter insertion sites every 4-8 hours; watch for signs of inflammation (e.g., redness, swelling, increased temperature, tenderness); remove suspected catheter and reinsert new sterile catheter.
- Cleanse meatus and area around urinary catheter insertion every 8 hours.
- Change IV tubing/dressings per hospital protocols.
- Monitor temperature every 4 hours for increase.
- Administer prophylatic antibiotics on time to ensure adequate blood levels; monitor for desired and toxic effects.

☐ EVALUATION CRITERIA/DESIRED OUTCOMES

The Patient
- Has a normal body temperature
- Is free from inflammation at catheter insertion sites

NURSING DIAGNOSIS #5

a. **Anxiety** related to pain, dyspnea, unfamiliar surroundings, procedures
b. **Fear** of dying related to severity of condition
c. **Knowledge deficit** regarding disease process, diagnostic procedures, proposed treatments

Rationale: *Anxiety associated with CHF is precipitated by feelings of breathlessness, pain, or dyspnea. Indeed, concern about these feelings probably caused the patient/family to seek medical attention. During the diagnostic workup and admission to the nursing unit, additional procedures will need to be performed, possible increasing the patient's/family's anxiety. In the acute phase, fear about the possibility of death may be expressed by the patient/family. These feelings need to be modified as the associated stress further increases the workload of the failing heart and hinders recovery. Interventions may need to be directed towards family members as the patient may become more anxious/fearful because of their responses to the situation.*

☐ GOAL

The patient/family will express reduced feelings of anxiety or fear; will indicate understanding of proposed procedures/treatments; the patient will experience a reduction of fear.

☐ IMPLEMENTATION

- Explain the physical setting (e.g., ICU or high acuity nursing unit), monitoring equipment, and unit routines to patient/family; stress that continuing assessments by nursing staff do not necessarily reflect a deteriorating condition.

- Keep patient/family informed of progress/procedures; assess how much information is wanted at this time; recall that giving information is an effective way of reducing anxiety, but that during the acute phase, giving too much information may increase rather than decrease anxiety.
- Stay with patient during acute episodes of anxiety/fear (unless constant presence is more anxiety provoking) or permit family to stay with patient as much as possible without tiring patient.
- Explain to family members the effect of family anxiety/fear on patient's status; encourage family members to take time to eat and sleep; provide the nursing unit's telephone number, urging the family to call at any time for an update; inform family that nursing staff will call family if condition changes.
- Encourage patient/family to ventilate fears, apprehensions, ask questions; explain that these feelings are normal.
- Point out signs of improvement (e.g., positive changes in vital signs, edema, circulation) but do not give false reassurance.
- Explain use of relaxation techniques (e.g., meditation, imaging, distraction) as a means of decreasing anxiety; encourage their use if patient agrees.
- Assess previously effective coping strategies; explore their usefulness in the present situation; encourage the use of successful stress-reducing mechanisms.
- Offer to contact spiritual advisor if patient/family desires. Initiate referral to social services if available.
- Refer to *The Patient Experiencing Anxiety*, page 250, for additional interventions if needed.

☐ EVALUATION CRITERIA/DESIRED OUTCOMES

The Patient/family

- Indicates decreased anxiety/fear
- Describes procedures/treatments

The Patient

- Displays vital signs consistent with decreased stress (e.g., decrease in respiratory or heart rates, less dyspnea/restlessness when compared to baseline)

The Patient with Epilepsy

Definition/Discussion

Epilepsy is a disorder of the nervous system, characterized by seizures. The seizures are a result of excessive neuronal discharge of uncontrollable and paroxysmal nature. The causes of epilepsy include genetic disorder, problems before birth, difficult birth, head injury, nutritional or toxic disorder, hypoglycemia, brain tumor, and stroke. In some cases the causative factor may be unknown.

Nursing Assessment

☐ PERTINENT HISTORY

Medical and surgical history, head injury, cerebral vascular accident, intracranial tumor or vascular abnormalities, infections, ingestion of toxic substances, family history of seizures, current medications

☐ PHYSICAL FINDINGS

Blood/urine chemistries; drug screen; if seizure occurs: aura, behavior during seizure (e.g., movement, loss of consciousness, biting tongue, incontinence), duration of seizure, behavior after seizure (e.g., confusion, aphasia, localized weakness, headache, memory)

☐ PSYCHOSOCIAL CONCERNS/ DEVELOPMENTAL FACTORS

Age, sex, role in family, socialization skills, available coping strategies, life-style, available support systems

☐ PATIENT AND FAMILY KNOWLEDGE

Disease condition and treatment, chronic conditions, readiness and willingness to learn

Nursing Care

☐ LONG-TERM GOAL

The patient will be free from seizures due to continuing medication and avoidance of precipitating stimuli; the patient will verbalize and demonstrate an understanding and acceptance of the reality of a probably chronic condition; the patient will demonstrate coping strategies that effectively deal with the diagnosis.

NURSING DIAGNOSIS #1

Potential for injury related to seizure activity

Rationale: *During a seizure, abnormal movements and/or an altered level of consciousness place the person at risk for bodily harm.*

☐ GOAL

The patient will be free from physical injury.

☐ IMPLEMENTATION

- Institute seizure precautions including side rails up, padded side rails, padded tongue blade and oral airway at bedside, bed in low position, and suction available.
- Monitor for seizure activity.
- Determine level of consciousness and behavior every 2-4 hours since seizures may be manifested by changes in behavior such as staring into space.
- Administer anticonvulsants as ordered.
- Provide for privacy if seizure occurs; insert padded tongue blade if teeth are not clenched, loosen restrictive clothing; guide but do not restrain movements, establish a

patent airway; observe for warning signs or aura; determine where the seizure began and how it proceeds, what body parts and movement are involved; change in pupils or gaze, incontinence, duration of the seizure, level of consciousness.

- Position on side after the seizure, allow to sleep; reorient as needed; observe for any weakness or paralysis; evaluate behavior.
- Document observations in chronologic sequence including time; onset of unusual behavior; environmental stimulants or other possible preseizure factors (e.g., photosensitivity, chill, fatigue, stressors); description of ictal phase; location and type of tonic or clonic contractions; presence of incontinence; skin color and condition, automisms (eye fluttering, lip smacking); eye movements and pupillary changes; duration of seizure; description of postictal phase and progress of patient's condition; sensorium; level of awareness; speech difficulty; weakness; pain; and length of time it takes for patient to be reoriented and stabilized.
- Notify physician immediately if seizures are repetitive without periods of consciousness.

☐ EVALUATION CRITERIA/DESIRED OUTCOMES

The Patient

- Maintains physical integrity following any seizure activity

NURSING DIAGNOSIS #2

a. **Ineffective individual coping** related to social stigma associated with epilepsy, feelings of helplessness regarding seizures, chronic nature of disease
b. **Anxiety/fear** related to disease

Rationale: *Coping with the diagnosis of epilepsy requires the successful management of medications, general health, and interventions during a seizure. Emotional/environmental stressors can contribute to seizures. Inability to handle these stressors may lead to social isolation and/or noncompliance.*

☐ GOAL

The patient will demonstrate coping strategies that effectively deal with the diagnosis of epilepsy.

☐ IMPLEMENTATION

- Determine patient's continuing emotional status, appearance and behavior to determine reaction to diagnosis.
- Promote and facilitate an open discussion of feelings, attitudes, and beliefs among patient, family, and nurse or physician.
- Encourage verbalization and questions regarding misconceptions, fears, and social stigma of epilepsy.
- Discuss the concept of stress and its relationship to seizures.
- Provide information about local and national epilepsy organization.
- Refer to social services, counselors, others as needed.

☐ EVALUATION CRITERIA/DESIRED OUTCOMES

The Patient

- Verbalizes anxieties, fears, and concerns
- Demonstrates identification of coping strategies (verbally, behaviorally)

NURSING DIAGNOSIS #3

Knowledge deficit regarding new diagnosis, frequency of seizures, age/developmental status

Rationale: *Patients with a new diagnosis or history of epilepsy require information focusing on simple pathology; medications including schedule, toxic and side effects; triggering factors; occupational considerations; followup; and public awareness. The patient may lack all or part of this knowledge.*

☐ GOAL

The patient/family will verbalize and demonstrate understanding of disease, medications, and life-style adjustments.

☐ IMPLEMENTATION

- Determine patient's/family's present knowledge of epilepsy, learning ability, and readiness to learn.
- Explain all necessary information about each medication including name, dosage, frequency, toxic and side effects to observe and report, stressing importance of taking daily

medication as ordered to maintain therapeutic blood levels.

- Monitor drug blood levels to determine therapeutic range.
- Emphasize common side effects of anticonvulsants (e.g., blood dyscrasias, anemia, rash/skin eruptions, drowsiness, GI irritation, and gingival problems); provide guidelines to deal with side effects.
- Instruct regarding factors that may trigger a seizure (e.g., abrupt withdrawal of medication, alcohol, constipation, fatigue, excessive stress, menstruation, fever, visual disturbances, large amounts of caffeine).
- Discuss with patient/family life-style considerations such as engaging in strenuous physical activity, occupation and occupational hazards, restrictions on driving, need for medical alert bracelet/necklace and wallet ID card.

☐ EVALUATION CRITERIA/DESIRED OUTCOMES

The Patient

- Discusses factors that trigger a seizure
- Verbalizes adequate knowledge of medication
- Verbalizes necessary life-style changes

The Patient with Esophageal Varices

Definition/Discussion

Esophageal varices are dilated tortuous veins usually found in the submucosa of the lower esophagus, which may extend into the esophagus and into the stomach. They are nearly always caused by portal hypertension secondary to cirrhosis of the liver.

Nursing Assessment

☐ PERTINENT HISTORY

Medical and surgical history, history of sudden loss of blood through mouth or rectum, hematemesis or melena; cirrhosis, hepatitis, alcohol abuse, ulcers, gastritis, portal hypertension

☐ PHYSICAL FINDINGS

Presence of blood in emesis/stool; hepatomegaly, splenomegaly, abdominal distention; ascites; signs of shock (i.e., decreased blood pressure, increased pulse, and respiratory rates, restlessness); altered mental status; hepatic encephalopathy; esophageal varices seen on esophagoscopy; hemorrhoids

☐ PSYCHOSOCIAL CONCERNS/ DEVELOPMENTAL FACTORS

Age, sex, occupation, usual coping mechanisms, available support system, roles and responsibilities

☐ PATIENT AND FAMILY KNOWLEDGE

Disease process, treatment modalities to maintain liver function, progression of disease, bleeding episodes; level of knowledge, readiness and willingness to learn

Nursing Care

☐ LONG-TERM GOAL

The patient will recover within the limitations of the prescribed medical regimen.

NURSING DIAGNOSIS #1

a. **Fluid volume deficit** related to hemorrhage, vomiting, diarrhea
b. **Potential for injury** (hemorrhage related to dilated esophageal vessels
c. **Alteration in cardiac output: decreased** related to hemorrhage

Rationale: *Obstructed blood flow from the diseased liver results in congestion of blood in the portal system causing portal hypertension. Collateral circulation develops in the gastrointestinal tract to compensate for this obstruction. As pressure increases, esophageal varices form and are subject to insidious or sudden hemorrhage because of their fragility and location.*

☐ GOAL

The patient will be free from injury; will maintain fluid volume at an acceptable level; will be free from complications associated with bleeding.

☐ IMPLEMENTATION

- Monitor for signs of insidious or sudden bleeding (e.g., hematemesis, hematochezia, melena, decreased blood pressure, increased pulse, increased respiratory rate, abdominal distention).
- Monitor hemoglobin and hematocrit.

- Assist with insertion of Sengstaken-Blakemore tube; provide emotional support during procedure.
- Ensure that tube is taped securely; keep tube taut to prevent it from moving into the main body of the stomach and to maintain pressure on the bleeding varices.
- Label each lumen carefully and accurately including the amount of pressure or volume in each and frequency of inflation/deflation; know that sufficient pressure must be maintained to retard the bleeding but pressure must be released periodically to prevent necrosis of the tissue surrounding the tube; document on the patient's chart.
- Know that a complication of tube placement is acute respiratory distress caused by occlusion of airway by the balloon or regurgitation of gastric contents into the lungs; if balloon occlusion should occur, cut tube lumens immediately; keep a pair of scissors taped in an obvious place at patient's bedside.
- Maintain nasogastric tube to low intermittent suction; observe for frank bleeding and report immediately.
- Ensure proper functioning of suction equipment; measure drainage carefully; chart color and amount of drainage to monitor progress of bleeding.
- Keep patient NPO while tube is in place; if foods or fluid are given through the tube, give slowly in order to avoid regurgitation.
- Provide emesis basin, cool wash cloths; suction posterior pharynx as necessary to prevent accumulation of secretions.
- Lavage with iced saline if ordered to promote local vasconstriction.
- Monitor vital signs every 15-30 minutes during bleeding episode; every 2-4 hours and as needed if no bleeding is observed.
- Maintain accurate intake and output; maintain patent IV infusions using large-bore needles in anticipation of transfusing blood and blood products to maintain circulating blood volume.
- Prepare and maintain vasopressin drip to promote constriction of bleeding varices.
- Anticipate magnesium sulfate, saline, or lactulose enemas to promote intestinal evacuation of blood and to maintain normal ammonia levels.
- Prepare patient for esophagoscopy or endoscopy to identify source of bleeding if ordered.

☐ EVALUATION CRITERIA/DESIRED OUTCOMES

The Patient

- Has bleeding controlled without complications
- Is free from subsequent bleeding

NURSING DIAGNOSIS #2

a. **Anxiety** related to fear of the unknown,
b. **Ineffective individual/family coping** related to disease process, lifestyle changes
c. **Alteration in family process** related to treatment modalities
d. **Powerlessness** related to treatment modalities
e. **Self-care deficit: total** related to imposed restrictions
f. **Knowledge deficit** regarding disease process, management, complications

Rationale: *Esophageal varices often bleed suddenly and without warning. Adherence to medical regimens, and life-style and behavior changes must be maintained to prevent complications. Knowledge of complications and factors that contribute to the disease process may assist patient to comply with medical regimens.*

☐ GOAL

The patient will understand the disease process, cause of esophageal bleeding, and treatment.

☐ IMPLEMENTATION

- Explain all procedures including rationales, expected discomforts, and results; be aware that giving information is an effective way to reduce anxiety but that giving too much may only increase it.
- Explain essential life-style changes to prevent progression of the disease; ask patient to discuss incorporating these into current life-style.
- Refer to community support group such as Alcoholics Anonymous or social worker.
- Refer to *The Patient with Cirrhosis,* page 83.

☐ EVALUATION CRITERIA/DESIRED OUTCOMES

The Patient

- Verbalizes rationale, expected discomforts, results of procedures
- Identifies necessary life-style changes
- Actively participates in care
- States plan to adhere to medical regimen

The Patient with Guillain-Barré Syndrome

Definition/Discussion

Guillain-Barré syndrome is a disease of the nervous system characterized by demyelination, which alters nerve conduction in the peripheral and cranial nerves, resulting in paralysis and paresthesias. The etiology is unknown but immunologic and viral or infective theories have been postulated. There is complete recovery in 75% of the cases.

Nursing Assessment

☐ PERTINENT HISTORY

Medical and surgical history; history of infection or recent illness; numbness/tingling, motor weakness, facial weakness, difficulty walking, pain; problems controlling bladder/bowel; abrupt onset of symptoms; distribution of motor/sensory disturbance (usually ascending, distal to proximal)

☐ PHYSICAL FINDINGS

Symmetrically weak or flaccid extremities; decreased or absent deep tendon reflexes; ataxia; cranial nerve involvement (e.g., facial weakness, difficulty swallowing, diplopia); decreased or absent sensation; cerebrospinal fluid abnormalities (usually increased protein count); electromyography/nerve conduction velocity abnormalities; decreased vital capacity; decreased breath sounds and depth of respirations; abnormal arterial blood gases; increased heart rate; postural hypotension

☐ PSYCHOSOCIAL CONCERNS/ DEVELOPMENTAL FACTORS

Age, sex, usual roles and responsibilities, occupation; fear/anxiety, motivation, usual coping strategies (past and present), available support systems

☐ PATIENT AND FAMILY KNOWLEDGE

Understanding of disease process including course, prognosis and treatment; readiness and willingness to learn

Nursing Care

☐ LONG-TERM GOAL

The patient will function at maximal level of independence and will demonstrate psychosocial adaptation to disease and functional abilities.

NURSING DIAGNOSIS #1

a. **Impaired gas exchange** related to immobility, pulmonary congestion, inability to deep breathe and cough
b. **Ineffective breathing pattern** related to respiratory muscle paralysis
c. **Ineffective airway clearance** related to inability to deep breathe and cough

Rationale: *Immobility can predispose a patient to the development of pneumonia, atelectasis, or a pulmonary embolism. If Guillain-Barré syndrome affects the cranial nerves, specifically the vagus nerve, the individual loses the ability to clear the lungs. If the paralysis affects the respiratory muscles, the patient's vital capacity decreases and mechanical ventilation may be required.*

☐ GOAL

The patient will demonstrate effective air exchange.

☐ IMPLEMENTATION

- Ensure that vital capacity is measured every 2 hours; report decreasing vital capacity.
- Auscultate lungs every 4 hours.
- Monitor respiratory rate, rhythm, and depth every 1-4 hours.
- Assess for subjective complaints of shortness of breath or dyspnea.
- Encourage coughing and deep breathing every 1-2 hours.
- Monitor arterial blood gases for acid-base abnormalities and decreased oxygen saturation.
- Take temperature every 4 hours (an increased temperature together with lung congestion, abnormal chest x-ray, and lab studies indicates aspiration).
- Maintain a patent airway by correct positioning, suctioning, airway adjuncts (e.g., endotracheal, nasotracheal tubes).
- Maintain sterile technique when suctioning to prevent infection.
- Assess color, amount, consistency of pulmonary secretions.
- Keep head of bed elevated as able to reduce pressure on diaphragm and promote chest expansion.
- Apply antiembolic hose to prevent venous stasis; remove every 8 hours for 15 minutes and assess skin/circulation.
- Administer anticoagulants as ordered for actual/potential blood clot; monitor appropriate laboratory tests.

☐ EVALUATION CRITERIA/DESIRED OUTCOMES

The Patient

- Has blood gases within normal limits
- Maintains vital capacity within acceptable limits
- Exhibits adequate bilateral lung aeration, clear lung sounds upon auscultation

NURSING DIAGNOSIS #2

Impairment of skin integrity related to altered sensation, immobility, altered nutritional status, incontinence

Rationale: *An adequate blood supply delivering oxygen and nutrients to the skin and maintenance of a clean, dry environment is essential to promote healing and to preserve skin function. The paralysis and paresthesias associated with Guillain-Barré syndrome place the patient at risk for skin breakdown since the person cannot feel pressure/pain or move self to keep skin intact.*

☐ GOAL

The patient will maintain skin integrity.

☐ IMPLEMENTATION

- Monitor patient's ongoing motor and sensory function.
- Observe patient's skin (i.e., intactness, color, temperature, dry/moistness, turgor) every 4 hours and as necessary.
- Monitor nutritional intake to determine adequacy of food and fluids; consult with dietician.
- Keep skin clean and dry as a moist environment creates a medium for breakdown.
- Massage skin and bony prominences to promote circulation after each position change.
- Utilize pressure-prevention aids (e.g., cushions, devices, pads).
- Monitor temperature of bath water to prevent burns.

☐ EVALUATION CRITERIA/DESIRED OUTCOMES

The Patient

- Maintains dry, intact skin
- Is free of erythema at pressure points

NURSING DIAGNOSIS #3

Impaired physical mobility related to weakness, paralysis, ataxia

Rationale: *Disruption of nerve conduction results in musculoskeletal problems that significantly affect an individual's ability to perform motor activities. Prolonged paralysis may lead to atrophy and contracture deformities.*

☐ GOAL

The patient will actively or passively participate in mobilization.

☐ IMPLEMENTATION

- Monitor ongoing motor function to establish abilities and limitations.

- Assess degree of independent/dependent activities.
- Assist with activities as needed, maintaining patient safety.
- Encourage maximum possible independence.
- Reposition or encourage position change every 2 hours.
- Perform/instruct family to perform range-of-motion (ROM) exercises every 2-4 hours.
- Maintain therapeutic body alignment of shoulders, arm, hips, and legs.
- Utilize trochanter roll to maintain neutral position of hip, avoiding external and internal rotation, to help prevent pain and discomfort.
- Brace feet against footboard, in line with legs, heels off mattress and protected from pressure to prevent footdrop and skin breakdown.
- Support arms and hands in functional anatomic positions: flexed slightly at elbow, wrists extended and a hard hand roll or rubber ball to keep fingers in "grasp" position; use splints if necessary.
- Coordinate efforts with physical and occupational therapists for continuity of care.

☐ EVALUATION CRITERIA/DESIRED OUTCOMES

The Patient

- Changes position at least every 2 hours
- Participates in independent activities within physical limitations

NURSING DIAGNOSIS #4

a. **Alteration in nutrition: less than body requirements** related to difficulty in chewing or swallowing, fatigue, inadequate intake

b. **Impaired swallowing** related to disease effects

Rationale: *If Guillain-Barré syndrome affects the trigeminal (V), facial (VII), vagus (X), or hypoglossal (XII) cranial nerves, the patient will have difficulties chewing and swallowing. Fatigue, associated with inadequate caloric intake or increased demands as the patient progresses in rehabilitation, can contribute to a nutritional deficit. This deficit can lead to muscle atrophy and decreased energy. Sufficient nutrients are required to prevent muscle wasting.*

☐ GOAL

The patient will maintain optimal nutritional status, fluid intake, and electrolyte balance.

☐ IMPLEMENTATION

- Assess patient's gag reflex, ability to swallow, presence of facial paralysis, motor and sensory function of upper extremities prior to each eating attempt.
- Monitor electrolytes, as poor oral intake and fluid deficit can cause sodium, potassium, and chloride electrolyte imbalances.
- Ensure that IV fluids are given on time, that line is patent, and that site is free of redness, swelling.
- Monitor intake and output and dietary intake.
- Assist with oral intake as needed; coordinate efforts with speech and occupational therapies related to swallowing and ability to feed self.
- Advance diet as tolerated (full liquids, soft or pureed, regular) and give liquids with solids if oral secretions are decreased.
- Provide high-calorie, high-protein liquid supplements between meals; consult with dietician.
- Provide oral hygiene before/after each oral feeding to facilitate taste of food.
- Maintain patient in sitting position or with head of bed elevated during and 1 hour after eating/feeding to prevent regurgitation and aspiration.
- Administer nasogastric feedings as ordered; determine tolerance by checking residual every 4 hours.
- Administer hyperalimentation therapy as ordered; refer to *The Patient Receiving Total Parenteral Nutrition,* page 229.
- Weigh patient at least every 3 days at same time, on same scale, in same clothing.

☐ EVALUATION CRITERIA/DESIRED OUTCOMES

The Patient

- Swallows soft food without aspiration
- Tolerates parenteral or tube feedings with minimal residual, no diarrhea, balanced electrolytes

- Maintains weight within 10% of admission weight

NURSING DIAGNOSIS #5

Impaired communication: verbal related to paralysis of facial nerve and extremities, tracheostomy

Rationale: *Paralysis of the facial nerve can alter an individual's ability to communicate. Paralysis of the upper extremities can compound this problem. If the patient's respirations are compromised, requiring mechanical ventilation, a tracheostomy creates an additional barrier to verbal communication until the tube can be plugged.*

☐ **GOAL**

The patient will maintain/establish a means of communication.

☐ **IMPLEMENTATION**

- Assess patient's ability to communicate (verbal and nonverbal).
- Adapt call light for patient use.
- Ask questions that can be answered with "yes" or "no".
- Establish individual means of communication with patient (e.g., eye blinks).
- Consult speech therapist as necessary.
- Inform patient of staff's understanding/empathy of communication problem.
- Encourage family participation in care.

☐ **EVALUATION CRITERIA/DESIRED OUTCOMES**

The Patient

- Expresses self verbally or nonverbally
- Communicates wants and needs to staff/visitors

NURSING DIAGNOSIS #6

Sensory-perceptual alteration: tactile, visual related to paresthesia, diplopia

Rationale: *Sensory disturbances alter the individual's ability to perceive incoming stimuli such as touch and movement of extremities. Involvement of cranial nerve III (oculomotor) in Guillain-Barré syndrome results in diplopia, causing visual discomfort.*

☐ **GOAL**

The patient will be able to interpret incoming tactile and visual stimuli with or without assistance.

☐ **IMPLEMENTATION**

- Monitor ability to sense touch as well as numbness or tingling to determine deficit or improvement.
- Assess ongoing visual function.
- Provide a safe environment with adequate lighting, bed in low position, uncluttered area, call light within reach, instructions to call for assistance when ambulating; orient as needed.
- Provide with an eye patch to help with diplopia.
- Explain each test and procedure before it is begun, utilizing phrases such as "I'm going to exercise your left leg now."

☐ **EVALUATION CRITERIA/DESIRED OUTCOMES**

The Patient

- Reports limitations (feeling/seeing)
- Is free from physical injury

NURSING DIAGNOSIS #7

Alteration in bowel elimination: constipation, diarrhea, incontinence related to inadequate fluid and dietary intake, loss of voluntary control, impaired communication, decreased peristalsis, intolerance to tube feedings, immobility

Rationale: *Bowel elimination problems can be caused by the inabilities to communicate the need to defecate, to ambulate to the bathroom or commode, or to feed self. Neurologic damage to the bowel or the inability to swallow and chew can compound the problem. Impaired mobility can slow down the process of peristalsis causing constipation.*

☐ GOAL

The patient will establish/maintain regular bowel elimination.

☐ IMPLEMENTATION

- Assess whether patient is aware of need to defecate.
- Assess and record character of bowel movements.
- Observe for incontinence regularly.
- Provide privacy and a comfortable position to stimulate evacuation.
- Assess for impaction as necessary.
- Offer patient fluids if able to tolerate.
- Administer stool softeners, bulk-forming laxatives, suppositories and enemas; monitor effectiveness.
- Monitor patient's intake of high-fiber foods, roughage.

☐ EVALUATION CRITERIA/DESIRED OUTCOMES

The Patient

- Evacuates soft, formed, bowel movements at least every 3 days
- Is free from diarrhea when on tube feedings

NURSING DIAGNOSIS #8

Powerlessness related to inability to perform activities of daily living (ADL) and role responsibilities, hospital restrictions

Rationale: *Impaired motor and sensory function in Guillain-Barré syndrome does not allow an individual to perform daily tasks as easily and independently as before. Restrictions such as being confined to bed, having to call for assistance when getting up, limited visitors, etc., contribute to feelings of lack of control.*

☐ GOAL

The patient will participate in care within limitations of illness.

☐ IMPLEMENTATION

- Instruct regarding tests, procedures, routines, etc., and their rationales in order to avoid misunderstanding; be aware that increased knowledge leads to an increased sense of control.
- Encourage patient to express view of impending events (e.g., test/procedures, transfer, rehabilitation).
- Reassess patient's physiologic stability/gains; share with patient and point out positives.
- Allow patient choices and decision-making opportunities when possible.
- Help to participate in care within limitations of illness; give positive reinforcement for doing so.
- Ensure environmental *powerfulness* by putting call light, telephone, and other desired items within reach.
- Utilize familiar objects such as pictures of self/family, personal hygiene items and clothes when feasible in an effort to bridge the gap between the past, present, and future.

☐ EVALUATION CRITERIA/DESIRED OUTCOMES

The Patient

- Participates in care as able
- Expresses understanding of situation

NURSING DIAGNOSIS #9

a. **Grieving** related to actual/perceived loss of function
b. **Anxiety** related to fear of unknown
c. **Disturbance in self-concept: body image, role performance, personal identity** related to loss of body functions, physical changes, role changes, dependence
d. **Fear** related to unknown prognosis

Rationale: *Reactions to hospitalization are compounded by individual differences in disease progression and recovery. As the paralysis increases, loss of function and questionable return to full function increase levels of anxiety. The patient is part of a family unit and the disease ramifications can touch all members of the family. Alterations in motor and sensory function place the patient in a dependent position for even the most basic needs. With adequate information and support, patient and family coping strategies can effectively deal with the situation.*

GOAL

The patient/family will grieve adaptively; will adapt to altered roles/resoponsibilities.

IMPLEMENTATION

- Observe patient's/family's verbal and nonverbal behavior.
- Encourage patient/family to talk about their concerns/fears, to ask questions; provide as much information as they need and want.
- Keep patient/family fully informed.
- Encourage family to assist with patient care whenever possible and to spend as much time with patient as possible.
- Provide for financial and spiritual counseling if necessary.
- Provide patient/family with information about local/national Guillain-Barré support groups.
- Refer to *The Patient Experiencing Grief and Loss,* page 272, and *The Patient Experiencing a Body-Image Disturbance,* page 253.

EVALUATION CRITERIA/DESIRED OUTCOMES

The Patient/family

- Verbalizes feelings related to fears, changes
- Asks questions related to coping with effects of disease
- Utilizes others for support

NURSING DIAGNOSIS #10

Knowledge deficit regarding disease process/treatment, prognosis/outcomes

Rationale: *It is difficult to determine the course of this disease for any particular patient. Many patients never develop the respiratory paralysis that requires a tracheostomy or mechanical ventilation. Neurologic deterioration usually covers a period from a few days to several weeks, while rehabilitation is much more variable, extending from 2 weeks to 2 years. The uncertainty of time and extent of paralysis makes teaching and learning difficult.*

GOAL

The patient/family will demonstrate adequate knowledge of Guillain-Barré syndrome.

IMPLEMENTATION

- Provide with verbal and written information abut the disease.
- Offer reassurance and encouragement concerning recovery.
- Reinforce teaching provided by other therapies (e.g., physical, speech, occupational, respiratory).
- Begin to teach patient about medications.
- Provide with written instructions regarding exercises, follow-up appointment, and therapies.
- Consult with patient/family and make appropriate referrals to local community agencies for home assistance. (Early referral is desirable.)

EVALUATION CRITERIA/DESIRED OUTCOMES

The Patient

- Describes disease process in own words
- States adequate knowledge of prescribed drugs
- Develops a beginning plan for care after discharge

The Patient with a Head Injury

Definition/Discussion

Head injuries occur as a result of a direct impact, such as an object hitting the head or the head hitting a stationary object like the windshield of a car. Indirect forces from activities such as jumping from a height and landing on the feet can also cause cerebral trauma by transmitting force up to the brain. A *closed,* blunt, or nonpenetrating injury implies that the skull is intact. An *open* or penetrating injury disrupts the integrity of the scalp and skull. Types of injury include

- scalp injury
- skull fracture (linear, basal and depressed are the most common)
- dural tear
- concussion and contusion
- intracranial hemorrhage including epidural, subdural, subarachnoid, intracerebral, and brainstem bleeding
- secondary damage to the brain or brainstem as a result of edema, ischemia, or infection

(*Head injury puts the patient at risk for increased intracranial pressure and intracranial surgery. Refer to those guides as needed for additional nursing care.*)

Nursing Assessment

☐ **PERTINENT HISTORY**

Medical and surgical history; cause of injury; alcohol, medication use; use of protective equipment (seatbelts, helmets)

☐ **PHYSICAL FINDINGS**

Level of consciousness (LOC), pupils, neuromotor function; cerebrospinal fluid (CSF) leakage or bleeding from ears, nose, etc.; palpable bumps and skull fractures; bruising; skull films indicative of fracture; computerized tomography (CT) scan showing bleeding, edema, skull fracture; respiratory status; headache, vomiting, amnesia, aphasia, dysphasia

☐ **PSYCHOSOCIAL CONCERNS/ DEVELOPMENTAL FACTORS**

Age, personality, life-style, role in family, family's emotional reaction to injury, usual family coping strategies

☐ **PATIENT AND FAMILY KNOWLEDGE**

Level of knowledge, understanding of condition, treatment, prognosis, expected outcome; readiness and willingness to learn

Nursing Care

☐ **LONG-TERM GOAL**

The patient will return to roles in home, family, occupation with minimal possible residual effects of acute head injury; OR the patient will maintain stable vital functions with/without moderate complications and neurologic deficits throughout lengthy rehabilitation and convalescence; OR the patient will be sustained with compassion and dignity until life-support systems have been disconnected.

NURSING DIAGNOSIS #1

Alteration in tissue perfusion: cerebral related to increased intracranial pressure (ICP)

Rationale: *Intracranial bleeding, direct injury to brain tissue, and the development of edema alter the intracranial volume ratio of brain tissue, blood volume, and cerebrospinal fluid. The result is an increase in ICP resulting in cerebral perfusion pressure changes; see also*

The Patient with Increased Intracranial Pressure, page 122.

GOAL

The patient will demonstrate adequate cerebral perfusion.

IMPLEMENTATION

- Assess patient's LOC, behavior, motor/sensory function (symmetry, movement [spontaneous/to command/to painful stimuli]), pupillary signs (symmetry, size, reactivity, deviation) every 1-2 hours and as necessary.
- Monitor vital signs (heart rate, blood pressure, temperature) every 15 minutes to 1 hour and as necessary; a change in respirations is an early sign of increased ICP and of hypoxia and/or hypercapnia.
- Monitor arterial blood gas values for acid-base abnormalities and decreased oxygen saturation as hypercapnia causes cerebral vasodilation, which increases cerebral edema.
- Hyperventilate before suctioning; limit suctioning to 10-15 seconds to reduce carbon dioxide levels, increase oxygenation, and prevent hypoxia.
- If ICP monitoring device is in place, monitor ICP every 15 minutes to 1 hour and as needed.
- Maintain proper functioning of ICP monitoring device (i.e., closed system, positioning of transducer, recalibration, system free of air).
- Maintain venous outflow from the brain by elevating head of bed and properly aligning head/neck.
- Monitor intake and output, electrolytes, and specific gravity as ordered to determine potential fluid imbalance contributing to cerebral edema.
- Administer fluids within fluid restriction (usually 1,400 cc/24 hours) to prevent cerebral edema.
- Instruct patient to refrain from activities that increase intrathoracic or intra-abdominal pressure (e.g., straining for bowel movement, isometric exercises, holding breath when turning in bed, hip flexion, coughing, blowing nose).
- Utilize restraints only when absolutely necessary because agitation will increase ICP.
- Assess patient's level of comfort (e.g., headache, nausea, vomiting) since these complaints indicate increased ICP.
- Administer PRN medications as ordered (e.g., stool softeners, antiemetics, analgesics); evaluate results.
- Administer steroids as ordered to prevent cerebral edema.
- Organize nursing care to allow optimal rest periods for patient.
- Employ optimal aseptic technique and infection control measures regarding tubing and dressing changes (infection increases metabolic rate, cerebral blood flow, and cerebral edema).
- Notify physician immediately of significant changes in vital signs or neurologic status.
- Institute measures to treat increased ICP as ordered: administer diuretics (mannitol, furosemide), barbiturates, or short-acting narcotics to decrease brain metabolism and oxygen demand, therefore blood flow to brain; implement hypothermia to reduce metabolism, body's oxygen requirements, and cerebral blood flow; drain CSF via intraventricular drain; prepare patient/family for surgical interventions.

EVALUATION CRITERIA/DESIRED OUTCOMES

The Patient

- Has ICP of 0-15 mm Hg, cerebral perfusion pressure greater than 50 mm Hg
- Maintains neurologic status

NURSING DIAGNOSIS #2

a. **Ineffective breathing pattern** related to increased ICP, alteration in LOC
b. **Ineffective airway clearance** related to increased ICP, alteration in LOC
c. **Impaired gas exchange** related to increased ICP, alteration in LOC

Rationale: *There are a number of abnormal respiratory patterns associated with increased ICP. As pressure increases, vital centers located in the brainstem are affected. Cheyne-Stokes breathing consists of waxing and waning respirations with periodic apnea. Central neurogenic hyperventilation, associated with lesions in the lower midbrain and upper pons, is hallmarked by continuous, regular, rapid, deep respiration. Pressure in the mid to lower* *pons region causes prolonged inspiration followed by prolonged expiration and a pause (apneustic breathing). Cluster breathing or irregular spurts of breathing interspersed with apnea is associated with lesions in the lower pons and upper medulla. Finally, a completely irregular pattern of breathing (ataxic, or Biot's breathing) that may progress to apnea is indicative of pressure on the medulla.*

Loss of consciousness is the earliest and most sensitive indicator of increased ICP. A change in consciousness or responsiveness may impair an individual's ability to clear pulmonary secretions or aerate adequately, causing an acid-base disturbance in arterial blood gases.

☐ GOAL

The patient will demonstrate effective air exchange.

☐ IMPLEMENTATION

- Assess LOC, ability to maintain open airway.
- Maintain a patent airway by correct positioning, suctioning, utilizing airway adjuncts.
- Monitor respiratory rate, rhythm, and depth every 15 minutes to 1 hour.
- Auscultate breath sounds every 2-4 hours for adequate aeration and to detect adventitious sounds.
- Assess circulatory status (i.e., pulse, blood pressure, skin color) every hour to detect hypoxia.
- Monitor arterial blood gas values for acid-base abnormalities and decreased oxygen saturation.
- Administer oxygen as ordered.
- Encourage deep breathing and limited coughing every 1-2 hours.
- Assess color, amount, consistency of pulmonary secretions to determine need for sputum culture, treatments to break up secretions.

☐ EVALUATION CRITERIA/DESIRED OUTCOMES

The Patient

- Has arterial blood gases within normal limits
- Maintains regular respiratory rate of 12-24/minute
- Maintains clear breath sounds to auscultation

NURSING DIAGNOSIS #3

a. **Potential for injury** related to inadequate stabilization of cervical column, seizures, altered level of responsiveness, drug therapy (steroids)

b. **Potential for infection** related to impaired integrity of cranium

Rationale: *Cervical injury must be ruled out in any situation associated with trauma. Inadequate stabilization, particularly in the emergency setting, may cause secondary damage to the spinal column. Cerebral injury may alter neuronal functioning leading to the development of seizures. An individual may sustain physical injury during the clonic-tonic period of seizure activity. Restlessness and confusion in a patient with a head injury puts the person at risk for physical injury. Secondary brain/brainstem damage can occur as a result of an infectious process if bacteria are introduced via a CSF leak. Finally, corticosteriods (e.g., dexametasone [Decadron]), used to treat or prevent cerebral edema irritate the gastrointestinal tract and can cause bleeding.*

☐ GOAL

The patient will be free from infection, hemorrhage, or secondary damage.

☐ IMPLEMENTATION

- Maintain head and neck stability until spinal injury has been ruled out in order to prevent secondary injury.
- Monitor for seizure activity; refer to *The Patient with Epilepsy,* page 93.
- Protect from injury caused by restless movements, disorientation, and seizures (e.g., bed in low position, padded side rails up, reorientation to environment, allowing family to be at the bedside); avoid the use of physical restraints unless absolutely necessary.
- Assess for otorrhea or rhinorrhea to detect CSF leak.
- Do not pack ear or nose if CSF leak suspected (may increase ICP); rather, provide a sterile field to collect drainage and notify physician.
- Monitor temperature every 4 hours for presence of infection.
- Administer medications (anticonvulsants, an-

tibiotics); evaluate effect; administer antacids and cimetidine when patient on steroids.

- Monitor for gastric bleeding if patient is receiving steroids.
- Assess patient's LOC every 1-2 hours and as needed to anticipate behavior that may cause physical injury.

☐ EVALUATION CRITERIA/DESIRED OUTCOMES

The Patient

- Is free from further injury
- Maintains neurologic status
- Is free from blood in vomitus or stools, complaints of stomach pain

> **NURSING DIAGNOSIS #4**
>
> a. **Alteration in fluid volume: excess** related to steroid therapy, syndrome of inappropriate antidiuretic hormone (SIADH)
>
> b. **Fluid volume deficit** related to diuretic therapy, fluid restriction, diabetes insipidus, decreased oral intake
>
> ***Rationale:*** *Management of cerebral edema or increased ICP with drug therapy and/or fluid restriction can result in fluid and electrolyte imbalances. Alterations in ADH secretion as a result of head injury cause fluid overload or deficit.*

☐ GOAL

The patient will maintain adequate fluid intake and output.

☐ IMPLEMENTATION

- Monitor intake and output to determine source of deficit or excess.
- Report urinary output less than 30 cc/hour or over 200 cc/hour for 2 consecutive hours.
- Monitor laboratory findings indicative of fluid imbalance (e.g., electrolytes, osmolarity, BUN, creatinine).
- Monitor weight daily.
- Take vital signs every 1-2 hours to measure hemodynamic response to fluid imbalance.
- Monitor central venous pressure, pulmonary artery pressure, and pulmonary capillary wedge pressure if present every 1-2 hours and as necessary for hemodynamic response to fluid imbalance.
- Assess skin turgor and presence of edema every 4 hours.
- Administer replacement fluids and medications if necessary; evaluate effectiveness.

☐ EVALUATION CRITERIA/DESIRED OUTCOMES

The Patient

- Maintains serum electrolytes, osmolarity, urine specific gravity within normal limits
- Has urinary output within normal range
- Demonstrates good skin turgor, moist mucous membranes

> **NURSING DIAGNOSIS #5**
>
> **Impaired physical mobility** related to deficits in motor/sensory function, decreased LOC
>
> ***Rationale:*** *Cerebral damage as a result of head injury can result in contralateral hemiparesis, hemiplegia, or decorticate or decerebrate posturing.*

☐ GOAL

The patient will actively or passively participate in mobilization.

☐ IMPLEMENTATION

- Monitor LOC, behavior every 1-2 hours and as needed to determine neurologic status as well as abilities and limitations in regard to mobility.
- Monitor motor/sensory function (symmetry; movement [spontaneous/to command/to painful stimuli]) every 1-2 hours and as needed to determine neurologic status as well as abilities and limitations.
- Perform passive range of motion every 2-4 hours to prevent contractures and atrophy.
- Reposition every 2 hours to relieve pressure.
- Utilize bed board, foot board, etc., to prevent contractures.
- Coordinate activities with occupational and physical therapists.
- Inspect skin for redness, breakdown when turning and bathing patient.
- Massage bony prominences, heels, elbows every 2-4 hours to promote circulation.

- Utilize decubitus-prevention measures (e.g., heel protectors, elbow protectors, egg-crate mattress, alternating pressure mattress).

☐ EVALUATION CRITERIA/DESIRED OUTCOMES

The Patient

- Is repositioned, up in chair, or ambulated regularly
- Retains mobile joints
- Is free from contrctures, muscle atrophy

NURSING DIAGNOSIS #6

a. **Ineffective individual coping** related to physical disabilities, memory loss, postconcussion syndrome, dependence
b. **Ineffective family coping** related to loss and grief
c. **Fear** related to uncertain future

Rationale: *Sequelae of head injury may include limitations in movement, speech, cognition, and vision requiring assistance with activities of daily living. Short-term memory loss is also very common following head trauma. Headache, irritability, inability to concentrate, insomnia, and fatigue characterize the postconcussion syndrome, which may last a few weeks to a few years. These conditions may place the individual in a dependent state. The family is forced to cope with the unexpectedness of the injury, treatment including possible surgery, an uncertain prognosis, and actual physical or cognitive deficits in addition to the disruption in family roles and lifestyle. These concerns can all generate fear.*

☐ GOAL

The patient/family will demonstrate adaptive, effective, coping patterns that deal with loss and/or grief.

☐ IMPLEMENTATION

- Assess patient's/family's coping strategies; are they effective? adaptive?
- If needed, work with patient/family to identify and try new ways to cope adaptively with current situation.
- Consider referrals to family/social services, counseling as needed.
- Provide information related to tests/procedures, progress, prognosis, treatment.
- If appropriate, help family/patient concentrate on positive attributes, retained abilities.
- Encourage family to assist with patient care whenever possible and to spend as much time with patient as possible, talking, reading, playing favorite music.
- Help to express feelings, ask questions about current situation.
- Provide for financial and spiritual counseling as desired.

☐ EVALUATION CRITERIA/DESIRED OUTCOMES

The Patient/family

- Verbalizes feelings related to loss and grief
- Utilizes each other for support
- Expresses confidence in coping abilities

NURSING DIAGNOSIS #7

Knowledge deficit regarding treatment, prognosis, outcome

Rationale: *The family is unprepared for the traumatic nature of head injury. Information shared with the family regarding the patient's condition may need to be continually reinforced due to high levels of stress and life-and-death concerns.*

☐ GOAL

The family will demonstrate adequate knowledge of patient's condition.

☐ IMPLEMENTATION

- Continue to assess family's knowledge and understanding of the situation daily.
- Inform family of patient's progress, prognosis, and plan of care focusing on realistic expectations.
- Encourage verbalization and questions if possible.
- Utilize resources (written materials, clinical specialist, pastoral care, social services) to assist with teaching.
- Assist family decision-making regarding discharge plans and long-term needs.

☐ EVALUATION CRITERIA/DESIRED OUTCOMES

The Family

- Describes patient's status accurately
- Has realistic expectations of patient's rehabilitation potential

The Patient Requiring Hemodialysis

Definition/Discussion

Hemodialysis removes toxic waste products and fluids from the systemic circulation to maintain the body in homeostasis when the kidneys are not functioning adequately.

Time involved for hemodialysis is approximately 3-5 hours, depending on the patient's condition and the type of machine used. It is usually done 3 times a week.

The artificial kidney machine contains a semipermeable membrane that separates the patient's blood from the dialyzing solution. Hemodialysis is based upon three principles of fluid and particle movement, diffusion, osmosis, and ultrafiltration. Through diffusion and osmosis, molecules and ions of waste products pass from the area of higher concentration (the patient's blood) to the area of lower concentration (the dialyzing solution) until a degree of equilibrium between the two is achieved. Molecules may also pass from the dialyzing solution into the blood, thus the electrolyte content of the dialysate can be manipulated to meet the patient's needs based on blood chemistries and clinical evaluation. Ultrafiltration involves movement of fluid across a semipermeable membrane as a result of an artificially created pressure gradient. Types of access to the patient's circulation include

- *external arteriovenous shunting (cannulization):* a silastic-Teflon cannula is surgically inserted and fixed in an artery (usually the radial artery of the nondominant arm or the posterior tibial artery of either leg); another cannula is fixed in a nearby vein. Arterial blood is shunted through the artificial kidney and returned to the patient via the venous cannula. After dialysis is completed, both cannulae are connected so that the flow of blood from artery to vein through the "shunt" is continuous.
- *internal arteriovenous fistulization:* a tiny opening is surgically created between an artery and a nearby vein; this enables the arterial blood to enter into and engorge the vein, which is then easily punctured at time of dialysis. Two needles are inserted: one to carry the blood to the artificial kidney, and one to return the blood to the patient. The needles are removed and reinserted for each treatment. No external device is used and problems of clotting and infection are minimized. Patency of the fistula is achieved by the rapid flow of blood.
- *arteriovenous graft*: permanent access device created by suturing a bovine artery graft material to the patient's own vessel when the patient's own vessels are not suitable.
- *femoral or subclavian vein catheterization* for emergency or temporary (acute) hemodialysis

Public law 92-603 of July 1973 provides financial assistance to all persons covered by Social Security, or their dependents, who have end-stage renal disease and who require dialysis (and/or kidney transplantation). Approximately 80,000 persons in the US are being maintained on permanent dialysis.

Nursing Assessment

☐ PERTINENT HISTORY

High and rising serum potassium level; acute renal failure, end-stage renal disease; severe fluid/electrolyte imbalance; severe pulmonary edema or congestive heart failure (CHF); chemical or drug toxicity

☐ PHYSICAL FINDINGS

Lethargy, restlessness; confusion; pallor; anorexia, oliguria or anuria; general edema, possible cardiac dysrhythmias (indicative of related electrolyte imbalances, especially hyperkalemia); elevated BUN, creatinine, serum proteins; decreased hematocrit, hemoglobin (blood products may be administered during dialysis)

☐ PSYCHOSOCIAL CONCERNS/ DEVELOPMENTAL FACTORS

Anxiety/fear regarding treatment/disease, especially if acute dialysis or initial session; body-image disturbances; depression/powerlessness with long-term condition; possible hopelessness/fear of dying in patients with end-stage renal disease

☐ PATIENT AND FAMILY KNOWLEDGE

Purpose/expected effects of procedure; postdischarge regimen (e.g., diet, medications, scheduled dialysis sessions); evaluation procedure for renal transplant; community resources

Nursing Care

☐ LONG-TERM GOAL

The patient will adhere to prescribed regimen to aid recovery from the acute renal failure and to return to usual roles OR the patient will adapt to the reality of long-term dialysis and will live within its accompanying limitations.

NURSING DIAGNOSIS #1

a. **Anxiety** related to limited understanding of hemodialysis procedure, expected course of renal dysfunction
b. **Powerlessness** related to perceived lack of control over disease/treatment
c. **Disturbance in self-concept: body image** related to loss of renal function, use of external device to achieve bodily function

Rationale: *Lack of knowledge and fear of the unknown cause high anxiety and stress levels. Depending upon the precipitating indication for hemodialysis, the patient/family may have had little time to prepare for the procedure.*

Dialysis patients usually have many conflicts regarding being dependent on a machine and health team for life, and these may be expressed by a variety of feelings and emotions. During the first few weeks, the patient often feels increasingly better physically. Next, s/he may become discouraged and easily depressed. Finally, most patients achieve some degree of acceptance of medical condition and imposed limitations, display fewer negative feelings, and plan for changes in life-style. Acceptance of patient's feelings by the nurse will often keep the patient from acting them out by refusing to cooperate, going off fluid and dietary regimens, etc.

Changes in physical appearance may result in a lessened sense of self; this is often increased by changes in usual role functioning. Intervention may need to be directed at family members to decrease the patient's feelings of dependency and promote a sense of control over at least some aspects of the prescribed regimen. Some patients may grieve for the loss of their kidneys and may require assistance in accepting the necessity for dialysis. Other dialysis patients can become very attached to "their" machine and incorporate it into their body image.

☐ GOAL

The patient/family will indicate decreased level of anxiety; will identify those aspects of the disease process/treatment regimen s/he can control; will incorporate new body image into self-concept.

☐ IMPLEMENTATION

- Assess level of anxiety before dialysis begins (sad? happy? feeling helpless or hopeless? anxious?); validate your observations with the patient ("You seem down today; are you?") as a way of getting patient to express feelings; provide empathic listening.
- Encourage patient/family questions regarding disease process, treatment; accept and acknowledge all verbalizations; indicate that these are usual and expected feelings for dialysis patients; if prognosis is that chronic renal failure (CRF) is not likely, emphasize the temporary nature of the procedure to promote hopeful attitude.
- Initiate measures to prevent communication breakdown by setting up family, patient, and staff conferences with psychiatric clinical specialist, psychiatrists, social worker, or other mental health person; ensure that all care givers are aware of health team decisions.
- Acknowledge that weight loss, pallor, loss of energy, shunts, and venipuncture scars are

all reminders to patient that body integrity is interrupted by illness and treatment.

- Help to adjust to body-image changes by giving recognition for any involvement in planning and managing own care, by eliciting feelings and listening carefully to what patient says, and by reminding patient of previously successful coping mechanisms for stressful situations (this reaffirmation of ability to cope should help revive patient's sense of self-worth and promote feelings of control).
- Provide opportunities for patient to exert some degree of control over own life (e.g., planning and managing own care via scheduling of medications, fluids, foods); involve patient as much as possible; reassure that increasing independence from the health team is a sign of progress, and not rejection by staff.
- Explain to family the importance of allowing patient to perform own self-care tasks as much as possible.
- Encourage spouse and children to attend a support group, if available, in hospital or community (family members may need help in coping with a variety of feelings in related to the dialysis).

☐ EVALUATION CRITERIA/DESIRED OUTCOMES

The Patient

- Participates in decision making regarding plan of care
- Expresses acceptance of need for dialysis
- Reaffirms self-worth
- Verbalizes decreased anxiety concerning dialysis and prognosis

NURSING DIAGNOSIS #2

a. **Fluid volume deficit** related to rapid volume depletion

b. **Alteration in cardiac output: decreased** related to dysrhythmias, effects of CHF

c. **Impaired gas exchange** related to decreased cardiac output, effects of CRF (anemia), the dialysis procedure itself (hemolysis)

Rationale: *When the osmolarity of the dialysate is significantly higher than the patient's blood, there is a risk of rapid volume depletion because too much fluid is removed in too short a time period. Rapid fluid reduction may cause hypotension with resultant hypoxia.*

Even when the fluid volume remains stable, the patient may show signs of a decreased cardiac output if there are electrolyte imbalances (especially potassium) that cause cardiac dysrhythmias. Hyperkalemia causes changes in cardiac conduction that may result in cardiac standstill. A too-rapid reduction in potassium can also cause dysrhythmias secondary to hypokalemia (refer to Table 1, Common Fluid and Electrolyte Imbalances, *page 14.*

Patients with CRF often have developed chronic CHF. Fluid congestion within the pulmonary circulation causes an alteration of the ventilation/perfusion ratio and results in impaired gas exchange (refer to The Patient with Congestive Heart Failure, *page 88). The patient should demonstrate improved exchange after dialysis as the excess fluid removed from the systemic circulation will decrease the workload and increase the efficiency of the heart as a pump, improving pulmonary as well as the systemic circulation.*

Anemia may be secondary to CRF as decreased red blood cell production results from decreased erythropoietin production in the diseased kidneys. Turbulent blood flow through the dialysis machine may cause destruction of red blood cells. As a result of both anemia and hemolysis, the oxygen-carrying capacity of the patient's blood is diminished and the patient develops symptoms reflecting impaired gas exchange.

☐ GOAL

The patient will maintain fluid and electrolyte balance and a cardiac output sufficient to promote normal gas exchange.

☐ IMPLEMENTATION

- Review ECG pattern and vital signs before initiating dialysis to establish baseline data.
- Inform physician of predialysis laboratory results (serum electrolytes, BUN, hematocrit/hemoglobin) for instructions as to composition of dialysate and administration of medications/blood products.
- Monitor blood pressure, pulse, and respira-

tions every 5-10 minutes during the first half hour of dialysis and every 15-30 minutes throughout the procedure; watch for signs of fluid volume deficit (e.g., decreased blood pressure, increased pulse); inform physician and decrease rate of dialysis, adjust concentration of dialysate, or administer blood components (refer to Table 2, *Blood and Blood Components*, page 17) as ordered.

- Administer volume expanders or vasopressors as ordered; continue to monitor blood pressure and pulse every 15 minutes; watch for indications of effectiveness or signs of fluid overload (with volume expanders) or hypertension (with vasopressors); if untoward effects noted, discontinue infusion and contact physician.
- Position flat in bed if hypotensive; if dyspneic, elevate head 15°-30° and administer oxygen as ordered.
- Assess throughout dialysis for symptoms of decreased cardiac output and related hypoxia (e.g., irregular or weak pulse, dizziness, labored respirations, mental confusion).
- Monitor cardiac rhythm as ordered; report/record presence of dysrhythmias and related symptoms; administer medications as ordered; watch for expected effectiveness and toxicity.
- Auscultate lungs for presence of rales (indicative or CHF/fluid volume excess) every hour.
- Monitor arterial blood gases as ordered; watch for decreased pO_2 and acidosis; assess for symptoms of respiratory insufficiency (e.g., increased respiratory rate, shallow or labored respirations, irritability/agitation, loss of consciousness) and inform physician; prepare for possible intubation and mechanical ventilation (refer to *The Patient with Asthma*, page 32).

☐ EVALUATION CRITERIA/DESIRED OUTCOMES

The Patient

- Has stable blood pressure and pulse and normal lab values (serum electrolyes, hematocrit, hemoglobin, arterial blood gases)
- Experiences regular cardiac rhythm or has dysrhythmias controlled
- Has normal respirations and breath sounds

NURSING DIAGNOSIS #3

a. **Potential for injury** (hemorrhage) related to heparinization, vulnerability for dislodgment of vascular access equipment
b. **Potential for injury** (air embolism) related to air entering hemodialysis tubing
c. **Potential for infection** related to impaired skin integrity at vascular access site, increased susceptibility for hepatitis and AIDS through frequent blood transfusions
d. **Potential for injury** related to seizures secondary to fluid volume excess, related electrolyte imbalances

Rationale: *Hemorrhage may occur by accidental needle dislodgment, disconnection of the shunt, or rupture of a machine coil during the procedure. Heparin, which requires about 4 hours to metabolize postdialysis, is used to prevent clotting of the blood as it is cycled through the dialysis machine. The risk for bleeding continues until the heparin has been metabolized.*

Any opening in the hemodialysis system can become a port of entry for air. When an air bolus greater than 50 cc enters the patient's vascular space, there is the risk of air embolism developing. Perhaps even more significant than the amount of air necessary to cause an air embolism is the rate of entry. Given the large vessels used for cannulization and the active pumping action of the machine, it can be expected that air entering through the dialysis system would reach the heart and lungs faster than air entering through an ordinary peripheral or central IV line.

Infection at the access site is a potential problem if strict asepsis is not maintained. Local infection may lead to systemic infection, especially for patients with CRF whose immune system is compromised. When frequent transfusions are required to treat anemia secondary to renal failure and hypovolemia during dialysis, the patient is at increased risk for developing hepatitis and AIDS as the viruses causing these conditions can be transmitted through blood from an infected donor. Hospital staff are also at risk when administering transfusions and should exercise caution when performing venipunctures and handling blood.

Fluid volume excess may occur between dialysis treatments because of retention of sodium and water. If the fluid volume overload is severe, cerebral edema and resultant seizures may develop. While dialysis rapidly removes fluid volume excess from systemic circulation, cerebral edema requires additional time to resolve; therefore, the patient being dialyzed continues to be at risk for seizures during and after the procedure.

☐ GOAL

The patient will remain free from injury and infection.

☐ IMPLEMENTATION

- Inspect access site every 15-30 minutes during dialysis for patency and signs of bleeding or infection; notify physician of significant findings; administer protamine sulfate to counteract effects of heparin as ordered.
- Check patency of shunt or fistula every 4 hours when patient not being dialyzed; observe fluid fluctuation in external shunt; auscultate for bruit and palpate for thrill in internal fistula; notify physician if patency not verified.
- Initiate measures to prevent introduction of air into dialysis system; tape all connections securely; avoid kinks in the tubing and negative pressures between the pump and the patient.
- Monitor coagulation and hematology studies according to orders or unit protocol; inform physician of significantly prolonged times or decreased hematocrit and hemoglobin.
- Ensure that no punctures are made in external shunt; do not take blood pressure nor withdraw blood from access extremity; post a sign (at bedside or by door to patient room) to remind all members of the health team to observe these precautions; explain reasons to patient.
- Watch for signs of air embolism (e.g., chest pain, cyanosis, decreased blood pressure, weak, rapid pulse, coughing, loss of consciousness); if present, turn patient onto left side in Trendelenburg's position to isolate air embolus in the right atrium; notify physician immediately; discontinue dialysis, administer oxygen, and prepare for possible intracardiac aspiration by physician.
- Monitor for signs of systemic infection (e.g., increased temperature, pulse, and respirations; decreased blood pressure; changes in skin color or mental status).
- Administer antibiotics as prescribed; watch especially for toxicity (with impaired renal functioning, the liver is primarily responsible for clearing drugs from the body).
- Monitor liver function studies (SGOT, SGPT, LDH) for elevations indicative of hepatitis; monitor serology reports for positive hepatitis associated antigens (HAA); assess for signs of hepatitis (e.g., fatigue, jaundice, fever); institute isolation precautions as ordered; explain purpose to patient/family.
- Monitor hematology studies for indications of immunosuppression (decreased white blood cell count and lymphocytes) and serology studies for positive AIDS antigen (HTLV/III); confer with physician in interpreting test results; initiate protective isolation precautions as ordered; explain purpose to patient/family.
- Maintain seizure precautions (refer to *The Patient with Epilepsy,* page 93); administer antiseizure medications as ordered; monitor for effectiveness and toxicity; record/report seizure activity.
- Monitor serum electrolytes before and after dialysis; inform physician of abnormal post-dialysis levels.
- Assess for signs of increased intracranial pressure (e.g., widening pulse pressure, bounding pulse, headache, restlessness, respiratory pattern changes); administer mannitol as ordered, titrating according to orders or hospital protocol; monitor for effectiveness and toxicity.

☐ EVALUATION CRITERIA/DESIRED OUTCOMES

The Patient

- Has stable vital signs, is afebrile
- Has normal lab values (hematology, liver function studies, serology, electrolytes)
- Is free from seizure activity

NURSING DIAGNOSIS #4

a. **Alteration in comfort** (headache) related to fluid volume excess

b. **Alteration in comfort** (angina) related to myocardial ischemia secondary to hypoxia

Rationale: *Fluid overload experienced between dialysis sessions may cause cerebral edema (which may in turn cause headache) or CHF. With CHF there is hypoxia because of impaired gas exchange (see Nursing Diagnosis #2). When the heart attempts to contract in the hypoxic state, myocardial ischemia (manifested as anginal pain) develops.*

☐ GOAL

The patient will be comfortable; will be free from headache or angina.

☐ IMPLEMENTATION

- Assess regularly for signs of discomfort; implement measures to promote relief.
- Administer prescribed analgesic for headache and/or vasodilator or calcium-channel blocker prescribed for angina; monitor for effectiveness and toxicity.
- Explain reasons for discomfort to patient/family (understanding cause may decrease anxiety that intensifies discomfort).
- Assist patient in using distraction/imagery to control discomfort (refer to *The Patient Experiencing Pain,* page 180).

☐ EVALUATION CRITERIA/DESIRED OUTCOMES

The Patient

- Expresses relief from headache and/or angina

NURSING DIAGNOSIS #5

Knowledge deficit regarding care of shunt or fistula

Rationale: *To promote compliance with the hemodialysis schedule and transplant procedure postdischarge regimen, the patient/family requires sufficient information about care of the shunt or fistula and schedule for hemodialysis sessions. When applicable, the patient may need information concerning the evaluative procedure for renal transplantation.*

☐ GOAL

The patient/family will demonstrate proper shunt care; will describe dialysis schedule; will discuss evaluative procedure for renal transplantation.

☐ IMPLEMENTATION

- Assess knowledge and ability to carry out skin-cleansing technique at shunt site using aseptic technique; correct and teach as necessary, following hospital protocol.
- Instruct to check for patency by palpating the thrill and listening for the bruit in the internal fistula.
- Teach to check external shunt site for swelling, coolness, redness, or other discoloration of skin that might suggest infection or leak in shunt, and to report these to dialysis team.
- Teach necessary restrictions for bathing, swimming when external shunt is used; ensure patient has 2 bulldog clamps at all times in case of accidental separation of cannulae, and ensure patient/family knows how to use them.
- Teach to protect shunt from injury; to avoid any constrictions on arm (e.g., blood pressure cuff, tourniquet, tight clothing); not to carry purse or packages on affected arm; to avoid sleeping on arm; to avoid pressures or weights.
- Reinforce what physician has told patient/family concerning anticipated dialysis sessions after discharge; ensure that patient has a written schedule for outpatient dialysis appointments.
- Confer with physician before discussing possible renal transplantation with patient; answer questions and refer to local chapter of National Kidney Foundation for additional information as needed; refer to *The Patient Undergoing Renal Transplantation,* page 216.

☐ EVALUATION CRITERIA/DESIRED OUTCOMES

The Patient

- Demonstrates proper shunt care
- States indications for notifying physician
- Describes schedule for dialysis sessions
- Discusses possible renal transplantation procedure, if applicable

The Patient Requiring Hemodynamic Monitoring

Definition/Discussion

Pulmonary artery catheterization is an invasive procedure in which a catheter is inserted via a major vein (subclavian or femoral) and threaded into the heart. Once in the right atrium, this balloon-tipped catheter is inflated to permit the catheter to float forward with the flow of blood until it reaches the pulmonary artery (PA). The pressures at the catheter tip are reflected back through tubing to a transducer where they are viewed on an oscilloscope (monitor). As the catheter is moved forward through the right atrium (RA), right ventricle (RV), and pulmonary artery (PA), characteristic waveforms are seen. Once in the PA, the balloon is deflated and PA pressures (PAP) are continuously monitored. Pulmonary capillary wedge pressures (PCWP) may also be taken by periodic balloon inflation. This multilumen catheter has a proximal port for RA pressure and cardiac output measurement, a distal port for PA pressure, and balloon inflation. Some catheters permit IV fluid administration.

A central venous pressure (CVP) line is a catheter placed in the superior vena cava (SVC) to measure pressure of blood returning to the heart. It indicates fluid volume and the function and pumping ability of the right side of the heart.

Nursing Assessment

☐ **PERTINENT HISTORY**

Medical and surgical history; medical diagnoses; reason for insertion of CVP line; illness preventing use of certain veins (e.g., mastectomy, lymph node dissection), history of IV drug abuse resulting in sclerosed veins; reason for insertion of CVP or PA line

☐ **PHYSICAL FINDINGS**

Baseline vital signs (blood pressure, pulse, respirations, temperature) and breath sounds; presence of pain, redness, or swelling in anticipated area of insertion; preprocedure chest x-ray results, if done; history or current occurrence of ventricular dysrhythmias

☐ **PSYCHOSOCIAL CONCERNS/ DEVELOPMENT FACTORS**

Age; sex, occupation, usual coping mechanism; available support; roles and responsibilities; past experience with CVP or PA catheter insertion; anxiety level

☐ **PATIENT AND FAMILY KNOWLEDGE**

Reason for procedure, function of line; patient role in preventing complications during insertion and in catheter maintenance; readiness and willingness to learn

Nursing Care

☐ **Long-Term Goal**

The patient will undergo central venous and/or pulmonary artery catheterization and pressure monitoring free from ill effects.

NURSING DIAGNOSIS #1

a. **Potential for infection** related to invasive procedure
b. **Potential for injury** (air embolus) related to injection of air during catheter insertion

Rationale: *Air embolism and contamination of the catheter or insertion site are the major complications to be avoided. Lines threaded into central blood vessels and cardiac chambers provide access for microorganisms. Manipulation of lines by many different* *personnel increases the opportunities for breaks in the systems and introduction of microorganisms. In addition, the critically ill patient is at high risk for infection due to loss of normal defense mechanisms.*

☐ GOAL

The patient will be free from injury (e.g., embolus, treatment errors) and infection associated with use of CVP and/or PA lines.

☐ IMPLEMENTATION

- Prepare skin with povidone iodine and alcohol before catheter insertion; ensure that person inserting catheter maintains strict aseptic technique including wearing mask, sterile gown, and gloves; catheter must be kept sterile.
- Flush all air out of IV line before procedure.
- Place patient in Trendelenburg's position to distend jugular or subclavian vein; this also increases venous pressure and decreases likelihood of air embolus.
- Have patient perform Valsalva maneuver (bear down) during catheter insertion to decrease chance of air embolus with inspiration; know that this may be contraindicated in patient with heart disease as the maneuver may cause vagal stimulation and bradycardia.
- Secure catheter to skin with tape to prevent migration of the catheter with movement; physician may suture catheter to skin.
- Apply povidone iodine ointment and a sterile, air-occlusive dressing to the insertion site to prevent bacterial infection; label dressing with date, time, and nurse's initials; securely tape catheter connection sites.
- Assess breath sounds immediately after the procedure and every 1-2 hours thereafter to detect development of pneumothorax; ensure that postprocedure x-ray is done to determine catheter placement or presence of pneumothorax; notify physician immediately if symptoms of pneumothorax are present; refer to *The Patient With a Pneumothorax*, page 197.
- Change dressing every 48 hours according to hospital protocol; wear sterile gloves and mask, cleanse site with povidone iodine and alcohol, apply povidone iodine ointment and a sterile air-occlusive dressing; if the catheter appears to have been pulled out of vein, do not push it back in since reinsertion could introduce microorganisms; retape catheter in position to prevent further slipping; note any redness, swelling, or discharge from the insertion site; document condition of site.
- Change IV tubing and flush solutions every 24 hours; when changing tubing, place patient in Trendelenburg's position and tell to do Valsalva maneuver or hold breath to avoid air embolus; use sterile technique; label new tubing with date, time, and nurse's initials.

☐ EVALUATION CRITERIA/DESIRED OUTCOMES

The patient

- Is free from redness, swelling, or discharge from insertion site
- Is free from chest pain, shortness of breath, diminished breath sounds, altered mental state related to catheter

NURSING DIAGNOSIS #2

Potential for injury related to unknown etiology

Rationale: *Proper medical treatment is dependent on correct pressure readings. The nurse must be experienced in manipulation of the equipment and interpretation of the waveforms to ensure accurate readings.*

☐ GOAL

The patient will receive appropriate and timely medical treatment based on accurate hemodynamic pressure readings.

☐ IMPLEMENTATION

- Ensure proper functioning of PA monitoring equipment by calibrating transducer to air every 8 hours
  - with transducer at 4th intercostal space (ICS) mid-axillary line (MAL), open transducer to air by turning stopcock between patient and transducer off to patient and uncapping open port to air
  - follow manufacturer's specifications as to what monitor calibration buttons to use and desired digital waveform readouts
  - when appropriate calibration criteria have

been achieved, reestablish system by turning stopcock off to the open port and flushing pressure system between transducer and distal catheter (normal PA waveform should appear on monitor)

- Take all readings with transducer at 4th ICS at MAL; take all readings in same position as possible; level transducer at each reading.
- Record pressures, patient position, and whether patient was on or off ventilator on appropriate forms to ensure consistency in conditions for readings.

To take PAP reading

- Keep distal (PA) port of catheter of catheter open to transducer.
- Turn pressure trace to *full scale.*
- Observe digital readout as well as graphic waveform.
- Record systolic/diastolic pressure.

To take PCWP reading

- Keep distal port open to transducer.
- Attach a 3-cc syringe to inflation lumen port with valve or stopcock.
- Turn valve to the "on" position.
- Remove syringe and draw up 1.5 cc of air.
- Turn monitor to *mean* pressure and *full scale.*
- Gently and slowly instill air only until wedged waveform appears; if no resistance is felt, stop insertion of air and notify physician)balloon may have ruptured).
- Observe digital readout as well as graphic waveform; do not wedge balloon longer than 30 seconds.
- Record pressure as well as amount of air needed to wedge balloon.
- Remove syringe and let air passively flow out of balloon (pulling air out of balloon puts additional stress on balloon and leads to premature balloon rupture).
- Observe for reappearance of PAP waveform.
- Turn patient to right side and have him/her cough as you flush the line if catheter remains wedged; if still wedged, repeat on left side; if still wedged, notify physician.

To take an RA pressure reading

- Follow procedure for PAP readings using this transducer if proximal port is connected to its own transducer, but turn monitor to *mean* pressure rather than systolic/diastolic.
- If proximal port shares distal port transducer
  - turn stopcock between transducer and distal port off toward patient
  - turn stopcock between transducer and proximal port off toward IV solution
  - set monitor display to *mean* pressure and *full scale*
  - observe digital readout and graphic waveform; record mean pressure
  - turn stopcocks back to original positions to reestablish continuous PAP monitoring; flush distal line with in-line flush device; observe for return of PAP waveform on monitor; reset monitor to systolic/diastolic pressure monitoring
  - reestablish prescribed flow rate for proximal IV solution

To obtain a cardiac output (CO)/cardiac index (CI)

- Follow the specific directions of the equipment manufacturer.
- Observe steps common to most types of equipment
  - connect in-line temperature probe to CO machine
  - set CO computer for size of PA catheter (e.g., 7 French) and volume of injectate (5 cc or 10 cc); set height and weight for calculation of body surface area (BSA) if indicated
  - prepare 3 syringes of injectate (normal saline or 5% dextrose in water); be sure to expel all air bubbles
  - prepare stopcock port in proximal line for injectate; in choosing stopcock port, note it is best to instill injectate in a straight line through stopcock rather than at a 90° angle (this may require temporarily disconnecting IV infusion and capping IV tubing with sterile needle)
  - connect syringe with injectate to stopcock and turn so proximal port is open to injectate
  - instill injectate as rapidly as possible at signal specified by CO computer manufacturer; note CO/CI readings as displayed (display may also include blood and injectate temperatures and BSA)
  - repeat procedure with 2nd and 3rd syringes of injectate
  - record average of 3 COs and 3 CIs
  - reestablish IV in proximal line

To take CVP reading using CVP catheter

- Use port with largest lumen for CVP monitoring when there is more than 1 lumen in CVP catheter; do not measure CVP in port through which viscous solutions (e.g., blood, albumin, hyperalimentation) are infused as these will make reading inaccurate.
- Use correct procedure when doing central venous pressure readings
  - place patient flat in bed without a pillow under head if possible (ensure that legs are not dangling as this will decrease pres-

sure); document the position used in nurse's notes and use this position for all subsequent readings
- place zero point on manometer at midaxillary line (level of right atrium); mark chest with pen at midaxillary line to ensure consistent readings
- turn stopcock off to patient and allow IV fluid to flow into manometer; use only a standard isotonic or hypotonic solution for CVP measurement so that the pressure is in centimeters of water; fill to a few centimeters above anticipated reading
- turn stopcock off to IV solution, allowing fluid in manometer to fall until it equalizes with pressure in SVC; fluid should fluctuate with respiration, going down with inspiration and up with expiration; level at which fluid stops falling is CVP reading; if patient is on a ventilator, disconnect briefly during this step; if patient must remain on ventilator, document this and perform all subsequent readings on ventilator
- turn stopcock off to manometer, briefly flush the IV line, and resume the IV flow at the prescribed rate
- record CVP reading and any special conditions under which it was taken in chart; know that a normal CVP is 5-15 cm H_2O; 15 cm or above may indicate heart failure, fluid volume overload; 5 cm or below may indicate fluid volume depletion

- Notify physician of significant changes in pressure readings so that medical therapy can be adjusted as needed.

☐ EVALUATION CRITERIA/DESIRED OUTCOMES

The Patient

- Has readings reported accurately on prescribed schedule
- Has results reported to physician
- Has appropriate changes in therapy instituted

NURSING DIAGNOSIS #3

Alteration in cardiac output: decreased related to ventricular dysrhythmias, pulmonary artery catheter displacement

Rationale: *As catheter passes through the RV, it further irritates myocardial muscle, resulting in PVCs, ventricular tachycardia, or ventricular fibrillation. A catheter may move about abnormally in cardiac chambers with contractions of the heart, and striking cardiac tissue already irritated from hypoxia. Loose connections, blood or clots in the line, improper technique in measurements can damage the delicate catheter and balloon, and result in inaccurate results and therapy. Delays or incorrect treatment in an unstable patient could have serious effects.*

☐ GOAL

The patient will be free from ventricular dysrhythmias; will respond rapidly to pharmacologic therapy/catheter repositioning if dysrhythmias occur.

☐ IMPLEMENTATION

- Monitor ECG rhythm continuously to detect dysrhythmias early.
- Keep lidocaine for IVP administration ready at bedside for rapid treatment of dysrhythmias according to standard protocol.
- Have resuscitation equipment readily available.
- Monitor PA waveforms to detect movement of catheter into RV, abnormal waveforms (see Table 3; page 121).
- Maintain normal patient oxygenation to decrease hypersensitivity of myocardium due to hypoxia.

☐ EVALUATION CRITERIA/DESIRED OUTCOMES

The Patient

- Has no ventricular dysrhythmias
- Has waveforms indicating correct placement of PA catheter
- Responds within seconds to drug therapy to decrease ectopy
- Has patent, intact catheter
- Has normal waveforms for chamber being monitored
- Receives appropriate therapy based on accurate pressure readings

NURSING DIAGNOSIS #4

Knowledge deficit regarding insertion procedure, catheter maintenance

Rationale: *Complications during catheter insertion can be minimized by patient cooperation with health team instructions. Once CVP line is established, the patient needs to avoid activities that could dislodge the line. The patient who understands the reason for a procedure is better able to cooperate with care.*

☐ GOAL

The patient will understand and cooperate with CVP line insertion and maintenance.

☐ IMPLEMENTATION

- Explain reason for insertion of CVP line to the patient/family.
- Tell about any expected pain, discomfort, or sensations during catheter insertion (e.g., wetness of cleansing solution on skin, needle prick when local anesthetic is given, pressure when catheter is inserted, and temporary discomfort at insertion site).
- If not contraindicated, have patient practice doing Valsalva maneuver or hold breath before insertion.
- Tell to avoid sudden movements after insertion to avoid dislodging the catheter; normal movements will be possible.
- Instruct patient about procedures (e.g., CVP readings, dressing changes, fluid administration).
- Tell to report any chest pain or difficulty breathing to the nurse.

☐ EVALUATION CRITERIA/DESIRED OUTCOMES

The Patient

- States reasons for CVP line
- Demonstrates maneuvers to be used during insertion
- States intention to avoid sudden movements that could dislodge catheter
- Knows to reports any pain or difficulty breathing promptly

Table 3 Troubleshooting the PA Catheter

Problem Noted	Possible Cause	Nursing Interventions
No wave form	Loose connections Stopcock position incorrect Clot in catheter	• Tighten all connections. • Check that catheter is open to transducer. • Aspirate clot and irrigate catheter
Damped waveform	Catheter tip against vessel wall Occlusion with blood or clot Pressure bag low	• Cough and deep breathe. • Reposition patient. • Flush system continuously. • Maintain 300 mmHg pressure in pressure bag.
Inability to wedge	Balloon rupture due to —overinflation of balloon —aspiration of air from balloon —absorption of blood protein —decreased elasticity	• Use less than 1.5 cc air; record amount used. • Remove air from balloon passively. • Use catheter for 2-3 days only. • Seal off inflation port if rupture occurs to prevent inadvertent introduction of air into PA.
Spontaneous wedging	Catheter migrates forward to peripheral branch Balloon was left inflated	• Move patient side to side. • Cough and deep breathe. • Obtain daily CXR to check position. • Notify physician. • Always deflate balloon and note return to PAP waveform.

The Patient with Increased Intracranial Pressure

Definition/Discussion

Increased intracranial pressure (ICP) is a rise above normal of the pressure of the cerebrospinal fluid (CSF) in the subarachnoid space. Normal intracranial pressure ranges between 0 and 15 mm Hg.

Nursing Assessment

☐ PERTINENT HISTORY

Conditions that cause an *increase in brain size:* tumor; surgical manipulation; infarction; anoxic event (e.g., drowning, asphyxia, smoke inhalation, accidents, cardiac or respiratory arrest); head injury; brain abscess; metabolic disorder (e.g., chemical toxicity, diabetic acidosis); Reye's syndrome; conditions that *increase intracranial blood volume:* hypercapnia, hypoxemia, or hyperthermia causing cerebral vasodilation; tumor; cerebral hemotoma; an aneurysm or arteriovenous malformation; subarachnoid hemorrhage causing intracerebral bleeding; conditions that *increase CSF volume:* tumors of the choroid plexus; subarachnoid hemorrhage meningitis, or cerebripseudotumor causing decreased CSF absorption; hydrocephalus, tumor, or trauma causing a blockage of CSF flow

☐ PHYSICAL FINDINGS

Altered level of consciousness (LOC)/responsiveness; pupillary changes; motor/sensory changes in extremities; vital sign changes (Cushing's triad: increased blood pressure, decreased heart rate, and widening pulse pressure); changes in depth, rate, and pattern of respirations; patient complaints of headache, vomiting, and/or papilledema; increased ICP readings via an ICP monitor (epidural, intraventricular, or subarachnoid)

☐ PSYCHOSOCIAL CONCERNS/ DEVELOPMENTAL FACTORS

Age, sex, usual coping strategies; acceptance of condition, usual roles and responsibilities

☐ PATIENT AND FAMILY KNOWLEDGE

Etiology, treatment, outcomes, signs and symptoms of increased ICP; level of knowledge, readiness and willingness to learn

Nursing Care

☐ LONG-TERM GOAL

The patient will maintain stable vital functions with minimum complications through the period of actual or potential increased intracranial pressure; the patient will experience reduction of increased intracranial pressure with no residual neurologic deficits.

NURSING DIAGNOSIS #1

Alteration in tissue perfusion: cerebral related to an increase in brain tissue, intracranial blood volume, CSF volume

Rationale: *ICP is indicative of the balance in the intracranial volume (brain tissue, blood, and CSF). An alteration in either the arterial pressure or intracranial volume alters cerebral perfusion. Cerebral perfusion pressure (60-90 mm Hg) is the amount of pressure needed in the cerebral vasculature to supply oxygen and nutrients to the brain. A cerebral perfusion* *pressure (CPP) of 50 mm Hg is minimum for adequate cerebral perfusion. CPP equals the mean arterial blood pressure minus the mean ICP.*

GOAL

The patient will demonstrate adequate cerebral perfusion.

IMPLEMENTATION

- Assess patient's LOC, behavior, motor/sensory function (symmetry; movement: spontaneous, to command, to painful stimuli), pupillary signs (symmetry: size and reactivity; deviation) every 1-2 hours and as necessary.
- Monitor vital signs every 15 minutes to 1 hour and as necessary; a change in respirations is an early sign of increased ICP and hypoxia/hypercapnia.
- Monitor arterial blood gas values (ABGs) for acid-base abnormalities and decreased oxygen saturation.
- Hyperventilate before suctioning; limit suctioning to 10-15 seconds to reduce carbon dioxide levels, to increase oxygenation, and to prevent hypoxia.
- Maintain venous outflow from the brain by elevating head of bed and properly aligning head/neck.
- Monitor intake and output, electrolytes, and specific gravity to determine potential fluid imbalance contributing to cerebral edema.
- Administer fluids within fluid restriction (1,400 cc/24 hours) to prevent cerebral edema.
- Instruct to refrain from activities that increase intrathoracic or intra-abdominal pressure (e.g., straining for bowel movement, isometric exercises, holding breath when turning in bed, hip flexion, coughing, blowing nose).
- Utilize restraints only when absolutely necessary because agitation will increase ICP.
- Assess patient's level of comfort (headache, nausea, vomiting) since these complaints indicate increased ICP.
- Administer PRN medications as ordered (e.g., stool softeners, antiemetics, analgesics); evaluate effectiveness.
- Administer steroids to prevent cerebral edema as ordered.
- Organize nursing care to allow optimal rest periods for patient.
- Employ optimal aseptic technique and infection control measures regarding tubing and dressing changes (infection increases metabolic rate, cerebral blood flow, and cerebral edema).
- Notify physician immediately of neurologic and other significant changes (e.g., vital signs).
- Institute measures to treat increased ICP as ordered
  - administer diuretics (mannitol, furosemide), barbiturates, or short-acting narcotics to decrease brain metabolism and oxygen demand, therefore blood flow to brain
  - implement hypothermia to reduce metabolism, body's oxygen requirements, and cerebral blood flow
  - drain CSF via intraventricular drain
  - prepare patient/family for surgical interventions
- If ICP monitoring device (e.g., subarachnoid screw, intraventricular catheter, or epidural sensor)
  - assist with insertion as needed, maintaining sterility, obtaining equipment, and monitoring patient's clinical status.
  - maintain covered insertion site; do not change dressing; notify physician if dressing becomes wet.
  - allow adequate length of tubing to prevent dislodgement when patient moves.
  - maintain a closed system with tight connections and proper position of stopcocks to prevent infection, inadvertent loss of CSF, or herniation.
  - balance or zero the system every 4-12 hours and as necessary; maintain proper level of transducer to obtain accurate measurements
  - measure ICP every 15 minutes to 1 hour and as necessary
  - report and record increases in pressure and changes in waveform, especially plateau waves (A waves or Lundberg waves) of 50-100 mm Hg lasting approximately 5-20 minutes
  - check the system for air, blood, tissue, or kinks if waveform becomes damped
  - drain intraventricular catheter according to physician orders
  - assess the color, clarity, consistency, and amount of CSF drained
  - record the amount of CSF drained at the

end of each shift and mark the collection bag
  - change and label the drainage bag according to hospital policy (at least every 24 hours or when 3/4 full)
  - send tip of catheter to lab for culture and sensitivity after removal
  - cover site with sterile dressing after catheter is removed and notify physician of any persistent drainage

☐ EVALUATION CRITERIA/DESIRED OUTCOMES

The Patient

- Has ICP 0-15 mm Hg, CPP greater than 50 mm Hg
- Maintains or improves neurologic status

NURSING DIAGNOSIS #2

a. **Ineffective breathing pattern** related to increased ICP, alteration in LOC
b. **Ineffective airway clearance** related to increased ICP, alteration in LOC
c. **Impaired gas exchange** related to increased ICP, alteration in LOC

Rationale: *There are a number of abnormal respiratory patterns associated with increased ICP. As pressure increases, vital centers located in the brainstem are affected. Cheyne-Stokes breathing consists of waxing and waning of respirations with periodic apnea. Central neurogenic hyperventilation, associated with lesions in the lower midbrain and upper pons, is hallmarked by continuous, regular, rapid, deep respirations. Pressure in the mid to lower pons region causes prolonged inspiration followed by prolonged expiration and a pause (apneustic breathing). Cluster breathing or irregular spurts of breathing interspersed with apnea is associated with lesions in the lower pons and upper medulla. Finally, a completely irregular pattern of breathing that may progress to apnea is indicative of pressure on the medulla and termed ataxic, or Biot's, breathing.*

Loss of consciousness is the earliest and most sensitive indicator of increased ICP. A change in consciousness or responsiveness may impair an individual's ability to clear pulmonary secretions or aerate adequately, causing an acid-base disturbance in ABGs.

☐ GOAL

The patient will demonstrate effective air exchange.

☐ IMPLEMENTATION

- Assess patient's LOC, ability to maintain open airway.
- Maintain a patent airway by correct positioning and suctioning, utilizing airway adjuncts as needed.
- Monitor respiratory rate, rhythm, and depth every 15 minutes to 1 hours.
- Auscultate breath sounds every 2-4 hours for adequate aeration and to detect adventitious sounds.
- Assess circulatory status (pulse, blood pressure, skin color) every hour to detect hypoxia.
- Monitor ABGs for acid-base abnormalities and decreased oxygen saturation.
- Administer oxygen as ordered.
- Encourage deep breathing and limited coughing every 1-2 hours.
- Assess color, amount, consistency of pulmonary secretions as necessary to determine need for possible sputum culture, treatments to break up secretions.

☐ EVALUATION CRITERIA/DESIRED OUTCOMES

The Patient

- Has ABGs within normal limits
- Maintains regular respiratory rate of 12-24/minute
- Has adequate bilateral lung aeration

NURSING DIAGNOSIS #3

a. **Alteration in fluid volume: excess** related to steroid therapy, syndrome of inappropriate antidiuretic hormone (SIADH)
b. **Fluid volume deficit** related to diuretic therapy, fluid restriction, diabetes insipidus

Rationale: *Management of cerebral edema or increased ICP with drug therapy and/or fluid restriction can result in fluid and electrolyte imbalances. Syndrome of inappropriate secretion of antidiuretic hormone (SIADH) can occur with a variety of brain disorders, the stress of surgery, anesthesia, and certain medications.*

GOAL

The patient will demonstrate adequate fluid balance.

IMPLEMENTATION

- Monitor intake and output; notify physician of urinary output less than 30 cc/hour for 2 consecutive hours.
- Monitor laboratory findings (e.g., electrolytes, osmolarity, BUN, creatinine).
- Check specific gravity every 1-4 hours for SIADH and diabetes insipidus.
- Weigh patient daily for weight gain associated with fluid retention.
- Monitor vital signs every 1-2 hours for hemodynamic response to hypo/hypervolemia (tachycardia, hypo/hypertension).
- Monitor central venous, pulmonary artery, and pulmonary capillary wedge pressures (if pulmonary artery catheter is in place) every 1-2 hours and as necessary for hemodynamic response to hypo/hypervolemia.
- Assess patient's skin turgor and presence of edema every 4 hours.
- Administer fluids and medications as ordered.
- Evaluate effectiveness of interventions (fluid increase or decrease, electrolyte replacement).
- Review Table 1, *Common Fluid and Electrolyte Imbalances,* page 17.

EVALUATION CRITERIA/DESIRED OUTCOMES

The Patient

- Excretes at least 30 cc urine/hour
- Maintains electrolytes, osmolarity, specific gravity within normal limits
- Is free from indications of fluid excess, deficit

NURSING DIAGNOSIS #4

Impairment of skin integrity related to immobility, hypothermia therapy

Rationale: *An increase in ICP alters an individuals's LOC or responsiveness, putting the person at risk for developing pressure sores. If hypothermia is utilized to treat increased ICP, the patient is at risk for skin breakdown because of the direct contact with the hypothermia mattress and decreased tissue perfusion. In addition, barbiturate coma, another strategy to decrease ICP, renders an individual immobile and at risk for skin problems.*

GOAL

The patient will maintain intact skin.

IMPLEMENTATION

- Assess patient's skin turgor, presence of edema every 4 hours and as needed.
- Assess patient's peripheral circulation every 4 hours.
- Keep patient's skin clean and dry.
- Reposition every 2 hours; utilize supports such as pillows, sheepskin, foam.
- Promote circulation by rubbing bony prominences when turning.
- Assess patient's nutritional status.

EVALUATION CRITERIA/DESIRED OUTCOMES

The Patient

- Maintains intact skin
- Is free from skin redness
- Has adequate peripheral circulation

NURSING DIAGNOSIS #5

Potential for injury related to seizure activity, drug therapy (steroids), decreased level of responsiveness

Rationale: *Cerebral edema may alter neuronal functioning leading to the development of seizures. An individual may sustain physical injury during the clonic-tonic period of seizure activity. Corticosteriods such as dexamethasone (Decadron) used to treat/prevent increased ICP, irritate the gastrointestinal (GI) tract, and cause bleeding. As ICP increases and applies pressure on the brainstem (midbrain, pons, and medulla), the trigeminal nerve (cranial nerve V) responsible for the corneal reflex may be absent. The patient is at risk for corneal abrasion in this situation.*

GOAL

The patient will be free from physical injury.

☐ IMPLEMENTATION

- Monitor for seizure activity; refer to *The Patient with Epilepsy*, page 93.
- Administer medications (anticonvulsants, antacids, cimetidine) as ordered; evaluate effectiveness.
- Monitor for gastric bleeding by assessing GI secretions for color and presence of blood.
- Assess patient's neurologic status including cranial nerves.
- Apply artificial tears and/or eye patches as needed to lubricate and protect the eyes.

☐ EVALUATION CRITERIA/DESIRED OUTCOMES

The Patient

- Is free from seizure activity injury
- Exhibits no signs of GI bleeding
- Has no corneal abrasions

NURSING DIAGNOSIS #6

Alteration in nutrition: less than body requirements related to NPO status, nausea and vomiting, fluid restriction, altered LOC

Rationale: *Increased ICP causes an alteration in the patient's LOC that may limit ability to ingest food or fluids orally. The nausea and vomiting associated with increased ICP may require a nasogastric (NG) tube and restriction of oral intake. The treatment for increased ICP often includes fluid restriction to prevent cerebral edema.*

☐ GOAL

The patient will maintain optimal nutritional status and fluid intake.

☐ IMPLEMENTATION

- Assess patient's LOC and comfort level to determine ability to handle food and fluids.
- Monitor intake and output and dietary intake to determine deficit and ongoing status.
- Insert NG tube for nausea/vomiting; attach to low intermittent suction if ordered.
- Administer tube feedings as ordered.
- Administer hyperalimentation as ordered; refer to *The Patient Receiving Total Parenteral Nutrition*, page 229).
- Monitor electrolytes since poor oral intake, NG suction, and fluid restriction can cause imbalances.
- Monitor daily weights.
- Auscultate bowel sounds every 4-8 hours to determine presence or absence of peristalsis.
- Record and monitor number and character of bowel movements.

☐ EVALUATION CRITERIA/DESIRED OUTCOMES

The Patient

- Maintains weight within 10% of admission weight
- Increases oral intake without nausea/vomiting
- Tolerates parenteral or tube feedings

NURSING DIAGNOSIS #7

Sensory-perceptual alteration related to sensory overload/deprivation, sensory deficits, altered LOC

Rationale: *The patient's ability to interpret own environment may be altered by putting the patient into a coma in an attempt to control increased ICP. The ability to see, hear, and feel may be altered as a result of the condition contributing to the increased ICP (e.g., a tumor pressing on the auditory nerve, hemiparesis). The patient with actual or potential increased ICP will often be hospitalized in a critical care setting where constant monitoring, extensive equipment, and numerous personnel contribute to sensory overload/deprivation.*

☐ GOAL

The patient will be able to interpret incoming stimuli.

☐ IMPLEMENTATION

- Assess patient's neurologic status including LOC, cranial nerve function, motor and sensory function to determine abilities and deficits.
- Reorient to environment frequently.
- Explain all tests, procedures, and routines.
- Allow for uninterrupted rest periods to prevent sleep deprivation.
- Modify approach to patient based on present

- deficits (e.g., approach patient from unaffected side, utilize touch, talk to patient).
- Increase/decrease stimuli as appropriate to correct sensory deprivation/overload.
- Avoid talking about meaningless subjects or about the patient in his/her presence as if patient does not exist.

☐ EVALUATION CRITERIA/DESIRED OUTCOMES

The Patient

- Is oriented to environment
- Obtains adequate rest

> **NURSING DIAGNOSIS #8**
>
> a. **Fear** related to uncertain future
> b. **Ineffective individual coping** related to actual or perceived loss of well-being
> c. **Alteration in family process** related to actual or perceived loss of well-being of patient
>
> ***Rationale:*** *Increased ICP causes an alteration in the patient's neurologic status, either temporary or permanent. This uncertainty and stress can inhibit the coping abilities of the patient/family.*

☐ GOAL

The patient/family will effectively adapt to actual or potential altered abilities.

☐ IMPLEMENTATION

- Assess understanding of increased ICP, treatment, and outcomes.
- Explain tests, procedures, need for frequent assessments, treatments.
- Keep family informed of patient's progress.
- Encourage verbalization of feelings and concerns.
- Assess family's emotional reaction to patient's condition and their coping strategies.
- Utilize other personnel to assist patient/family in coping with patient's condition (e.g., pastoral care, clinical nurse specialist, support group members).

☐ EVALUATION CRITERIA/DESIRED OUTCOMES

The Patient/family

- Verbalizes feelings related to fears
- Discusses ways to adapt to patient's changed status

> **NURSING DIAGNOSIS #9**
>
> **Knowledge deficit** regarding disease process, treatment, prognosis
>
> ***Rationale:*** *Inadequate preparation regarding increased ICP may be due to the unexpected and sudden hospitalization related to a head injury, cardiac arrest, or similar traumatic event. Inadequate pre-op teaching may also be a contributing factor.*

☐ GOAL

The patient/family will demonstrate adequate knowledge of ICP (potential and actual).

☐ IMPLEMENTATION

- Assess present knowledge of potential/actual ICP.
- Assess learning ability and readiness to learn.
- Correct any misinformation, fill in gaps of needed information.
- Ask patient/family to repeat information to ensure understanding.
- Inform about patient's progress, prognosis, and plan of care.
- Encourage verbalization and questions about current situation.

☐ EVALUATION CRITERIA/DESIRED OUTCOMES

The Patient/family

- Verbalizes cause of present condition
- Knows treatment procedures and rationale

The Patient Requiring an Intra-aortic Balloon Pump

Definition/Discussion

The intra-aortic balloon pump (IABP) is a mechanical device that works to decrease afterload and increase coronary perfusion pressure by counterpulsation. It is used primarily for patients in cardiogenic shock. The balloon catheter is inserted via the femoral artery and positioned in the descending thoracic aorta below the bifurcation of the subclavian artery and above the renal arteries. During ventricular diastole, just after the aortic valve closes, the balloon is inflated with helium or carbon dioxide (diastolic augmentation). This causes 2 things to happen.

1. Blood between the balloon and the heart is forced upward and back toward the heart. Because the aortic valve is closed, blood flows down the coronary arteries bringing oxygen and nutrients to the myocardium. Blood also flows via the subclavian, vertebral, and carotid arteries to the head and upper parts of the body.
2. Blood below the balloon is forced toward the lower part of the body and increases perfusion to the kidneys.

Prior to ventricular systole, the balloon is deflated. This rapid deflation decreases resistance in the aorta, thus decreasing impedance to ventricular ejection (afterload) and making it easier for the heart to eject its contents. Less workload on the hert results in less myocardial oxygen demand.

Nursing Assessment

☐ PERTINENT HISTORY

- Medical problems necessitating IABP therapy: myocardial infarction (MI) with cardiogenic shock; MI complicated by mechanical problems such as mitral regurgitation, ventricular septal defect, and papillary muscle dysfunction; MI with intractable angina or dysrhythmias; unstable angina; severe coronary artery disease postcatheterization and while waiting for surgery, left ventricular failure
- Medical problems definitely contraindicating IABP therapy: significant aortic regurgitation, dissecting aortic aneurysm, irreversible brain damage, chronic end stage heart disease
- Medical problems probably contraindicating IABP therapy: severe peripheral vascular disease, grossly irregular cardiac rhythm.

☐ PHYSICAL FINDINGS

Heart rate and rhythm (balloon is timed based on heart rhythm); blood pressure (patients in cardiogenic shock typically have systolic BP less than 90 mm Hg); pulmonary capillary wedge pressure (usually over 18 mm Hg); cardiac index (usually less than 1.9 liter/min/M^2); respiratory characteristics, coagulation studies, pain

☐ PSYCHOSOCIAL CONCERNS/ DEVELOPMENTAL FACTORS

Age, sex, developmental level, suddenness of acute illness, desire for extraordinary life support, family support, usual coping mechanisms, usual roles and responsibilities

☐ PATIENT AND FAMILY KNOWLEDGE

Understanding of how treatment may help, potential complications and possible need for cardiac surgery, need to remain immobile during treatment, readiness and willingness to learn

Nursing Care

☐ LONG-TERM GOAL

Patient will become hemodynamically stable and be successfully weaned from IABP therapy; will remain

free from complications such as bleeding, embolism, and infection.

NURSING DIAGNOSIS #1

Alteration in cardiac output: decreased related to changes in preload, afterload, contractility, and cardiac rhythm

Rationale: *Prior to IABP therapy, cardiac output is severely reduced due to one or more factors including: increased fluid volume that the heart cannot handle (preload); decreased contractile force secondary to muscle damage; increased vasoconstriction—a compensatory measure to shunt blood toward vital organs that also increases impedance to left ventricular ejection (afterload); ventricular dysrhythmias due to hypoxic irritability of myocardium; atrial dysrhythmias due to mitral valve disease. Effective counterpulsation should reverse these problems. However, improperly timed pumping, the occurrence of dysrhythmias that cannot be suppressed pharmacologically, the continued overload of the heart with fluid, or improper use of inotropes may cause ineffective pumping and possible further decreased cardiac output.*

☐ GOAL

Patient will experience an increase in cardiac output and cardiac index and a decrease in pulmonary capillary wedge pressure.

☐ IMPLEMENTATION

- Assess cardiac output (CO) and cardiac index (CI) at least hourly with a pulmonary artery catheter with CO/CI monitoring capabilities; expect a gradual increase in values toward normal ranges.
- Assess left ventricular function with pulmonary capillary wedge pressures (PCWP) at least hourly; expect a gradual decrease in pressures as the left ventricle works more effectively in ejecting contents.
- Calculate systemic vascular resistance (SVR)

$$SVR = \frac{MAP - RAP}{CO} \times 80$$

- expect gradual reduction in SVR; know tht an increased SVR may indicate need for supplemental treatment with sodium nitroprusside.
- Administer dopaminergic drugs and nitrates to increase contractility (dopamine, dobutamine), decrease preload (nitroglycerin), and decrease afterload (nitroprusside) as ordered; monitor blood pressure with indwelling arterial line every 5-15 minutes.
- Monitor cardiac rhythm; administer prescribed antidysrhythmic drugs continuously to suppress ectopic foci.
- Assess patient's mentation, skin color, temperature, peripheral pulses, and urine output hourly to note changes in peripheral perfusion secondary to low cardiac output.
- Assess lung sounds to detect improvement in congestive heart failure (CHF); expect to find rales and rhonchi diminishing.
- During the weaning process, assess all of the above parameters frequently (within 20 minutes of augmentation change, every 30 minutes × 4, then every hour) to identify a continued failing heart with withdrawal of IABP therapy (weaning may need to be discontinued if signs of deterioration [e.g., hypotension, increased PCWP, decreased urine, decreased level of consciousness, angina, change in heart rate/rhythm, ST-T wave changes] occur).

☐ EVALUATION CRITERIA/DESIRED OUTCOMES

The Patient

- Has cardiac output of 4-7 liter/min
- Has cardiac index between 2.5-4 liter/min/M^2
- Has PCWP between 8-12 mm Hg
- Maintains regular cardiac rhythm
- Has warm and dry skin, pink nailbeds, clear mentation, urine output of at least 30 cc/hr
- Has SVR of 800-1200 dynes
- Is successfully weaned from IABP without return to cardiogenic shock or CHF

NURSING DIAGNOSIS #2

Alteration in tissue perfusion: peripheral related to clotting or bleeding secondary to large invasive device in vascular system

Rationale: *The IABP catheter requires a larger than normal puncture wound to accommodate its size. The catheter remains in the aorta for several days and, as a foreign object, is prone*

to platelet adhesion and clot formation with subsequent embolism. Dextran and heparin are administered to prevent this. Thus when the catheter is removed, there may be extensive bleeding from the site. Patients with long-term CHF may have liver dysfunction that could further reduce normal clotting factors. Both abnormal clotting and bleeding interfere with perfusion to the extremities with oxygen and nutrient-rich blood for cellular metabolism. Embolism, due to the possibility of a dislodged atherosclerotic plaque during inflation and deflation of the balloon, may occur.

☐ GOAL

The patient will have normal peripheral tissue perfusion during and after IABP therapy.

☐ IMPLEMENTATION

- Assess and chart peripheral circulation at least hourly (e.g., pulses, color and temperature of skin, capillary refill); pay particular attention to the affected leg.
- Administer dextran to decrease platelet adhesiveness and heparin to decrease fibrin deposition as ordered; monitor clotting profiles (prothrombin time, activated partial thromboplastin time) to assess effectiveness of heparin; have protamine at bedside to reverse effects of heparin as needed.
- Check dressing over arterial puncture site every hour for bleeding.
- Keep at least 2 units of blood on hand during and immediately after IABP therapy.
- Apply direct manual or mechanical pressure to arterial puncture site for at least 30 minutes after catheter is removed, then apply small transparent dressing to allow easy observation of the site. Observe site and extremity frequently and report hematoma formation, bleeding, or decreased circulation to the extremity; reapply pressure if evidence of bleeding.

☐ EVALUATION CRITERIA/DESIRED OUTCOMES

The Patient

- Has strong pedal, tibial, popliteal, femoral pulses bilaterally
- Has warm and dry legs and feet with pink nailbeds and normal sensation
- Experiences no bleeding following removal of balloon catheter
- Exhibits no signs of arterial embolization (e.g., decreased level of consciousness, renal insufficiency, gastrointestinal distress)

NURSING DIAGNOSIS #3

a. **Impaired physical mobility** related to need to keep leg straight, head of bed down, and connection to numerous mechanical devices
b. **Alteration in comfort: pain** related to impaired physical mobility, incisions, and numerous attachments

Rationale: *Patient must remain relatively immobile to prevent dislodging of mechanical devices such as IABP catheter, pulmonary artery catheter, IV, Foley catheter, mechanical ventilation. In addition s/he must keep the affected leg straight and head of bed down to prevent kinking of balloon catheter. When permitted to turn, range of motion is limited by equipment and s/he may not be able to assume the most comfortable position. The patient may also not be fully alert and able to follow directions about maintaining specified positions and will need restraints, further interfering with mobility and comfort.*

☐ GOAL

Patient will be as comfortable as possible within the limitations imposed by therapy.

☐ IMPLEMENTATION

- Do not allow patient to sit up more than 30° (to prevent kinking of catheter); if possible, disconnect bed controls to prevent patient from accidentally raising head of bed.
- Teach patient to keep affected leg straight to prevent kinking of catheter; when turning patient side-to-side, keep leg straight and pay attention to all tubings; use soft restraints as needed.
- Explain reason for limited movement to the alert patient to increase chances of cooperation.
- Do passive ROM to all unaffected joints at least every 4 hours to decrease painful stiffness.
- Allow the patient as much freedom of move-

ment as possible (e.g., one arm may be free of invasive lines and could be left unrestrained; the arm with lines could be unrestrained while nurse is in room and only loosely restrained to allow lateral movement on the bed at other times).

- Turn side-to-side every 2 hours keeping affected leg straight; give back rubs and straighten linens regularly.
- Medicate for pain as needed if vital signs are stable; provide noninvasive pain relief (e.g., distraction with conversation, visitors, TV; guided imagery if patient can concentrate and is willing to try it; application of heat or cold to painful muscles) as needed.
- Remove lines that are no longer needed; convert extra IVs to heparin locks as possible to decrease number of attachments.

☐ EVALUATION CRITERIA/DESIRED OUTCOMES

The Patient

- Experiences relief of muscle aches with noninvasive measures
- Has pain relieved within 30 minutes of analgesic administration
- Moves unrestrained extremities freely and safely

NURSING DIAGNOSIS #4

Potential for infection related to invasive lines (Refer to Diagnosis 1, *The Patient with Hemodynamic Monitoring*, page 117.)

NURSING DIAGNOSIS #5

Sensory alteration related to intensive nursing care, multiple mechanical devices, and interrupted sleep cycles. (Refer to Diagnosis 1, *The Patient Experiencing Sensory Alteration*, page 275.)

The Patient Undergoing Intracranial Surgery: Craniotomy, Craniectomy, or Cranioplasty

Definition/Discussion

***Craniotomy* is an opening in the skull to form a bone flap.** *Craniectomy* is the removal of part of the skull to form a hole or holes of varying size. *Cranioplasty* is the placement of a bone graft or synthetic plate to repair a defect or opening in the skull. Intracranial surgery relieves intracranial pressure (ICP) by removing hematomas, fluid, tissue, or an arteriovenous malformation (AVM); repairing an aneurysm; clipping an AVM; redirecting fluid via a shunt; or repairing fracture injuries.

Nursing Assessment

☐ PERTINENT HISTORY

Past medical and surgical history; condition mandating surgery (e.g., hematoma following head injury, tumor, AVM, aneurysm, hydrocephalus; pre-op neurologic deficits; seizures); history of coagulation disorder; respiratory or cardiac problems; diagnostic tests and findings (CT scan, angiography, skull films)

☐ PHYSICAL FINDINGS

Level of consciousness (LOC), motor and sensory function, pupils, cranial nerve function, vital signs, respiratory status, head dressing and drainage, intracranial pressure, seizure activity, fluid status

☐ PSYCHOSOCIAL CONCERNS/ DEVELOPMENTAL FACTORS

Age, sex, occupation, roles and responsibilities, usual coping strategies, acceptance of condition, anxiety/fears

☐ PATIENT AND FAMILY KNOWLEDGE

General and neurosurgical pre- and post-op care; probable and possible anticipated results (e.g., deficits, rehabilitation); readiness and willingness to learn

Nursing Care

☐ LONG-TERM GOAL

The patient will remain neurologically stable postoperatively; the patient will resume pre-op neurologic function or participate in rehabilitation as fully as possible within limitations; the patient will resume normal or adjusted roles in family/home/society; OR the patient will maintain vital functioning and sustain life with comfort and dignity until death.

NURSING DIAGNOSIS #1

Alteration in tissue perfusion: cerebral related to increased ICP

Rationale: *Edema, bleeding, hydrocephalus, or cerebral infarction can cause cerebral ischemia. Increased drowsiness 24-96 hours postoperatively indicates cerebral edema. De-*

pending on the site and nature of the procedure, bleeding can occur in the meninges, cerebrum, cerebellum, or ventricles. Hypotension (intraoperatively or postoperatively) as well as thrombotic or air emboli can cause an infarction in the brain. In addition, vasospasm associated with an aneurysm clipping 4-11 days postoperatively contributes to an alteration in cerebral perfusion.*

☐ GOAL

The patient will demonstrate adequate cerebral perfusion.

☐ IMPLEMENTATION

- Refer to *The Patient with Increased Intracranial Pressure,* page 122, and *The Patient with a Head Injury,* Nursing Diagnosis #1, page 105.
- Monitor vital signs (heart rate, blood pressure, temperature, respiratory pattern) every 15 minutes to 1 hour and as necessary.
- Monitor ICP hourly and as necessary. Refer to *The Patient with Increased Intracranial Pressure,* page 122.
- Calculate cerebral perfusion pressure (CPP) by subtracting ICP from mean arterial pressure (MAP).

(MAP–ICP = CPP)

- Elevate head of bed 30°-45° unless otherwise specified.
- Position patient to maintain venous outflow from the brain; (position may need to be flat following subdural evacuation, turning may be limited when bone flap removed or with posterior fossa surgery); maintain head/neck in proper alignment.
- Assess head dressing and/or drain for amount and type of drainage every 1-4 hours.

☐ EVALUATION CRITERIA/DESIRED OUTCOMES

The Patient

- Maintains ICP of 0-15 mm Hg
- Has cerebral perfusion pressure (CPP) greater than 50 mm Hg
- Maintains or improves neurologic status

NURSING DIAGNOSIS #2

a. **Ineffective breathing pattern** related to increased ICP, alteration in LOC
b. **Ineffective airway clearance** related to alteration in LOC
c. **Impaired gas exchange** related to shallow respirations

Rationale: *Refer to* The Patient with Increased Intracranial Pressure, *Nursing Diagnosis #2, page 122. The long operative time required for some surgical procedures increases the risk for post-op complications. Shallow respirations lead to atelectasis, which may be indicated by a fever within the first 24-48 hours postoperatively.*

☐ GOAL

The patient will demonstrate effective air exchange.

☐ IMPLEMENTATION

- Refer to *The Patient with Increased Intracranial Pressure,* Nursing Diagnosis #2, page 122.
- Monitor temperature and pulse every 2-4 hours (elevations that may indicate atelectasis).
- Assess LOC, ability to maintain open airway.
- Maintain a patent airway by correct positioning, suctioning, utilizing airway adjuncts.
- Monitor respiratory rate, rhythm, and depth every 15 minutes to 1 hour.
- Auscultate breath sounds every 2-4 hours for adequate aeration and to detect adventitious sounds.
- Assess circulatory status (i.e., peripheral pulses, blood pressure, skin color) every hour to detect hypoxia.
- Monitor arterial blood gas values for acid-base abnormalities and decreased oxygen saturation.
- Administer oxygen as ordered.
- Determine need for ventilator. Refer to *The Patient Who is Ventilator-Dependent,* page 239.
- Encourage deep breathing and limited coughing every 1-2 hours.
- Assess color, amount, consistency of pulmonary secretions to determine need for sputum culture, treatments to break up secretions.

☐ EVALUATION CRITERIA/DESIRED OUTCOMES

The Patient

- Maintains arterial blood gases within normal limits
- Breathes regularly 12-24 times per minute
- Has normal breath sounds

NURSING DIAGNOSIS #3

a. **Alteration in fluid volume: excess** related to steroid therapy, syndrome of inappropriate antidiuretic hormone (SIADH)

b. **Fluid volume deficit** related to diuretic therapy, diabetes insipidus, blood loss, undertransfusion in surgery, fluid restriction, inadequate intake

Rationale: *Management of cerebral edema or increased ICP with drug therapy and/or fluid restriction can result in fluid and electrolyte imbalances. An altered LOC or loss of the gag reflex (cranial nerves IX and X) can contribute to problems with oral intake. SIADH can occur with a variety of brain disorders, the stress of surgery, anesthesia, and certain medications. Surgery in the pituitary-hypothalamic area can alter ADH secretion and cause diabetes insipidus.*

☐ GOAL

The patient will maintain adequate fluid intake and output.

☐ IMPLEMENTATION

- Refer to *The Patient with Increased Intracranial Pressure,* Nursing Diagnosis #3, page 124.
- Assess patient's LOC and cranial nerve function (gag reflex) before attempting oral intake
- Notify physician of urinary output less than 30 cc/hour or over 200 cc/hour for 2 consecutive hours.
- Monitor intake and output to determine source of deficit or excess.
- Monitor laboratory findings indicative of fluid imbalance (e.g., electrolytes, osmolarity, BUN, creatinine).
- Monitor weight daily.
- Obtain vital signs every 1-2 hours to measure hemodynamic response to fluid imbalance.
- Monitor ICP, central venous pressure, pulmonary artery pressure, and pulmonary capillary wedge pressure if present every 1-2 hours and as necessary for hemodynamic response to fluid imbalance.
- Assess skin turgor and presence of edema every 4 hours.
- Administer replacement fluids and medications if necessary; evaluate effectiveness.

☐ EVALUATION CRITERIA/DESIRED OUTCOMES

The Patient

- Maintains electrolytes, osmolarity, specific gravity within normal limits
- Excretes at least 30 cc and less than 200 cc urine every hour

NURSING DIAGNOSIS #4

a. **Potential for injury** related to seizure activity, drug therapy (steroids), cranial nerve V dysfunction, absence of bone flap, cerebrospinal fluid (CSF) leak/infection

b. **Potential for infection** related to surgical incision, CSF leak, CSF infection

Rationale: *Cerebral edema may alter neuronal functioning, leading to the development of seizures. Individuals requiring surgery for abscesses, arteriovenous malformations (AVM), intracerebral hemorrhages, and aneurysms are likely to experience seizures. Metabolic imbalances such as hypoxia, hypoglycemia, and electrolyte imbalances pre- or postoperatively can contribute to the development of seizures. An individual may sustain physical injury during the clonic-tonic period of seizure activity. Corticosteroids such as dexamethasone (Decadron), used to treat/prevent increased post-op ICP, irritate the gastrointestinal (GI) tract and cause bleeding. Cranial nerve V dysfunction resulting from increased ICP or direct injury places the person at risk for corneal abrasion. Increased ICP may also necessitate the bone flap not being replaced to allow the brain to expand. Communication with the subarachnoid space as a result of surgery or a basilar skull fracture can cause a CSF leak and a potential infection. Secondary brain/brainstem damage can occur as a result of the infectious process.*

☐ GOAL

The patient will be free from physical injury or secondary brain/brainstem injury, will be free from infection.

☐ IMPLEMENTATION

- Monitor for seizure activity; refer to *The Patient with Epilepsy*, page 93.
- Protect from potential injury related to seizures (e.g., keep bed in low position, side rails up and padded).
- Monitor for gastric bleeding by assessing GI secretions for color and presence of blood.
- Administer medications (anticonvulsants, antibiotics, antacids, cimetidine) as ordered; evaluate effectiveness.
- Assess cranial nerve V function every 3 hours.
- Apply artificial tears and/or eye patches as needed to lubricate and protect the eyes.
- Position to avoid pressure on flap site; use donut ring as necessary to avoid undue pressure on the area.
- Observe incision site and change or reinforce dressing as necessary, maintaining sterility.
- Assess for otorrhea or rhinorrhea indicating CSF leak.
- Do not pack ear or nose if CSF leak suspected since this may cause an increase in ICP.
- Monitor temperature every 4 hours.
- Assess patient's LOC every 1-2 hours and prn to determine changes.

☐ EVALUATION CRITERIA/DESIRED OUTCOMES

The Patient

- Exhibits no indications of GI bleeding
- Is free from corneal abrasions
- Is free from signs and symptoms of infection
- Maintains neurologic status

NURSING DIAGNOSIS #5

a. **Impaired physical mobility** related to decreased LOC, paresis/plegia
b. **Impairment of skin integrity** related to limitations in mobility
c. **Self-care deficit: total** related to loss of mobility

Rationale: *Mobility may be limited postoperatively as a result of alterations in wakefulness/arousal, motor/sensory function. Immobility or limitations in mobility caused by an altered LOC and motor/sensory deficits places the person at risk for the development of skin problems. Patients who are immobilized as a result of intracranial surgery or have a decreased LOC may be unable to perform activities of daily living.*

☐ GOAL

The patient will actively or passively participate in mobilization; will be free from injury.

☐ IMPLEMENTATION

- Assess LOC, motor/sensory functions to determine abilities and limitations.
- Perform range-of-motion exercises every 4 hours while patient is confined to bed.
- Reposition or assist with repositioning every 2-4 hours to relieve pressure over bony prominences.
- Coordinate nursing efforts with physical therapy.
- Encourage patient participation in activities as appropriate.

☐ EVALUATION CRITERIA/DESIRED OUTCOMES

The Patient

- Maintains joint mobility
- Sits in chair, ambulates as able
- Is free from pressure sores

NURSING DIAGNOSIS #6

Impaired communication: verbal, related to dysphasia

Rationale: *Expressive or receptive aphasia may become evident postoperatively as a result of surgical manipulation of brain and/or cerebral edema.*

☐ GOAL

The patient will demonstrate improved ability to express self or increased ability to understand.

☐ IMPLEMENTATION

- Assess patient's ability to express self and to understand verbal and written communication.
- Speak in short, simple sentences in a calm, unhurried manner.
- Acknowledge understanding of patient's difficulty with communication.
- Utilize alternative methods of communication (e.g., magic slate, alphabet board) as able and needed.
- Utilize family members to help understand patient's needs and communication abilities.

☐ EVALUATION CRITERIA/DESIRED OUTCOMES

The Patient

- Communicates basic needs

NURSING DIAGNOSIS #7

Knowledge deficit regarding disease process, treatment, prognosis

Rationale: *Inadequate preparation in regard to intracranial surgery may relate to insufficient pre-op teaching if surgery is sudden and unexpected. Prior to discharge from unit, the individual with minimal or no deficits will require basic information related to drug therapy and follow-up care.*

☐ GOAL

The patient/family will demonstrate adequate knowledge related to surgery, pre-op and post-op interventions.

☐ IMPLEMENTATION

- Inform patient/family about shaving of the head, head dressings, frequency of nursing assessments, use of invasive equipment, and the probable and possible anticipated results, including potential rehabilitation.
- Encourage verbalization and questions if possible.
- Inform patient/family of progress, prognosis, and plan of care.
- Prior to discharge from unit, instruct regarding medications; and need for therapy (speech, occupational, physical).

☐ EVALUATION CRITERIA/DESIRED OUTCOMES

The Patient/family

- States type of surgery to be done and rationale
- Knows what to expect in immediate post-op period

NURSING DIAGNOSIS #8

Alteration in comfort: pain related to increased ICP, surgical manipulation

Rationale: *Manipulation of intracranial tissue during surgery causes edema resulting in increased ICP; the patient may subsequently complain of a headache. Preoperatively, the pathology alters the intracranial contents and pressure causing a headache.*

☐ GOAL

The patient will be free from or have a reduction in pain.

☐ IMPLEMENTATION

- Assess the patient's level of discomfort using a 0-10 point self-rating scale, if possible.
- Administer analgesics; evaluate effectiveness.
- Promote a quiet, restful environment; position for comfort with head of bed elevated to promote venous drainage.
- Evaluate effectiveness of comfort measures.
- Assess for factors contributing to the pain experience (e.g., anxiety, increased blood pressure, increased ICP, inadequate rest); provide alternate interventions (e.g., guided imagery, distraction).

☐ EVALUATION CRITERIA/DESIRED OUTCOMES

The Patient

- Verbalizes reduction or absence of pain following interventions

NURSING DIAGNOSIS #9

Alteration in nutrition: less than body requirements related to NPO status, IV fluid restriction, altered LOC, dysphagia, difficulty chewing

Rationale: *Postoperatively the patient may exhibit an altered LOC or cranial nerve dysfunction as a result of cerebral edema or direct surgical manipulation which can prohibit or reduce oral intake. In an effort to control ICP, fluids may be restricted. An IV will be necessary to keep the patient NPO until the neurologic and GI status improves.*

☐ GOAL

The patient will maintain optimal nutritional status and fluid intake.

☐ IMPLEMENTATION

- Assess LOC and cranial nerves V, VII, IX, X, XII functions to determine ability to handle food and fluids.
- Monitor intake and output.
- Monitor electrolytes since lack of oral intake and fluid deficit can cause electrolyte imbalance.
- Administer IV fluids as ordered.
- Administer nasogastric feedings and water if ordered.
- Administer hyperalimentation as ordered.
- Provide oral hygiene before/after each oral feeding to facilitate taste sensation.
- Obtain and monitor daily weights.
- Auscultate bowel sounds every 4-8 hours to determine presence or absence of peristalsis.
- Record and monitor number and character of bowel movements.
- Assist with oral feedings when indicated.
- Advance diet as tolerated (i.e., full liquids, soft or pureed, regular).

☐ EVALUATION CRITERIA/DESIRED OUTCOMES

The Patient

- Maintains weight within 10% of normal
- Tolerates parenteral or tube feedings if applicable
- Has increased oral intake without aspiration

NURSING DIAGNOSIS #10

Sensory-perceptual alteration related to sensory deficits, altered LOC

Rationale: *The patient's ability to see, hear, and feel may be altered as a result of the condition necessitating surgery, (e.g., a tumor pressing on the auditory nerve, hemiparesis). The patient may be lethargic, confused, or disoriented pre- and postoperatively, limiting ability to accurately interpret the environment.*

☐ GOAL

The patient will be able to accurately interpret incoming stimuli.

☐ IMPLEMENTATION

- Assess patient's neurologic status (LOC, cranial nerve function, motor/sensory function) to determine abilities and deficits.
- Orient to environment every 1-2 hours.
- Explain all tests/procedures, routines to patient.
- Modify approach to patient based on present deficits (e.g., approach patient from unaffected side).
- Avoid talking about meaningless information or about the patient in his/her presence as if patient does not exist.

☐ EVALUATION CRITERIA/DESIRED OUTCOMES

The Patient

- Is oriented to environment

NURSING DIAGNOSIS #11

a. **Fear** related to uncertain future
b. **Ineffective individual coping** related to actual/perceived loss of well-being
c. **Alteration in family process** related to actual/perceived loss of well being of patient
d. **Anxiety** related to unknown prognosis/future
e. **Disturbance in self-concept: body-image, self-esteem, role performance, personal identity** related to actual/perceived loss of well-being
f. **Alteration in sexuality patterns** related to motor/sensory deficits, change in role, self-esteem, decreased LOC

Rationale: *The condition necessitating surgery may be causing a temporary or permanent alteration in the patient's neurologic status. This* *uncertainty stresses the coping abilities of the patient/family.*

GOAL

The patient/family will effectively adapt to actual or potential altered abilities.

IMPLEMENTATION

- Assess understanding of condition and anticipated post-op outcomes.
- Explain tests/procedures, frequent assessments, treatments.
- Keep family informed of patient's progress.
- Encourage verbalization of feelings, concerns, questions.
- Assess patient's/family's emotional reaction to patient's condition.
- Utilize other personnel to assist patient/family to cope with patient's condition (e.g., pastoral care, clinical nurse specialist, social services).

EVALUATION CRITERIA/DESIRED OUTCOMES

The Patient/family

- Verbalizes feelings related to fears
- Discusses ways to adapt to patient's changed status

The Patient Undergoing a Laryngectomy

Definition/Discussion

A laryngectomy is an excision of the larynx performed most commonly as a treatment for laryngeal cancer. There are several different types of procedures

- *partial laryngectomy:* performed for early stage or intrinsic cancer of the larynx (limited to the true vocal cords), involving creation of a laryngofissure or thyrotomy (an opening into the larynx through the thyroid cartilage for removal of affected portion of vocal cord). A temporary tracheostomy may be performed.
- *total laryngectomy:* performed for late stage or extrinsic cancer of the larynx (extension beyond the vocal cords), involving removal of the entire larynx including thyroid cartilage, epiglottis, hyoid bone, cricoid cartilage, and 2 or 3 rings of the trachea. The pharyngeal opening of the trachea is closed, resulting in the need for a permanent tracheal stoma. This procedure requires the removal of many structures essential to speech and also interferes with both olfactory and taste mechanisms because breathing is done directly into the trachea.
- *radical neck dissection:* may be performed in addition to total laryngectomy if there is metastasis to neck tissues and lymph nodes.

Nursing Assessment

☐ PERTINENT HISTORY

Hoarseness or alteration in voice, pain/burning in throat when drinking hot liquids and citrus juices, dysphagia, pain in laryngeal prominence (Adam's apple), malaise and fatigue, unplanned weight loss, chronic laryngitis, referred pain to ear, occupational voice straining or inhalation of noxious fumes, family history of laryngeal cancer, smoking, excessive alcohol intake

☐ PHYSICAL FINDINGS

Palpable lump in throat; enlarged cervical lymph nodes; cough; dyspnea, laryngeal stridor; halitosis; cachetic appearance, general debility

☐ PSYCHOSOCIAL CONCERNS/ DEVELOPMENTAL FACTORS

Life-style changes (more common in smokers, persons who have had long-term stress on vocal cords); previous coping patterns; support persons; most common in men ages 55-70

☐ PATIENT AND FAMILY KNOWLEDGE

Types of treatments (e.g., pre-op radiation therapy, possibility of hyperalimentation or tube feedings, types of surgical procedures); new means of communication, either temporary (with partial laryngectomy) or permanent

Nursing Care

☐ LONG-TERM GOAL

The patient will accept diagnosis and resultant body-image changes; the patient will positively perceive and utilize rehabilitation for communication skills, performance of activities of daily living (ADL), and other role responsibilities for return to appropriate level of functioning.

NURSING DIAGNOSIS #1

Anxiety related to surgical procedure, anticipated changes in physical appearance, ability to communicate

Rationale: *Preoperatively, the patient may have concerns about the disease process,* *prognosis, the anticipated surgery and changes in life-style.*

☐ GOAL

The patient will be prepared for the surgical procedure; will demonstrate verbal understanding of post-op expectations.

☐ IMPLEMENTATION

- Assess information needs of the patient including perceptions, misconceptions, and common fears (e.g., death, mutilation, lack of ability to communicate, loss of social acceptance, threat of cancer spread).
- Plan nursing care to provide time for the patient to express concerns and ask questions.
- Instruct regarding equipment, tubes, procedures, and the ICU environment if appropriate.
- Discuss changes in appearance resulting from specific surgery; prepare the patient/family for these alterations.
- Identify predictors of post-op depression (inevitable to some degree as evidenced by loss of control, powerlessness) and available support systems such as previous experience in health care systems, stress, and relations with others.
- Explain there will be a loss of sense of taste and smell immediately post-op but that they will return slowly to some degree.
- Identify rehabilitation potential by determining strengths, coping mechanisms, education level, speech and writing ability, acceptance by self and by family, life-style, and occupation.
- Refer to *The Patient Experiencing a Body-Image Disturbance,* page 253 for additional interventions.

☐ EVALUATION CRITERIA/DESIRED OUTCOMES

The Patient

- Expresses reduction in anxiety
- Displays nonverbal signs suggestive of relief of anxiety
- Identifies a plan for coping with physical and functional changes

NURSING DIAGNOSIS #2

Impaired communication: verbal related to temporary or permanent tracheostomy

Rationale: *Postoperatively, the patient will no longer be able to speak, (either temporarily or permanently) because the artificial airway created by the tracheotomy bypasses the vocal cords, which may have been removed; normal phonation is impossible.*

☐ GOAL

The patient will communicate by alternate methods while verbal communication is impaired.

☐ IMPLEMENTATION

- Preoperatively, discuss the predicted post-op inability to speak; agree on a method of communication to be used post-op and have patient/family/nursing staff practice (preplanned communication allows the patient some degree of control and independence); suggested methods include
  - writing on an erasable slate, clipboard, or notebook (make sure the surface is large enough and strong enough to be leaned on when writing)
  - board with words and pictures to which patient may point (may be an electronic board that will "speak" for the patient)
  - hand signals or signs
  - eye blinks for short answers to questions that may be answered "yes" or "no"
- Postoperatively, initiate previously agreed-upon communication as soon as patient is awake.
- Assist speech pathologist with initiation of speech training; usual methods include esophageal speech instruction or the use of an external or internal artificial larynx.
- Encourage and reinforce efforts in learning new speech method.
- Discourage adoption of bad communication habits (e.g., facial grimacing and whispering), which may call attention to disability rather than implementing adaptive ability.
- Consider having a successful laryngectomee visit the patient to demonstrate how successful speech rehabilitation can be.

☐ EVALUATION CRITERIA/DESIRED OUTCOMES

The Patient

- Successfully establishes and maintains post-op communication
- Demonstrates a positive response to speech rehabilitation regimen

NURSING DIAGNOSIS #3

Alteration in nutrition: less than body requirements related to anorexia, pre-existing difficulty in swallowing

Rationale: *It is likely that the candidate for laryngectomy had been unable to ingest a normal diet with essential nutritional needs prior to hospitalization, especially patients with a history of excessive alcohol intake/smoking, or those with a pre-op course of radiation therapy. Improved nutritional status will diminish the surgical risks. Postoperatively, a nasogastric tube may be in place for feedings (total parenteral nutrition may be considered, but is not usually ordered preoperatively).*

☐ GOAL

The patient will receive adequate intake to meet metabolic requirements.

☐ IMPLEMENTATION

- Preoperatively, assess patient's nutritional status; consider height, weight, and body frame, recent weight loss; condition of hair, skin, nails, mouth, and teeth; usual dietary pattern and favorite foods.
- Encourage full consumption of prescribed diet; arrange for soft, mechanical soft, or full liquid diet as tolerated; if indicated, arrange for frequent smaller meals rather than three standard meals; provide nutritional supplements between meals.
- Record nutritional intake; if intake is less than body requirements, contact the physician about tube feedings or total parenteral nutrition (TPN).
- Record daily weights.
- Postoperatively, continue accurate recording of intake and output and provide diet tube feeding
- Reassess nutritional status as post-op course progresses; inform physician of significant findings; initiate referral to dietician as appropriate.

☐ EVALUATION CRITERIA/DESIRED OUTCOMES

The Patient

- Maintains or gains weight
- Receives a caloric intake sufficient to meet daily requirements
- Exhibits improved appearance of skin, nails, hair, and mouth

NURSING DIAGNOSIS #4

Alteration in oral mucous membranes related to pre-op smoking, excessive alcohol intake, malnutrition, radiation therapy; surgical manipulation

Rationale: *The patient requiring a laryngectomy may have existing mouth lesions or may be at risk for developing mouth lesions. Poor oral hygiene will increase the risk of mouth lesions.*

☐ GOAL

The patient will regain/maintain integrity of oral mucous membranes.

☐ IMPLEMENTATION

- Demonstrate proper oral hygiene; assist the as needed in providing oral care before meals and at bedtime.
- Administer prescribed medications and record patient responses; know that any oral infection must be eliminated prior to surgery.
- Provide mouth care every 2 hours when patient is NPO.
- Continue oral hygiene regimen postoperatively; demonstrate and assist patient in learning how to irrigate the oral cavity with peroxide and water solution or mouthwash as ordered.

☐ EVALUATION CRITERIA/DESIRED OUTCOMES

The Patient

- Displays intact oral mucous membranes
- Demonstrates the ability to provide adequate oral hygiene to self

NURSING DIAGNOSIS #5

Ineffective airway clearance related to increased secretions secondary to tracheostomy

Rationale: *During the early post-op period the patient may be unable to clear own secretions.*

☐ GOAL

The patient will have a patent airway.

☐ IMPLEMENTATION

- Assess patient at beginning of shift and as necessary for need for suctioning; auscultate both lungs; inspect patient's color; observe respiratory rate and character; if patient is being ventilated by mechanical device, ensure that settings are as ordered and that all alarms are functioning (elevated pressure and decreased tidal volumes may indicate need for suctioning).
- Administer prophylactic antibiotics as ordered and monitor effects.
- Review *The Patient with a Tracheostomy,* page 236.

☐ EVALUATION CRITERIA/DESIRED OUTCOMES

The Patient

- Maintains patent airway with suctioning and/or coughing
- Experiences no post-op complications secondary to aspiration or pooling of secretions

NURSING DIAGNOSIS #6

Alteration in tissue perfusion: cardiopulmonary, cerebral related to carotid artery rupture

Rationale: *Carotid artery rupture may occur in those patients requiring extensive surgery, especially in those who may have had radiation therapy prior to surgery. Carotid artery rupture is a medical emergency requiring prompt recognition and initiation of treatment (e.g., ligation) to prevent hemorrhage and death.*

☐ GOAL

The patient will be monitored for early indications of severe bleeding.

☐ IMPLEMENTATION

- Carefully monitor and record post-op vital signs every 2-4 hours as ordered, reporting any significant changes.
- Gently palpate carotid pulses, one at a time, for strength and equality at least once a shift during the first 2-3 days postoperatively; record findings for future comparisons.
- Notify physician if carotid pulse is absent.
- If bleeding is detected at carotid area, remain with patient, apply pressure over the site, and call for assistance immediately.

☐ EVALUATION CRITERIA/DESIRED OUTCOMES

The Patient

- Demonstrates normal vital signs and carotid pulses
- Is free from carotid artery bleeding

NURSING DIAGNOSIS #7

Disturbance in self-concept: body image related to disfiguring surgery, the responses of others to the disfigurement

Rationale: *This diagnosis is more likely to present in the patient requiring extensive surgery, such as a radical neck disection, than in a patient with a laryngectomy. Because the individual's self-concept is integrally dependent on body image, which is internalized by interactions with others, it is possible for the patient to experience some difficulty in integrating the new body image and adapting self-concept accordingly.*

☐ GOAL

The patient will integrate the changes in physical appearance and resultant functional changes into self-concept.

☐ IMPLEMENTATION

- Assess for common reactions indicating disturbance in self-concept (e.g., refusal to look at stoma or in mirror, unwillingness to discuss changed appearance, refusal to participate in speech rehabilitation, denial of the existence of disfigurement, signs of grieving, self-neglect, withdrawal from social contact with family and friends).

- Realize that even though the patient may have expressed grief and discussed the meaning of loss preoperatively, time is still needed to adapt to the actual changes; continue to plan nursing care to allow time for the patient to ventilate feelings, concerns, and questions throughout hospitalization.
- Support/encourage positive efforts to cope/adapt.
- Maintain a positive, accepting attitude towards the patient because body image is formed through the patient's interactions with others; encourage and support visitors by allowing them the opportunity to express their concerns, feelings, and questions as well.
- Consider the normal developmental tasks (e.g., maintaining ego integrity, generativity, or establish identity) to be achieved by the patient when assessing adaptation to changed body image and when planning further interventions to resolve identified problems in adapting.
- Role play with the patient to practice expected experiences after discharge (e.g., shopping, interactions with children, returning to work setting).
- Describe clothing that will safely cover the stoma and camouflage structures removed.

☐ EVALUATION CRITERIA/DESIRED OUTCOMES

The Patient

- Displays positive attitudes towards physical self and speech rehabilitation
- Is free from signs of self-concept disturbance

NURSING DIAGNOSIS #8

Knowledge deficit regarding care of stoma and tracheostomy, modifications in daily self-care regimen, community resources

Rationale: *In order to successfully return to normal roles in the community, the patient/family must have sufficient information to provide daily stoma and tracheostomy care and to modify normal self-care activities.*

☐ GOAL

The patient/family will learn stoma and tracheostomy care and will be aware of available community resources for laryngectomees; the patient will learn how to ensure safety when providing daily self care.

☐ IMPLEMENTATION

- Instruct in stoma and tracheostomy self-care measures including daily cleaning, necessary alterations in daily activities (e.g., avoiding dust and pollen), and precautions (e.g., wearing protective scarf or clothing).
- Advise to cover stoma instead of mouth when coughing or sneezing; instruct to use handkerchief rather than tissue to avoid introducing lint into artificial airway.
- Explain precautions to take when bathing/showering to prevent inhalation of soap or excess water into the stoma (e.g., soap body up only to the chest; wash head and neck areas while standing before a mirror; shower using a handheld spray below stoma level or fashion a stoma protector by venting a plastic medicine cup and attaching ties to apply it as a protector around neck before showering).
- Inform that shaving, haircuts, and scalp shampoos create special problems as soap and hair should not enter the stoma; suggest applying petroleum jelly at the hairline to prevent dripping and wearing a towel or commercial device designed to prevent aspiration.
- Explain that swimming is generally forbidden for a person with a permanent stoma; wading or sitting in shallow water or hot tub may be permitted.
- Inform the patient/family that a person with a stoma produces about a pint or more secretions/day and thus requires 40% humidity in the air to prevent tracheitis sicca (crusting and scaling at the stoma and airway); suggest using commercial humidifiers, a pan of water on a stove or radiator, or a hot bath.
- Instruct the patient to keep the stoma covered at all times to protect it from dust, lint, insects, and sudden changes in temperature; clothing may effectively protect the stoma but the patient may wish to wear a stoma shield to protect clothing from secretions.
- Teach first aid interventions, especially giving artificial respiration to stoma rather than to nose or mouth.

- Begin instructions for self-care measures as soon as possible postoperatively (assess readiness) to promote more rapid acceptance and recovery during rehabilitative phase of treatment.
- Encourage to perform normal activities with necessary alterations (moderation in all normal activities, control of emotions, avoiding fatigue, to abstain from alcoholic beverages and smoking, to wear special identification such as Medic-Alert identification bracelet or card).
- Initiate referral to and be sure patient has name of community service agencies for rehabilitative support, educational programs, and social activities.

☐ EVALUATION CRITERIA/DESIRED OUTCOMES

The Patient/family

- Demonstrates the ability to perform home care tasks including mouth care, stoma and tracheostomy care, and modifications for bathing self
- Has received a documented referral to community service agency
- Knows how to effect a protective shield over stoma

The Patient with Meningitis and/or Brain Abscess

Definition/Discussion

Meningitis is an inflammation of the membranes of the brain and spinal cord. A brain abscess *or cerebral abscess* is a severe focal infection within the brain with a suppurative process. Encephalitis is an infection of the brain substance. Myelitis describes an inflammation or infection of the spinal cord. Overlap of these conditions is common and terms like meningo-encephalitis or encephalomyelitis may be used.

Nursing Assessment

☐ **PERTINENT HISTORY**

Past medical history for chronic illness (e.g., diabetes, alcoholism); neoplasm, sickle cell anemia, immunosuppression, splenectomy; recent respiratory infection, middle ear infection, mastoiditis, sinusitis; recent surgery, lumbar puncture, skull fracture, or head trauma; exposure to mumps, meningitis, or travel out of the country; crowded living/working conditions; ingestion of poisons/toxins/drugs; complaints of behavior changes, fever, nausea, vomiting, headache, stiff neck, photophobia, diplopia, painful ocular movement, arthralgia, sore throat, backache

☐ **PHYSICAL FINDINGS**

Altered level of consciousness (LOC), lethargy, confusion, seizures (focal, generalized), ataxia, positive Brudzinski's and Kernig's signs; nuchal rigidity, opisthotonus, nystagmus, ptosis, diminished hearing, tachycardia, dysrhythmia, elevated blood pressure; altered breathing patterns; vomiting; diarrhea, petechial rash

☐ **PSYCHOSOCIAL CONCERNS/ DEVELOPMENTAL FACTORS**

Age, sex, occupation, interaction with significant others, developmental level, behavior patterns, usual coping mechanisms, previous experience with illness and hospitalization, family roles, responsibilities, available support

☐ **PATIENT AND FAMILY KNOWLEDGE**

Level of comprehension, understanding of condition, pathophysiology, relationship to symptoms, communicability, treatment, readiness and willingness to learn

Nursing Care

☐ **LONG-TERM GOAL**

The patient will regain optimal health with minimal neurologic disability; the patient will resume former roles in home, family, and community.

NURSING DIAGNOSIS #1

a. **Alteration in tissue perfusion: cardiopulmonary** related to immobility
b. **Ineffective airway clearance** related to fatigue, weakness, altered LOC
c. **Ineffective breathing pattern** related to depressed respiratory effort
d. **Impaired gas exchange** related to depressed respiratory effort, immobility, weakened cough reflex

Rationale: *Immobility and dehydration result in pooling and thickening of respiratory secre-*

tions. Altered consciousness, depressed cough and gag reflexes predispose the patient to poor airway clearance and aspiration. Hypercapnia and hypoxia from increased intracranial pressure (ICP) result in reflex vasodilation further increasing pressure on sensitive brain tissue.

☐ GOAL

The patient will maintain adequate oxygenation.

☐ IMPLEMENTATION

- Auscultate breath sounds every 2-4 hours and report any adventitious sounds (crackles, wheezes)
- Monitor respiratory rate, pattern, patency, exchange; observe skin, nail beds, mucous membranes for cyanosis.
- Monitor arterial blood gases (ABGs) for hypoxia, chest x-rays for infiltrates.
- Ensure position change at least every 2 hours.
- Instruct to take 10 deep breaths an hour.
- Check for depressed gag reflex.
- Set up properly functioning suction equipment; suction gently to clear secretions.
- Utilize side-lying.
- Maintain patent airway utilizing suctioning, positioning, jaw thrust, head tilt.
- Administer oxygen as ordered; monitor effectiveness.
- Observe for increased confusion, restlessness; report any to physician.
- Encourage activity to tolerance as ordered (e.g., turning).
- Discourage smoking.

☐ EVALUATION CRITERIA/DESIRED OUTCOMES

The Patient

- Maintains ABGs within normal limits
- Has no adventitious breath sounds
- Is alert and oriented
- Has unlabored respirations with good air exchange

NURSING DIAGNOSIS #2

a. **Alteration in tissue perfusion: cerebral** related to inflammatory processes, increased ICP
b. **Potential for injury** related to disorientation, restlessness, seizures, unfamiliar environment
c. **Alteration in thought processes** related to changes in LOC
d. **Impaired communication: verbal** related to disorientation and confusion

Rationale: *Inflammatory processes cause tissue swelling that interferes with fluid movement within the cranium, increases ICP, and obstructs cerebral blood flow.*

☐ GOAL

The patient will maintain adequate tissue perfusion; will remain oriented with intact thought processes and communication; will be free from injury.

☐ IMPLEMENTATION

- Observe and record LOC on admission and with each patient contact (e.g., orientation to person/place/time/situation; memory, ability to attend, behavior, inappropriate response, subtle changes).
- Check neurologic status every 1-2 hours and as necessary until stable (e.g., pupil response, ability to follow commands, motor ability, hand grips, move and focus eyes, visual acuity, deep tendon reflexes, seizure activity, verbal response).
- Monitor for signs of ICP (e.g., increasing blood pressure, decreasing pulse, respiratory irregularities, restlessness, confusion, pupillary changes, focal deficits, seizures).
- Refer to *The Patient with Increased Intracranial Pressure,* page 122.
- Note any seizure activity; record affected body parts, length of seizure, and aura if any.
- Institute seizure precautions (side rails up and padded, bed in low position, oral airway at bedside, suction equipment ready, call bell within easy reach, night lighting, and rectal temperatures only).
- Administer anticonvulsants as ordered; monitor effectiveness.
- Elevate head of bed 30° if not contraindicated.
- Maintain head and neck alignment to facilitate venous return.
- Administer appropriate antibiotic therapy as ordered.

- Maintain quiet, restful environment (e.g., low lights, quiet hallway, avoid jarring the bed or unnecessary procedures).
- Minimize the number of caretakers.
- Teach patient to avoid Valsalva maneuver (e.g., straining, coughing, sneezing) and to change position slowly.
- Approach in a calm manner; be consistent, speak clearly and slowly to increase comprehension.
- Talk to patient while providing care; use therapeutic touch and listening techniques.
- Verbally orient to person/place/time/situation; provide calendar; allow clocks, radio, television, and other familiar objects, (e.g., photographs, books, hobbies); apply hearing aids and glasses.
- Use patient's name; encourage visitation by family/friends.
- Perform range-of-motion (ROM) exercises, (passive, active) as ordered; establish routines.
- Anticipate patient needs (e.g., toilet; oral care).
- Avoid restraints if possible.
- Monitor any signs/symptoms of septic shock (e.g., hypotension, elevated temperature, increasing respiratory rate, confusion, disorientation, peripheral vasoconstriction).

☐ EVALUATION CRITERIA/DESIRED OUTCOMES

The Patient

- Maintains orientation and alertness
- Is free from seizure activity
- Has vital signs within normal limits
- Is free from injury
- Verbalizes ability to rest
- Communicates needs

NURSING DIAGNOSIS #3

Fluid volume deficit related to decreased fluid intake, abnormal fluid loss

Rationale: *Hypermetabolic state of infectious processes combined with anorexia, nausea and vomiting results in increased sensible/insensible fluid losses, altering fluid and electrolyte balance. Increased ICP stimulates the anterior hypothalamus and vagus nerve, increasing secretion of hydrochloric acid and altering gastric mucosa, which potentiates ulcerative processes.*

☐ GOAL

The patient will maintain adequate fluid and electrolyte balance and blood volume.

☐ IMPLEMENTATION

- Measure vital signs every 2-4 hours.
- Monitor lab studies, specifically CBC and electrolytes.
- Test urine specific gravity every shift.
- Observe for signs of dehydration (e.g., tenting, dry mucous membranes, increasing pulse, increasing serum sodium, weight loss, increasing urine specific gravity, fluid loss greater than fluid intake).
- Record intake and output every shift and as necessary; note and report imbalances.
- Weigh on admission and daily; monitor for changes greater than 1-2 lb.
- Encourage oral fluids as ordered (e.g., water, soda, Popsicles, Jell-O).
- Serve fluids frequently in small amounts to minimize gastric distension.
- Maintain temperature less than 101°F (38.3°C); institute cooling measures as needed (e.g., light clothing and covers, tepid sponge baths, antipyretics as ordered).
- Administer IV therapy as ordered; record type and amount infused; refer to Table 1, *Common Fluid and Electrolyte Imbalances,* page 14.
- Maintain and monitor central venous pressure as ordered; refer to *The Patient Requiring Hemodynamic Monitoring,* page 117.
- Observe for signs of gastrointestinal bleeding (e.g., abdominal tenderness, pain, hematemesis, melena stools, decreased hematocrit) and report.
- Hematest urine, stool, emesis periodically and as necessary.
- Administer antacids, cimetidine (Tagamet) as ordered.
- Inspect for signs of fluid retention indicating syndrome of inappropriate antidiuretic hormone secretion (SIADH) (e.g., decreasing urine output, dependent edema, crackles on auscultation, increasing urine specific gravity, decreasing serum sodium concentration).

☐ EVALUATION CRITERIA/DESIRED OUTCOMES

The Patient

- Has vital signs within normal limits
- Maintains serum electrolytes values within normal limits

- Has moist skin with good turgor
- Maintains temperature below 101°F
- Excretes at least 30 cc urine/hour
- Maintains weight within 1-2 lb of normal
- Remains alert and oriented

NURSING DIAGNOSIS #4

Alteration in nutrition: less than body requirements related to anorexia, fatigue, nausea and vomiting

Rationale: *Infectious and healing processes increase metabolic and nutritional needs. Increased intracranial pressure stimulates nausea and vomiting.*

☐ GOAL

The patient will maintain an adequate nutritional level with minimal nausea and vomiting.

☐ IMPLEMENTATION

- Monitor changes in LOC which indicate increasing ICP (e.g., increased blood pressure, decreased pulse, widened pulse pressure).
- Measure and record quantity and characteristics of emesis.
- Interview patient/family for food preferences.
- Provide diet as ordered and tolerated.
- Serve small, frequent, nutritious meals.
- Instruct to eat slowly and to avoid lying flat for 1 hour after meals.
- Allow family-prepared foods when therapeutic.
- Keep accurate record of nutrients consumed.
- Weigh patient on admission and daily.
- Administer antiemetics one-half hour before meals; evaluate effect.
- Provide pleasant environment for eating (e.g., eliminate odors, unpleasant sights, and fresh air).
- Arrange for family member to eat with patient if appropriate.
- Limit fluid intake 1 hour before, during, and 1 hour after meals to minimize distension.
- Provide good oral care.
- Administer tube feedings as ordered for severe nausea/vomiting.

☐ EVALUATION CRITERIA/DESIRED OUTCOMES

The Patient

- Consumes 75% of food served
- Participates in food selection
- Maintains weight within 1-2 lb of normal

NURSING DIAGNOSIS #5

Impairment of skin integrity related to immobility, diaphoresis, neurologic deficits

Rationale: *Bedrest/immobility combined with poor nutritional intake and moist skin can result in breakdown from local irritation and ischemic changes over pressure-sensitive areas.*

☐ GOAL

The patient will maintain an intact skin.

☐ IMPLEMENTATION

- Keep skin clean and dry.
- Change soiled or moist linen.
- Encourage active/passive ROM exercises as ordered (may increase ICP).
- Instruct to turn frequently; remind or help with turning at least every 2 hours.
- Use light covers/clothing to avoid excess moisture.
- Maintain fluid/nutritional balance.
- Observe skin for signs of pressure injury (e.g., erythema, blanching, maceration, breakdown).
- Inspect bony prominences for signs of injury (e.g., occiput, heels, elbows, trochantors, scapula).
- Massage skin, especially bony prominences, at least twice/shift; use sheepskin, heel pads, etc., as needed.

☐ EVALUATION CRITERIA/DESIRED OUTCOMES

The Patient

- Retains intact skin
- Changes position frequently
- Complies with ROM guidelines

NURSING DIAGNOSIS #6

Alteration in comfort: pain related to bedrest, meningeal irritation

Rationale: *Meningeal irritation and increased ICP result in symptoms such as headache, photophobia, neck and back pain. Bedrest may aggravate existing back pain and cause muscle spasm/soreness.*

☐ GOAL

The patient will attain an adequate level of comfort.

☐ IMPLEMENTATION

- Assess level of discomfort using a 0-10 point self-rating scale for an objective measure of the pain.
- Evaluate indicators of pain (e.g., facial expression, movement), location, duration, radiation, intensity, precipitating/relieving factors.
- Implement comfort measures (e.g., dim lighting, gradual position changes, guided imagery, repositioning, distraction, pillows).
- Massage sore muscles, back gently with lotion.
- Administer analgesics as ordered; evaluate one-half hour later for effect.
- Teach patient to avoid movements that increase ICP (e.g., straining, coughing, sneezing, blowing nose).
- Apply cool moist compresses to forehead; minimize noise.
- Limit visitors to one at a time.
- Refer to *The Patient Experiencing Pain,* page 180.

☐ EVALUATION CRITERIA/DESIRED OUTCOMES

The Patient

- Verbalizes decreased pain
- Exhibits ability to rest
- Participates in activities as tolerated

NURSING DIAGNOSIS #7

a. **Ineffective individual coping** related to required adaptation to hospital environment
b. **Disturbance in self-concept: body image, role performance** related to disease condition
c. **Alteration in family process** related to interrupted roles, separation from significant others
d. **Anxiety** related to actual/potential changes in body functioning
e. **Fear** related to medical/nursing intervention, illness, risk of death
f. **Grieving** related to actual, potential, or perceived loss of body functioning

Rationale: *Illness produces changes in the body and its functioning. Separation from familiar surroundings and other significant individuals causes stress. Hospitalization disrupts normal routines and practices, and roles change. Fear and anxiety are expressed about the known and unknown. Incorporating these changes into the individual's self-concept, body image, and daily functioning promotes adaptation.*

☐ GOAL

The patient/family will demonstrate positive adaptation.

☐ IMPLEMENTATION

- Orient to hospital routines and unit.
- Explain all procedures and rationale.
- Describe the illness and relate symptoms to disease state.
- Answer questions honestly and completely; reinforce previous teaching.
- Institute listening techniques (e.g., open-ended questions; unrushed, quiet atmosphere).
- Allow verbalization of thoughts/fears.
- Share indications of improvement with patient/family.
- Involve patient/family in care and decision making as able.
- Observe present coping mechanisms; support/guide the patient/family to new ones as needed.
- Reinforce independence.
- Support patient/family in adaptive process (e.g., allow touch, overnight visitation, privacy, phone calls).
- As patient recovers, encourage diversional activities (e.g., hobbies, reading, radio).

☐ EVALUATION CRITERIA/DESIRED OUTCOMES

The Patient/family

- Participates in care and decision making
- Interacts appropriately with family/staff
- Talks of illness, its impact, and potential outcome

NURSING DIAGNOSIS #8

Knowledge deficit regarding illness, hospitalization, treatment

Rationale: *Patients/families harbor misinformation and misconceptions about body function, illness, and hospitalization. Understanding of the process, illness, and symptomology promotes compliance and adaptive behaviors.*

☐ GOAL

The patient/family will demonstrate adequate knowledge regarding the illness, hospitalization, and follow-up care.

☐ IMPLEMENTATION

- Determine understanding of illness and therapeutic interventions.
- Encourage questions.
- Discuss disease condition, symptoms, effect on body, and treatment.
- Explain all procedures/treatments and rationale.
- Involve family in teaching sessions.
- Use appropriate teaching techniques (e.g., limit session time, use terms easily understood, supply examples the patient/family can relate to, use reinforcement techniques).
- Discuss signs/symptoms of complications (e.g., headache, paresis/paralysis, seizures, hearing loss).
- Instruct patient/family about communicability (e.g., airborne, droplet, handwashing/secretion precautions).

☐ EVALUATION CRITERIA/DESIRED OUTCOMES

The Patient

- Relates information about illness and care
- Verbalizes complications requiring follow-up
- Relates specific information regarding home care and follow-up

The Patient with a Myocardial Infarction:

Definition/Discussion

A myocardial infarction (MI) is an area of necrotic tissue in the heart muscle caused by an inadequate blood supply from the coronary arteries or an imbalance in myocardial oxygen demand and coronary artery supply. The first part of this guide will provide outlines for care during the period immediately after the MI through transfer to nonacute status.

Once the patient has passed the acute phase of treatment for an MI and life-threatening complications have been avoided or resolved, the focus of medical and nursing management changes to rehabilitative efforts. The patient is now ready for gradually increasing activity while continuing to be monitored continuously, either by cable or telemetry devices. Prescribed modifications of life-style and resultant changes in role functioning/family dynamics require assessment, cooperative planning, intervention, and evaluation to prepare the patient for discharge with a health maintenance regimen that s/he will follow willingly.

Nursing Assessment

☐ **PERTINENT HISTORY**

Previous MI, cardiovascular disease or identified risk factors (e.g., elevated low-density lipoproteins; decreased high-density lipoproteins; elevated triglycerides; diet rich in calories, fats, cholesterol, refined sugars, salts; hypertension; cigarette smoking; abnormal glucose tolerance; sedentary living; familial history)

☐ **PHYSICAL FINDINGS**

Pain: sudden, constant, substernal, crushing, unrelieved by rest or sublingual nitroglycerin, frequently radiating down left arm, both arms, or up to neck; diaphoresis; jugular venous distension; peripheral edema; increased respiratory rate; normal heart sounds (S1 and S2) and possible rubs, murmurs, gallops (S3 and S4); vesicular, bronchovesicular, bronchial breath sounds with possible adventitious sounds (crackles, rhonchi, wheezes); chest wall pulsations; dysrhythmias, presence of CPK-MB cardiac isoenzyme; results of chest x-ray, cardiac catheterization; ECG, echocardiography; radioisotope studies

☐ **PSYCHOSOCIAL CONCERNS/ DEVELOPMENTAL FACTORS**

Age, sex, personality type, psychosocial stress; fear of death, disability; coping style, life changes, resource and support systems, educational level, occupation

☐ **PATIENT AND FAMILY KNOWLEDGE**

Disease process, risk factors, treatment; acceptance of treatment; level of knowledge, readiness and willingness to learn

Nursing Care

☐ **LONG-TERM GOAL**

The patient will maintain life functions and initiate cardiac healing; the patient will be free from complications and will seek convalescent and rehabilitation care.

NURSING DIAGNOSIS #1

a. **Alteration in cardiac output: decreased** related to impaired contractility, dysrhythmias
b. **Altered tissue perfusion: cardiopulmonary, cerebral, renal, and peripheral** related to decreased cardiac output

Rationale: *Myocardial muscle necrosis results in impaired cardiac contractility and ejection of blood. The hemodynamic consequences range from minimal to life-threatening decreases in cardiac output and blood pressure resulting in congestive heart failure, cardiogenic shock, and cardiac arrest. Injured and ischemic zones around the area of necrosis are electrically unstable and contribute to dysrhythmias, which decrease output and may cause cardiac arrest.*

Inadequate blood flow through the microcirculation is a direct result of decreased cardiac output. The outcome of hypoperfusion is cellular hypoxia (because of decreased perfusion through the lungs) and eventual cell death. The heart, brain, and kidneys, because of their high metabolic needs, suffer the most serious side effects. Extremities, although demonstrating clinical symptoms of hypoperfusion, will tolerate the effects of hypoxia longer.

☐ GOAL

The patient will maintain cardiac output adequate to perfuse heart, lungs, brain, kidneys, and extremities.

☐ IMPLEMENTATION

- Assess vital signs every 1-4 hours; measure hemodynamic pressures and cardiac output as ordered.
- Monitor for signs and symptoms of decreased cardiopulmonary perfusion (e.g., angina, dysrhythmias, tachycardia, tachypnea, hypotension, narrowing pulse pressure, decreased cardiac output).
- Monitor cardiac rhythm continuously; record a rhythm strip for the chart every 4 hours or more frequently if irregular; note premature beats, particularly ventricular.
- Palpate peripheral pulse to assess perfusion of premature beats; watch for signs and symptoms of decreased cardiac output (e.g., dizziness, fainting, pallor, hypotension) during dysrhythmias; document patient responses.
- Administer antidysrhythmics according to physician-prescribed protocol; monitor for expected actions; notify physician if ineffective or if signs of toxicity occur.
- Administer vasodilators and inotropic drugs as ordered: evaluate effectiveness according to improvement in perfusion; administer the smallest amount of medication required to produce desired effects without toxicity.
- Monitor for signs and symptoms indicating decreased cerebral perfusion (e.g, restlessness, confusion, somnolence, psychosis).
- Monitor for signs and symptoms indicating decreased renal perfusion (e.g., urine output less than 30 cc/hour, decreased specific gravity, lack of response to diuretics, elevated BUN or creatinine clearance, peripheral edema, pulmonary crackles).
- Monitor for signs and symptoms indicating decreased peripheral perfusion (e.g., cool, pale, moist, or clammy skin; cyanosis; absent or weak peripheral pulses; peripheral or dependent edema).
- Eliminate or reduce pressure points: change position every hour; discourage leg crossing; use sheepskins, elbow and heel protectors, egg-crate mattress as necessary; encourage patient to wiggle hands and feet every hour; remove antiembolus stockings for 15 minutes every 8 hours; inspect skin underneath before replacing; do not allow pillows behind knees or use knee gatch.
- Inform physician of patient's responses to medical regimen and/or signs and symptoms of complications.

☐ EVALUATION CRITERIA/DESIRED OUTCOMES

The Patient

- Has no complaints of chest pain
- Displays normal sinus cardiac rhythm with strong peripheral pulses
- Is oriented to time, place, person, self
- Has urine output greater than 30 cc/hour with BUN, creatinine within normal limits
- Has warm, dry skin with no pallor/cyanosis

NURSING DIAGNOSIS #2

Impaired gas exchange related to decreased cardiac output, fluid volume excess

Rationale: *When cardiac output is diminished, left ventricular end diastolic volume (LVEDV) rises. Because the injured left ventricle is less compliant, left ventricular end diastolic pressure (LVEDP) also rises. LVEDP is transmitted first to pulmonary vasculature and eventually*

to peripheral vasculature. Elevated vascular pressures result in pulmonary and peripheral edema. Pulmonary artery catheterization (e.g., with Swan-Ganz catheter) is used to guide the medical management of decreased cardiac output. The nurse is responsible for monitoring hemodynamic readings and informing the physician of significant findings.

Decreased cardiac output also triggers compensatory mechanisms including vasoconstriction, antidiuretic hormone release, and aldosterone production. Retention of salt and water and increased vascular pressure contribute to peripheral pulmonary edema, which impairs gas transport from the alveoli to the blood by increasing the distance for diffusion.

☐ GOAL

The patient will maintain gas exchange in lungs adequate to promote oxygenation of all body tissues.

☐ IMPLEMENTATION

- Auscultate breath sounds and monitor respiratory rate, depth, pattern, and effort every 1-4 hours.
- Assess for signs and symptoms of pulmonary edema (e.g., dyspnea related to exertion, paroxysmal nocturnal dyspnea, orthopnea; cough; blood-tinged or frothy sputum; tachypnea; diminished breath sounds; adventitious breath sounds, crackles; elevated pulmonary artery wedge pressure); measure hemodynamic pressures as ordered.
- Elevate head of bed; limit activities during periods of dyspnea; assist with changes of position as needed.
- Assess for signs and symptoms of hypoxia (e.g., changes in blood gases [i.e., decreased oxygen content/saturation and partial pressures]); tachycardia; rising systolic blood pressure; irritability, agitation, headache, confusion, angina; cyanosis of tongue and mucous membranes); modify environment to decrease oxygen needs (e.g., maintain bedrest); medicate for pain if assessed to be causative factor (see Nursing Diagnosis #3).
- Administer oxygen by nasal cannula (usually 4-6 liters/minute unless patient has chronic hypoxia, then 2 liters/minute) as ordered; maintain while on commode or in chair; contact physician if hypoxic symptoms persist.
- Administer agents that increase cardiac contractility, decrease preload (LVEDV) and afterload (peripheral vasoconstriction) as ordered; monitor effectiveness; be alert to possible side effects of medications; report patient responses to physician.
- Avoid fluid volume excess by using infusion pumps for each IV; mix IV drug concentrations to provide minimal flow rates; check for any IV drug incompatibilities; titrate dosage to effect desired.
- Give diuretics as ordered to decrease intravascular volume; report side effects (e.g., hyponatremia, hypokalemia, postural hypotension, muscle cramps, metabolic alkalosis, digitalis toxicity in presence of hypokalemia) to physician.
- Measure all sources of intake and output accurately; monitor daily weights.
- Maintain prescribed oral fluid restrictions.
- Ensure sodium-restricted diet if ordered; encourage foods high in potassium if not contraindicated.

☐ EVALUATION CRITERIA/DESIRED OUTCOMES

The Patient

- Regains normal respirations, vesicular breath sounds, is free from pulmonary crackles
- Has blood gases within normal limits for patient
- Has fluid output equal to or exceeding intake with no dependent edema or weight gain

NURSING DIAGNOSIS #3

a. **Activity intolerance** related to decreased cardiac output, pain
b. **Alteration in comfort: pain** related to myocardial ischemia

Rationale: *Muscles need nutrition and oxygenation from blood flow. When cardiac output is limited, oxygen supply to muscles and energy for muscle contraction are reduced. Pulmonary edema impairs gas exchange and the disabled lungs cannot supply the increasing oxygen demands. Dyspnea on exertion, which limits activity, is a result of the inability of the lung and heart to meet the increased demands of activity.*

Physical exercise also increases myocardial oxygen consumption at a time when coronary blood flow is reduced. This imbalance between supply and demand results in anginal pain or dysrhythmias. Pain, or the fear of pain, limits the patient's activity level. Dysrhythmias further decrease cardiac output and activity tolerance.

Angina is a manifestation of myocardial ischemia, which occurs whenever the metabolic demand on the myocardium disrupts the normal balance between myocardial oxygen supply and demand. Numerous factors influence myocardial oxygen consumption, but the most important are heart rate, ventricular wall tension, and myocardial contractility. Wall tension is related to blood pressure and chamber size. Myocardial oxygen demand rises with exercise, emotional stress, hypertension, tachycardia, and left ventricular outflow obstruction.

☐ GOAL

The patient will be free from pain while maintaining prescribed activity level.

☐ IMPLEMENTATION

- Organize nursing care and activities to provide periods of uninterrupted sleep and rest; minimize activity before and after treatments or meals; postpone activity during periods of pain.
- Provide physical assistance with repositioning, getting up to commode when required.
- Assess response to activity: note dysrhythmias, ST elevation, fatigue, dyspnea, pallor, cyanosis, confusion, dizziness, or angina; compare resting vital signs to vital signs immediately after and 3 minutes after activity.
- Assess, reduce or eliminate factors that influence activity tolerance (e.g., cardiac contractility [pulse, blood pressure], dyspnea secondary to pulmonary edema, hypoxemia, angina, pain medications, dysrhythmias, depression, sleep pattern disturbance).
- Teach methods to reduce precipitating factors
  - participate in cardiac rehabilitation program
  - reduce physical activity during stress
  - use nitroglycerin prophylactically
  - utilize stress-reduction techniques
  - adhere to diet, medication, exercise therapy
- Instruct patient to evaluate own response to activity: how and where to take pulse (before, immediately after, and 3 minutes after activity); to report (to nurse while hospitalized, to physician after discharge) pulse decreases with activity, pulse increases over 120, pulses that do not return to within 6 beats of resting pulse after 3 minutes; difficulty in breathing, chest pain, palpitations.
- Assess, document, and report patient's description of pain using a 0-10 point self-rating scale to obtain an objective measure of the pain; include onset, location and radiation, duration, characteristics, precipitating and aggravating/relieving factors, associated symptoms.
- Administer narcotic or analgesic medications as ordered and evaluate effectiveness; monitor for untoward effects.
- Monitor during exercise for chest pain, dyspnea, pallor or cyanosis, dysrhythmias, ST-T wave changes, excessive fatigue, dizziness, syncope, or cold sweat; stop activity if any occur; if symptoms do not subside with rest and prescribed medications, contact physician.
- Identify and reduce any factors that precipitate or aggravate pain (e.g., tachycardia, hypertension, diastolic hypotension, emotional stress, hypoxemia, exercise).
- Instruct regarding recognition of signs and symptoms of angina, medication treatment protocol for chest pain, when to call physician.
- Assess, document, and report to physician patient's ECG response to pain (e.g., ST segment depression; T wave; S3, S4 gallop; pulmonary crackles; dysrhythmias).
- Refer to *The Patient Experiencing Pain,* page 180.
- Assess after exercise for insomnia, excessive excitement, weakness, fatigue, muscle cramps, nausea/vomiting; work with patient to plan slightly decreased activity during next scheduled exercise period; reevaluate/modify plan as needed, working towards gradual increase in tolerance of activity
- Identify precipitating factors of activity intolerance during cold weather, after large meal, anger, grief, sexual intercourse; suggest strategies for modification.

- Teach energy conservation
  - encourage rest periods before and after exercise
  - avoid exercise following meals
  - sit rather than stand when performing activities of daily living
  - avoid smoking, alcohol, and caffeine before or after activity
- Avoid isometric exercise and Valsalva maneuver.
- Encourage advancement and adherence to a long-term exercise program; involve family in exercise program planning; provide information about existing community programs.

☐ EVALUATION CRITERIA/DESIRED OUTCOMES

The Patient

- Tolerates increasing activity as evidenced by
  - exercise heart rate less than 20 beats/minute over resting heart rate
  - pulse 3 minutes after exercise within 6 beats of resting pulse
  - systolic blood pressure increase less than 40 mm Hg and diastolic blood pressure increase less than 20 mm Hg after activity
  - regular cardiac rhythm without dysrhythmia or ST elevation
- Verbalizes absence of chest pain, discomfort, excessive fatigue, dyspnea, dizziness
- Describes at least 2 ways to conserve own energy
- States at least 4 precipitating factors of chest pain and ways to reduce them

NURSING DIAGNOSIS #4

a. **Fear** related to actual or perceived threat to life

b. **Anxiety** related to uncertainty of physical condition, possible effects of illness, unfamiliar environment

Rationale: *MI is a life-threatening disease. Emergency transportation, admission to CCU, and the multitude of monitoring devices, diagnostic procedures, and ongoing assessments reinforce the fears and anxieties. While these may be appropriate feelings, both fear and anxiety activate the autonomic nervous system causing additional stress to the already damaged myocardium. Family members' fears and anxieties can further increase the patient's emotional distress. Therefore, nursing measures to decrease fear and allay anxieties should be directed toward both patient and family.*

☐ GOAL

The patient/family will express fears/anxieties regarding the patient's MI, prognosis, treatment, and effects on life-style/family living; will use effective coping mechanisms; will relate decreased fear/anxiety.

☐ IMPLEMENTATION

- Provide brief explanations of admission and subsequent procedures/CCU routines; emphasize that frequent assessments by staff are part of the preventive purpose of the unit and do not indicate a deteriorating condition; indicate special training staff nurses have received as a means of instilling confidence.
- Allow patient some control over environment, personal care, visitors; decrease excess stimuli (e.g., avoid use of audio alarms unless required for safety); observe effect of visitors on patient and monitor visiting time accordingly.
- Encourage expression of feelings; listen attentively, acknowledging the validity of the concerns expressed; ask to recall past crises of this nature; suggest using similar coping strategies; offer to contact clergyman if patient/family desires; initiate referral to social services, if available.
- Reinforce/clarify physician's explanations (recall that attention span is decreased during severe stress); answer questions as best you can; if you do not know the answer, find someone who does.
- Remain with patient/family during periods of fear; use touch as tolerated to convey acceptance/support.
- Refer to *The Patient Experiencing Anxiety,* page 250.

☐ EVALUATION CRITERIA/DESIRED OUTCOMES

The Patient/family

- Identifies concerns and asks specific questions in order to problem solve
- Displays no physical cues of anxiety/fear
- Verbalizes feelings of decreased anxiety/fear

NURSING DIAGNOSIS #5

Alteration in bowel elimination: constipation related to decreased physical activity

Rationale: *Activity influences bowel elimination by stimulating peristalsis. The cardiac patient's reduced activity can result in constipation. With MI there is impaired pulmonary gas exchange and delivery of oxygenated blood to vital organs including the bowel, which loses normal peristaltic activity. Side effects of some medications used to treat infarction and its complications may also contribute to constipation. Changes of life-style demanded by hospitalization affect the elimination pattern of the patient. Diet restrictions, low-roughage foods, fluid restrictions, medications, and the disruption of normal elimination routine all contribute to the problem of constipation.*

☐ GOAL

The patient will demonstrate improved bowel elimination.

☐ IMPLEMENTATION

- Assess abdomen every 4-8 hours for distension, peristaltic waves, flatulence, bowel sounds; report significant findings/changes from baseline to physician.
- Establish regular bowel routine; provide privacy, close door, draw curtains; provide deodorizer; encourage rest before and after attempts to defecate to conserve energy.
- Tell to exhale during straining to avoid Valsalva maneuver; during defecation
  - assess for indications of vagal stimulation (e.g., bradycardia, dysrhythmias, dizziness)
  - assess for effects of increased myocardial oxygen consumption (e.g., angina, tachypnea, tachycardia)
  - intervene to relieve symptoms and to prevent possible life-threatening complications
- Promote high-bulk foods (e.g., cooked fruit, vegetables, fruit juices) and adequate fluid intake within restrictions; encourage to choose menu.
- Administer stool softeners PRN at a time of day compatible with patient's normal bowel routine.

☐ EVALUATION CRITERIA/DESIRED OUTCOMES

The Patient

- Passes soft, brown, formed stool daily or every other day
- Maintains regular cardiac rhythm, eupneic respirations, absence of angina during defecation
- Is free from abdominal discomfort

NURSING DIAGNOSIS #6

Sleep pattern disturbance related to pain, hospital environment

Rationale: *Illness and hospitalization have a great impact on the sleep cycle of the adult patient. Unfamiliar surroundings, noise, lights, closed-circuit observation, and interruptions for nursing care all make sleep difficult. The patient's normal presleep routine (familiar sleep clothes, personal hygiene habits, closing drapes and lights) is altered as is the normal sleep-wake cycle (instead of sleeping in large blocks of time, a patient sleeps at shorter intervals throughout the day). Pain, pain medication, loneliness, fear, and anxiety are additional contributors to sleep pattern disturbances.*

Sleep is necessary in the restructuring of neurophysiologic data so that new data can be integrated into the patient's character. Illness and hospitalization increase the the amount of incoming sensory data that need to be integrated, yet decrease necessary sleep time to integrate those data. Adaptability to change is diminished at a time when change is greatest.

☐ GOAL

The patient will receive adequate quantity and quality of sleep.

☐ IMPLEMENTATION

- Identify patient's normal presleep and sleep routines and adapt to hospital environment as you can.
- Assess presence of factors that contribute to sleep pattern disturbance (e.g., orthopnea,

paroxysmal nocturnal dyspnea, urinary frequency due to diuretic therapy, pain, fear, anxiety, loneliness, noise, lights, interruptions, medications)

- Initiate measures to modify causative factors (e.g., position for comfort with head of bed elevated; administer diuretic early in day; medicate for pain PRN; remain with patient).
- Reduce or eliminate environmental distractions (e.g., close drapes and turn out lights at night, reduce room alarms when safe to do so).
- Provide evening care (e.g., bedpan, back rub, mouth care, bath, fresh sheets, sufficient blankets and pillows, adequate room temperature).
- Organize nursing care to provide the fewest interruptions during sleep; rely on monitoring equipment for vital signs when possible.
- Administer prescribed sleep medication; if ineffective in combination with other interventions suggested, contact physician for possible additional order.

☐ EVALUATION CRITERIA/DESIRED OUTCOMES

The Patient

- Verbalizes feelings of rest upon awakening
- Relates feelings of a good night's sleep

NURSING DIAGNOSIS #7

Anxiety related to real or perceived restrictions on life-style

Rationale: *The patient in the convalescent phase of MI is asked to make many changes in life-style. The patient may view these changes as restrictions and be unsure of how/whether to comply and what effect they will have on the quality of life after discharge.*

☐ GOAL

The patient will reduce anxiety to at least a moderate level; will use effective coping mechanisms to incorporate life-style changes.

☐ IMPLEMENTATION

- Assess manifestations, level of anxiety, and coping patterns.
- Help to express concerns (e.g., "Many people in your situation are worried about discharge. What are your thoughts about going home?").
- Encourage to ask questions; answer them, but do not overwhelm with too much information at any one time.
- Emphasize positive aspects of changes, presenting realistic alternatives.
- Work with patient to plan rehabilitation program and to discuss the process and potential results with other cardiac rehabilitation patients.

☐ EVALUATION CRITERIA/DESIRED OUTCOMES

The Patient

- Maintains anxiety at a mild to moderate level
- Identifies benefits of cardiac rehabilitation program
- Verbalizes realistic methods of incorporating changes into life-style

NURSING DIAGNOSIS #8

Ineffective individual coping related to unresolved grief over actual or perceived loss of physical stamina

Rationale: *The patient in the convalescent phase of MI may be unable to make decisions regarding care because of active involvement in the grieving process. When the patient begins to put the losses into perspective and identifies both the positive and negative qualities of the loss, s/he may begin to participate in decision making but may still experience emotions of denial, anger, and depression. The stages of grief are not universal for all patients; one can alternate between stages many times before full resolution, acceptance, and problem solving is achieved. Until such time, unresolved feelings may interfere with rehabilitation as efforts at patient teaching may be unsuccessful.*

☐ GOAL

The patient will progress to resolution of grief; will participate in decision making for the future.

☐ IMPLEMENTATION

- Identify stage of grief and intervene accordingly; refer to *The Patient Experiencing Grief and Loss*, page 272.
- Assess contributing factors to grief (e.g., culture; social, economic status; prognosis of disease; current stage of health progress; degree of resolution in acute phase; support from family; locus of control over health progress; dependency, hopelessness, helplessness).
- Encourage to identify own strengths and support systems; ask to recall similar past events and identify previously effective coping strategies; explore ways of adapting previous strategies to current situation.
- Promote resolution of grieving process by assisting to gain control of own health (e.g., include in planning daily schedule; encourage to participate in decision making to problem solving regarding necessary changes in lifestyle).
- Answer questions about specific facets of rehabilitation regimen; proceed with predischarge teaching when you discern readiness to learn.

☐ EVALUATION CRITERIA/DESIRED OUTCOMES

The Patient

- Verbalizes feelings, asks questions about physical limitations
- Develops a plan for modifying lifestyle to adjust to physical limitations

NURSING DIAGNOSIS #9

Alteration in health maintenance related to lack of knowledge, denial of threat to health

Rationale: *MI is a result of a chronic atherosclerotic process. Because it is a chronic disease the patient must work to maintain health and achieve a higher level of wellness. Without knowledge of the changes required and an acceptance of their affect on personal health, the patient cannot incorporate favorable lifestyle changes.*

☐ GOAL

The patient will be restored to and maintain optimal physiologic, psychologic, social, vocational, and recreational status.

☐ IMPLEMENTATION

- Assess factors that contribute to alteration in health maintenance (e.g., cultural beliefs; locus of control, motivation; education; knowledge of disease and preventive behavior; social, economic status; religious beliefs; accessibility to health care services; degree of family support; alteration in self-image; depression; denial); modify interventions according to specific assessment.
- Establish a therapeutic relationship with patient/family so that health teaching is facilitated; answer any questions/concerns (e.g., community agencies, self-help programs).
- Teach to reduce risk factors of hyperlipidemia, obesity, diabetes, and hypertension by modifying diet
  - encourage verbalization of feelings about dietary restrictions
  - discuss effect of diet on health status
  - identify restricted foods
  - reinforce instructions of dietician
  - assist in menu planning and adapting diet restrictions to home menu
  - support any efforts to accept and work with diet
  - provide written guidelines for prescribed diet
- Assist to decrease stress
  - identify stressors and usual coping style
  - explain effects of stress on cardiovascular system
  - discuss methods of stress reduction; ask patient to identify those that can be incorporated into life-style
  - provide opportunity for practicing stress-reduction techniques
- Discuss effects of smoking on cardiovascular system and methods of smoking control; refer to available community programs.
- Work with patient to incorporate exercise into life-style
  - discuss relationship of activity and healing process
  - define purpose and beneficial results of hospital exercise program

☐ EVALUATION CRITERIA/DESIRED OUTCOMES

The Patient

- Plans menus that incorporate diet restrictions
- Plans and initiates home exercise program
- Identifies at least 2 stress-provoking situations and at least 1 option for coping with them

- Stops smoking or reduces number of cigarettes smoked daily

NURSING DIAGNOSIS #10

Knowledge deficit regarding cardiac rehabilitation regimen

Rationale: *Interventions in the convalescent/rehabilitative phase of treatment are new to the patient. The patient may have had some exposure to the information from public media or from friends and relatives. Knowledge must be clarified so that misconceptions and noncompliance do not occur.*

☐ GOAL

The patient will demonstrate adequate knowledge for health maintenance during the convalescent phase of treatment.

☐ IMPLEMENTATION

- Assess learning needs and readiness to learn; review pertinent history and psychosocial/developmental assessment for personal factors that influence learning (e.g., effect of illness on concentration, activity tolerance, age, intelligence/education, level of anxiety, denial, past experience or knowledge, locus of control, support systems, cultural background); plan individualized teaching program.
- Teach patient/family as needed
  - normal heart anatomy and function
  - coronary artery disease process
  - control of modifiable risk factors and subsequent benefits
  - sexual activity
  - medications (name, dosage, frequency, purpose or action, side effects)
  - provide specific instructions for hospital-based cardiac rehabilitation exercise program if ordered
  - develop plan for home exercise program; practice specific exercises while in hospital
  - give patient a written list of prescribed exercises
- Provide written guidelines for administration of medications.
- Encourage questions; repeat information as needed; ask for feedback to evaluate understanding.
- Discuss discharge plan including follow-up examinations, signs and symptoms to be reported to physician, procedure for handling emergency situations (e.g., pain unrelieved by nitroglycerin, palpitations, dizziness), cardiopulmonary resusitation training for family, available community resources.
- Evaluate patient's potential compliance with treatment plan.

☐ EVALUATION CRITERIA/DESIRED OUTCOMES

The patient/family

- Describes MI and healing process
- Identifies risk factors of coronary artery disease
- Describes medication regimen
- Identifies signs and symptoms to report to physician
- Verbalizes emergency protocol
- Is aware of available community resources

The Patient Undergoing a Nephrectomy

Definition/Discussion

A nephrectomy is the surgical removal of a kidney due to tumor (usually unilateral and malignant), irreparable damage, loss of function following infection or hydronephrosis, or for kidney donation. Partial nephrectomy is removal of a portion of a diseased kidney.

Nursing Assessment

☐ **PERTINENT HISTORY**

Renal history, urinary tract problems; hypertension, nephrosis, chronic nephritis, cancer, kidney stones; if kidney donor, note relationship to recipient

☐ **PHYSICAL FINDINGS**

Flank tenderness or pain, hematuria, CBC (may have anemia or require replacement of surgical blood loss), kidney function tests, chest x-ray

☐ **PSYCHOSOCIAL CONCERNS/ DEVELOPMENTAL FACTORS**

Family support system; meaning of kidney loss; relationship of kidney donor with recipient; feelings and concerns about planned post-op course

☐ **PATIENT AND FAMILY KNOWLEDGE**

Post-op fluid balance and renal function; measures to promote/maintain adequate kidney function

Nursing Care

☐ **LONG-TERM GOAL**

The patient will recover from the nephrectomy free from complications; the patient will be able to state plans for follow-up care.

NURSING DIAGNOSIS #1

Alteration in tissue perfusion: peripheral related to volume depletion postsurgery

Rationale: *The kidney is a very vascular organ. Excess surgical fluid loss may result in reduced blood volume leading to decreased cardiac output and shock. Decreased arterial supply to lower extremities may be evident after clamping of large vessels during surgery.*

☐ **GOAL**

The patient will maintain/regain adequate blood volume and peripheral tissue perfusion.

☐ **IMPLEMENTATION**

- Assess patient for signs of bleeding at surgical site.
- Monitor for changes in level of consciousness (LOC).
- Measure urinary output every 2 hours or as needed.
- Assess for indications of impending shock (e.g., excessive thirst, restlessness, disorientation, increased pulse, decreased blood pressure, narrowing pulse pressure, decreased urinary output).
- Monitor laboratory results for decreased hemoglobin, increased clotting time.
- Check peripheral pulses every 2-4 hours.
- Administer IV fluids and blood components as ordered, following hospital protocols; refer to Table 2, *Blood and Blood-Components*, page 17.

☐ **EVALUATION CRITERIA/DESIRED OUTCOMES**

The Patient

- Has hemoglobin within normal limits

- Excretes a normal urinary output
- Is free from signs of impaired circulation

NURSING DIAGNOSIS #2

Alteration in comfort: pain related to surgical incision, abdominal distension

Rationale: *In addition to expected general post-op pain, the patient may experience a "colicky" type of pain related to passage of clots down the ureter. Abdominal distension and paralytic ileus are common complications of kidney surgeries. They are thought to be caused by a reflex paralysis of intestinal peristalsis and to manipulation of the colon or duodenum during the surgical procedure.*

☐ GOAL

The patient will be comfortable.

☐ IMPLEMENTATION

- Assess the level of discomfort using a 0-10 point self-rating scale to obtain an objective measure of the pain.
- Medicate as ordered; evaluate effectiveness.
- Monitor for side effects of medication, especially for those detoxified in the kidneys.
- Change patient's position every 2 hours; splint incisional area with a small pillow when turning or coughing; maintain good body alignment.
- If nasogastric (NG) tube is inserted to decrease abdominal distension, maintain patency.
- Auscultate for bowel sounds (usually reappear 2-4 days postoperatively); ensure their presence prior to initiating oral feedings or removing NG tube.

☐ EVALUATION CRITERIA/DESIRED OUTCOMES

The Patient

- States effective pain relief after medication
- Changes position at least every two hours
- Has patent NG tube and return of bowel sounds

NURSING DIAGNOSIS #3

Ineffective breathing pattern (splinted/guarded respirations) related to incisional pain

Rationale: *The surgical incision for a nephrectomy is located in the subcostal, substernal, or posterior flank area; it may additionally injure the nerves of the diaphragm causing the patient severe pain on breathing and coughing.*

☐ GOAL

The patient will have normal respirations and breath sounds.

☐ IMPLEMENTATION

- Assess skin color, vital signs, chest excursion, dyspnea, stridor; place in semi-Fowler's position.
- Record respiratory rate and characteristics of least every hour and as necessary.
- Auscultate breath sounds every 2 hours.
- Monitor for changes in LOC.
- Turn, cough, and deep breathe every 2 hours or as ordered; avoid turning to operative side.
- Medicate for pain prior to position changes, coughing and deep breathing.

☐ EVALUATION CRITERIA/DESIRED OUTCOMES

The Patient

- Has normal respiratory pattern
- Is free from adventitious breath sounds

NURSING DIAGNOSIS #4

Fluid volume deficit related to decreased fluid intake

Rationale: *Adequate fluid intake is vital to maintaining a fluid volume that will keep the healthy kidney functioning normally.*

☐ GOAL

The patient will have fluid intake of 2,000-3,000 cc/day and a urinary output of at least 500 cc/day.

IMPLEMENTATION

- Maintain IV/oral intake of 2,000-3,000 cc/day.
- Observe, measure, and chart amount, color, odor, concentration, content, and specific gravity of urine; with adequate intake, output should be at least 500 cc/day.
- Maintain patency of Foley catheter to monitor output and to ensure remaining kidney remains free from infection; do not irrigate without surgeon's order; anchor catheter to patient to prevent pull and tension; pin to bed sheets so that tubing is not kinked, compressed, or bent and so urine will not pool in bladder or back up into kidney.
- Assess for signs and symptoms of fluid imbalance; refer to Table 1 *Common Fluid and Electrolyte Imbalances*, page 14.
- Monitor renal function study results.

EVALUATION CRITERIA/DESIRED OUTCOMES

The Patient

- Has a daily fluid intake of 2,000-3,000 cc
- Excretes at least 500 cc of urine daily
- Maintains electrolytes, BUN, and creatinine within normal limits

NURSING DIAGNOSIS #5

a. **Grieving** related to loss of kidney
b. **Anxiety** related to outcome of renal transplant

Rationale: *When a patient experiences loss of a body part it is normal for the patient to go through the grieving process and experience feelings of denial, anger, and sadness. The patient may have difficulty discussing the loss, and may experience alterations in physical activities. If the patient was a kidney donor, ambivalent feelings and anxiety may also be present whether or not they are manifested. Staff sometimes neglects the donor patient because s/he is free from disease; in reality, this patient needs a great deal of emotional support, especially if pressure has been put on patient to be a donor.*

GOAL

The patient will verbalize feelings about the loss of kidney and establish a positive self-image; will indicate decreased anxiety.

IMPLEMENTATION

- Plan care to permit time to encourage patient to express thoughts, feelings, and concerns over loss of kidney and about the kidney recipient.
- Allow patient to verbalize these feelings within acceptable limits; reinforce teaching regarding disease and prognosis.
- Distinguish adaptive from maladaptive behaviors and support accordingly; see *The Patient Experiencing Grief and Loss*, page 272.
- Provide accurate information, as ethically permitted, about the post-op status of the recipient.

EVALUATION CRITERIA/DESIRED OUTCOMES

The Patient

- Verbalizes feelings about loss of kidney
- States positive acceptance of change in body image
- Expresses decreased anxiety about the status of the recipient

NURSING DIAGNOSIS #6

Knowledge deficit related to postdischarge regimen

Rationale: *Knowledge about convalescent post-op course and future health maintenance leads to faster recovery from illness and prevention of future complications. Lack of knowledge can cause a high anxiety level.*

GOAL

The patient will verbalize understanding of follow-up care and health maintenance; will demonstrate proper wound care.

IMPLEMENTATION

- Assess patient's understanding of function of remaining kidney and reinforce or clarify information as needed.
- Instruct patient regarding wound care.
- Stress the importance of maintaining a fluid intake of 3,000 cc/day; explain that adequate fluid intake is important to excrete wastes, chemicals, and electrolytes, and to prevent urinary stasis and infection.

- Advise to exercise as physician orders, to avoid heavy lifting for 1 year, and to avoid activities that may lead to damaging the remaining kidney (e.g., contact sports, horseback riding).
- Explain the importance of avoiding persons with infections; review signs of symptoms of infection.
- Reinforce instructions as to when to notify physician and when to be seen for follow-up care.

☐ EVALUATION CRITERIA/DESIRED OUTCOMES

The Patient

- Verbalizes plans to comply with prescribed medical regimen
- Demonstrates proper wound care

The Patient with a Pacemaker: Permanent

Definition/Discussion

A permanent pacemaker is an implanted device used to provide electrical stimulation to the atria and/or ventricles in order to produce consistent cardiac contraction. It is an electronically-powered generator (usually via a lithium battery that lasts for 5 to 15 years) implanted beneath the skin and a catheter that extends from the generator through the superior vena cava and right atrium to the apex of the right ventricle of the heart. Current models can be programmed to pace continuously or on demand (i.e., if the patient's own heart rate falls below 60 beats/minute) and can trigger either atrial and ventricular contractions or both.

The most common indications for insertion of a permanent pacemaker are symptomatic bradycardia (i.e., patient becomes hypotensive or experiences dizziness, mental confusion, or loss of consciousness during bradycardic episode), various forms of heart block, sinus arrest without compensatory ectopic pacing, atrial flutter, and supraventricular tachycardia (Wolff-Parkinson-White syndrome).

Nursing Assessment

☐ **PERTINENT HISTORY**

Dysrhythmia necessitating pacemaker insertion, ECG demonstrating dysrhythmia; subjective description of symptoms associated with dysrhythmia

☐ **PHYSICAL FINDINGS**

Lightheadedness, dizziness, mental confusion, forgetfulness, fainting; palpitations, fatigue, activity intolerance; signs and symptoms of primary disease process (e.g., myocardial infarction, congestive heart failure, pulmonary edema); heart murmers and gallops; electrolyte imbalances, particularly potassium

☐ **PSYCHOSOCIAL CONCERNS/ DEVELPOMENTAL FACTORS**

Anxiety about procedure; effects of dysrhythmia on mentation and concentration; adaptation to possible changes in life-style, perception and acceptance of pacemaker

☐ **PATIENT AND FAMILY KNOWLEDGE**

Self-monitoring of pulse, telephone monitoring of pacemaker functioning; when to expect battery to require changing, follow-up care and indications for notifying physician; posthospitalization level of activity; readiness and willingness to learn

Nursing Care

☐ **LONG-TERM GOAL**

The patient will be able to resume and maintain usual activities and roles, understanding the limitations and precautions associated with this cardiac assistive device.

NURSING DIAGNOSIS #1

Alteration in cardiac output: decreased related to dysrhythmia secondary to impaired pacemaker function

Rationale: *When there is inadequate electrical stimulation to maintain regular cardiac contraction, a permanent pacemaker is needed to ensure pacing and sufficient cardiac output for permanent pacing for life maintenance. Any disruption in the expected function of the pacemaker will cause dysrhythmias and decreased cardiac output. Dysrhythmias such as premature ventricular contractions are not eliminated by the pacemaker but they can* *also alter cardiac output.*

GOAL

The patient will maintain hemodynamic stability with proper pacemaker function.

IMPLEMENTATION

- Assess baseline information of pacemaker function
  - date and location of pacemaker implant
  - pacemaker classification (chambers paced, chambers sensed, mode of response, programmable function, special tachydysrhythmia functions)
  - rate and internal settings (RR [ventricular spike to ventricular spike]; AA [atrial spike to atrial spike]; AV delay [PR interval], atrial output escape interval, ventricular escape interval).
- Assess cardiac monitor pattern
  - percentage of paced rhythm, type of pacing (e.g., artrial/ventricular)
  - maintenance of preset intervals and rates
  - paced P or QRS configuration
  - nonpaced P and QRS configuration
  - pacemaker capture
  - pacemaker sensing
  - pacemaker artifact
- Attach rhythm strip to chart at least every 4 hours.
- Check for consistency between documented settings and actual measurements; notify physician of discrepancies.
- Observe for signs of pacemaker electrode displacement (e.g., change in P-QRS configuration, failure to capture or sense).
- Observe for clinical symptoms of pacemaker failure (e.g., decreased blood pressure, decreased urine output; alteration in level of consciousness; palpitations, dizziness, chest pain, dyspnea).
- Observe for competing dysrhythmias (e.g., premature ventricular complexes, tachydysrhythmias).
- Treat dysrhythmias as ordered or per hospital protocols.

EVALUATION CRITERIA/DESIRED OUTCOMES

The Patient

- has blood pressure and peripheral pulses within normal limits
- Exhibits normal or improved orientation
- Is free of any threatening dysrhythmia

The Pacemaker

- is pacing, sensing, and capturing appropriately

NURSING DIAGNOSIS #2

a. **Alteration in comfort:** pain related to effects of surgical incision, restricted physical mobility
b. **Potential for infection** related to impaired skin integrity after surgical procedure

Rationale: *The patient with a permanent pacemaker implant experiences acute pain with the surgical incision. In addition to incisional pain, possible hematoma, swelling, infection, or sterile abcess at the incision site (usually right upper chest wall) increase discomfort. Temporarily restricted activities of the affected arm and shoulder further increase discomfort.*

GOAL

The patient will experience increased comfort.

IMPLEMENTATION

- Obtain patient's subjective description of pain or discomfort (onset, location, duration, frequency, pattern and quality of pain; intensity [use 0-10 scale]); ask what helps relieve pain or makes it worse.
- Reduce patient's fear of pain by explaining causes; estimate how long pain will last and assure patient that some discomfort is expected; discuss any misconceptions regarding pain or pain medications.
- Explain rationale for temporary activity restrictions.
- Give analgesics for pain relief; assess the response using intensity scale; contact physician for additional order if present medication ineffective.
- Inspect incision site every 8 hours for any signs of inflammation or infection, skin breakdown, hematoma, and condition of stitches.
- Check temperature every 4 hours; expect low-grade temperature during first 48 hours after insertion; inform physician if low-grade

temperature persists or if further elevation noted.
- If hemovac is present, measure every 8 hours and report any excessive bleeding.
- Begin range-of-motion (ROM) exercises to affected shoulder after checking with the physician, usually on the second post-op day; avoid raising arm above shoulder until ROM exercises have been ordered.
- Encourage patient to use affected arm and shoulder as soon as activities can be resumed to prevent frozen shoulder.

☐ EVALUATION CRITERIA/DESIRED OUTCOMES

The Patient
- Verbalizes feelings of increased comfort
- Has clean, healing wound
- Performs active ROM exercises with affected shoulder

> ### NURSING DIAGNOSIS #3
> **Disturbance in self-concept: body image** related to loss of body function and implanted device
>
> ***Rationale:*** *Body image is the person's mental idea and personal reaction to own body. The image is flexible and subject to change. After surgical implantation of a mechanical device, the patient may view the body differently because of changes in both appearance and function. Dependence on a mechanical device may change how the patient views own independence and body function.*

☐ GOAL

The patient will demonstrate adaptation to change and acceptance of loss.

☐ IMPLEMENTATION

- Refer to *The Patient Experiencing a Body-Image Disturbance,* page 253.
- Assess contributing factors to body image or self-concept (e.g., age; sex; how patient reacted to change, viewed self in past; usual coping behaviors; role responsibility [job, spouse]; value placed on lost body function; knowledge of disease and pacemaker function; reaction of family to illness; support systems; physiologic, psychologic health).
- Establish a trusting nurse-patient relationship; interact frequently and consistently; encourage patient to express feelings, ask questions; provide clear, concise, correct information; clarify misconceptions and avoid negative criticism.
- Encourage viewing/touching of insertion site.
- Allow patient to handle pacemaker model.
- Encourage self-care of operative site.
- Enlist assistance of support systems in providing positive interactions with patient.

☐ EVALUATION CRITERIA/DESIRED OUTCOMES

The Patient
- Shows signs of adaptive grief and mourning (e.g., describes feelings about necessity of pacemaker, touches insertion site, indicates plans after hospitalization)
- Participates in self care
- Continues social relationships and role responsibilities

> ### NURSING DIAGNOSIS #4
> **Knowledge deficit** regarding health maintenance with pacemaker
>
> ***Rationale:*** *Without previous experience, the patient may be unsure of how the implementation of a permanent pacemaker will change present life-style; the patient may experience feelings of uneasiness, irritability, and apprehension until adequate instruction is provided. In order to prevent misconceptions, to increase compliance, and to avoid complications, an effective individualized teaching program must be implemented.*

☐ GOAL

The patient will understand functioning of pacemaker; will identify indications for contacting physician; will actively participate in a health maintenance program.

☐ IMPLEMENTATION

- Assess understanding and knowledge of pacemaker function, priority of patient-identified learning needs, readiness to learn; delay teaching until you discern patient is ready.
- Reduce or eliminate barriers to learning by

meeting patient's physiologic needs; evaluate family's perception of disease and develop trust with frequent positive interactions.

- Reduce environmental distractions; concentrate on individualized, one-to-one teaching; include family in teaching program; provide opportunities and encourage patient/family to ask questions and become involved in making informed decisions.
- Develop and implement a teaching plan to give correct and relevant information; do not overwhelm patient with too much information; concentrate on priority information, expanding as patient tolerates
  - teach about natural pacing and conduction system; explain the relationship between electrical conduction and cardiac contractility
  - describe type of pacemaker patient has, how it works
  - explain need for physician follow-up, telephone checks
  - state expected battery life; tell where to obtain replacement
  - explain the importance of wearing an ID card, bracelet, pacemaker identification information card
  - teach how to take pulse (get return demonstration), keep pulse diary
  - discuss signs and symptoms to communicate to physician (e.g., dizziness, palpitations, changes in pulse rate or character), protection of pacemaker and electrical equipment
  - discuss present living patterns and effects pacemaker will make on them,(e.g., travel plans, return to normal activity)
- Encourage expression of feelings (usually involve dying, dependency, disability).
- Initiate referral to mental health nurse or psychologist if resolution of feelings not evident by time of discharge.

☐ EVALUATION CRITERIA/DESIRED OUTCOMES

The Patient

- Describes disease process, function of artificial pacemaker, and self-care routine
- Identifies indications for contacting physician
- Verbalizes confidence in maintaining self-care

The Patient with a Pacemaker: Temporary—External/Noninvasive

Definition/Discussion

A noninvasive/external pacemaker provides ventricular contraction through electrical stimulation as an alternative to temporary invasive devices. Large electrodes (5-10 centimeters/diameter) are placed on the anterior chest (apical area—V3) and on the back (between scapulae at heart level). These electrodes connect to the external pacemaker machine that delivers current through a cable to these pacing electrodes. Stimulation thresholds (the amount of current required to evoke an electrical ventricular response) usually range from 40-100 milliamps (mA). Capture is verified by both oscilloscope (electrical) and palpable pulse (mechanical). This temporary pacemaker provides ventricular pacing until a transvenous pacemaker can be inserted or until other definitive therapy becomes available (i.e., permanent pacemaker can be placed).

ECG electrodes are placed on the anterior chest and attached to leads and an ECG monitor to provide both a visible ECG display and to allow the pacemaker machine to sense the presence/absence of an R wave. Depending on the brand of machine used, the ECG cable connects directly to the pacemaker machine and is either viewed on the pacemaker's integral monitor or on any other available monitor (e.g., bedside monitor, portable monitor, monitor/defibrillator). The pacing rate is set on the pacemaker. Some pacers are asynchronous pacers. Others pace in both asynchronous and synchronous (demand) modes. In the demand mode, the pacer senses the presence/absence of R waves and the heart rate and paces if the R-to-R interval exceeds the set escape or pace rate. It will pace the heart at this selected rate and stop pacing only if the intrinsic heart rate rises above the demand pace rate.

In the fixed (asynchronous) mode, the pacemaker will provide a pacing stimulus at a set rate without regard to the underlying rhythm/rate. This is useful when no intrinsic rate has been confirmed and ECG is not available due to time constraints or possible noisy environment (e.g., operating room, electrocautery).

Criteria for patient eligibility for external pacing include: bradyasystole, symptomatic bradycardia refractory to medications, complete heart block, second degree AV block—Type II, asystole. Prophylactic uses include backup during elective or emergency cardioversion, drug toxicities, or during permanent pacemaker adjustments/failure, angiography/angioplasty, electrophysiologic studies, or surgery (especially in patients with a history of or tendency towards a suppressed conduction system). It may also be employed during clinical diagnostic or treatment procedures when bradyasystole is a possibility and/or temporary situations where invasive procedures are contraindicated or not preferred.

External pacing is continued until a temporary transvenous pacing wire can be inserted, until a permanent pacemaker can be implanted, or until normal cardiac electrical/mechanical activity is reestablished.

Nursing Assessment

☐ **PERTINENT HISTORY**

Medical history of cardiac disease including bradydysrhythmias, progressive heart block, suppressed conduction, cardiac arrest

☐ **PHYSICAL FINDINGS**

Hypotension less than 90 mm Hg, premature ventricular contractions, altered level of consciousness, chest pain, dyspnea, cardiac arrest, electrolyte imbalance (K^+), cardiac medication toxicity (e.g., digoxin, calcium channel blockers, beta blockers); cool, clammy skin, absent or weak peripheral pulses

☐ PSYCHOSOCIAL CONCERNS/ DEVELOPMENTAL FACTORS

Age, sex, developmental level, occupation, usual coping mechanisms, available support system, fear/anxiety related to potential discomfort, previous experience with illness and hospitalization

☐ PATIENT AND FAMILY KNOWLEDGE

Disease process and potential outcome, explanation of procedure, potential for discomfort, level of knowledge, acceptance of treatment, readiness and willingness to learn

Nursing Care

☐ Long-Term Goal

The patient will maintain hemodynamic stability and proper ventricular pacing during the acute emergency until definitive therapy is available.

NURSING DIAGNOSIS #1

a. **Alteration in cardiac output: decreased** related to ineffective cardiac activity (bradyasystolic arrest)
b. **Alteration in tissue perfusion: cardiopulmonary, cerebral, renal, peripheral** related to ineffective cardiac pumping activity, decreased cardiac output

Rationale: *When abnormalities of electrical impulse formation or conduction system failures cause slowing of the ventricular rate or absence of heart rate, cardiac output is decreased. When the amount of blood pumped by the heart is reduced, a compromised cardiac function results because the decreased pumping activity results in decreased circulation in capillary blood flow to all vital organs and tissues. Ventricular function must be restored by artificial/mechanical means to provide heart contraction to maintain cardiac output and circulation.*

☐ GOAL

The patient will have improved cardiac output and tissue perfusion.

☐ IMPLEMENTATION

- Position patient in supine or semi-Fowler's position.
- Apply noninvasive pacemaker rapidly when needed (the faster it is applied, the more chance of success, especially during asystole).
- Select demand or asynchronous mode (if pacemaker has option); demand mode is usually selected to ensure that spontaneous electrical activity will be sensed by the pacemaker.
- Attach ECG monitor to chest leads using any lead that provides a large R wave with either positive or negative deflection (e.g., lead II and other precordial leads); avoid interfering with location of pacing electrodes and possible defibrillation therapy.
- Apply anterior/posterior pacing electrodes; place the anterior electrode in the V3 position, and the posterior electrode in the center of the back. NOTE: Some modification of pacing electrode placement and/or size may be necessary in patients with large midline thoracic incisions to prevent electrode placement over dressings and/or metal skin staples, and in large breasted females.
- Check the pacemaker machine (most models have an R wave detector that flashes or beeps) to confirm that it is sensing a QRS (if the patient has electrical activity).
- If pacemaker fails to sense an R wave or paced beats, increase the sensitivity level and/or change the ECG lead placement.
- Select pace rate.
- Start pacemaker and increase current until capture (pacemaker causes ventricular contraction) is obtained (usually 40-100 mA are required to obtain capture).
- Verify capture
  - ventricular paced beat viewed on monitor display
  - R wave detector on pacemaker machine flashes or beeps
  - palpable pulse
- If monitor shows no capture, increase mAs until capture.
- If no pulse is generated at maximum mAs, initiate CPR; check for hemodynamic perfusion during pacing by obtaining viable blood

pressure (60-90 mm Hg systolic); obtain blood pressure in right arm: falsely elevated pressures have been noted in left arm with this pacing method.
- Attach rhythm strip to chart at least every hour.
- Assess monitor pattern and chart hourly for demand pacing, and more frequently if 100% paced; note percent paced rhythm, mA setting to capture and mA setting during pacing (should be increased 10mA above capture to maintain), rate setting (confirm that rate set on machine and patient's heart rate are consistent), if pacemaker is sensing properly (i.e., senses patient's intrinsic rhythm, if applicable, and senses paced beat).
- If 100% pacing is desired and patient's intrinsic rhythm is competing (i.e., pace rate is very close to the patient's intrinsic rate), increase the pace rate setting by 5-10 pulses per minute (ppm).
- Have emergency equipment and medications available, such as defibrillator, emergency cart, transvenous pacemaker.
- Observe monitor for pacer spike; the spike is artificially generated by the external pacemaker during current pulse; the spike typically ranges in length from 20-40 milliseconds; read product literature to determine expected spike duration since it will vary based on the manufacturer.
- When pacing and during set-up, know that a fall in current during the vulnerable period of T-wave is to be avoided, although the chances of inducing ventricular tachycardia/fibrillation are apparently small.
- Observe battery power indicator on machine and attach to wall-line power when possible to conserve battery.
- Secure pacemaker to a bedside cart or in bed with patient for transport from ER to critical care or if necessary to transport patient to procedure rooms.
- Monitor arterial blood gases every 2-4 hours to ensure adequate tissue perfusion.
- Monitor electrolytes to prevent life threatening dysrhythmias.
- Palpate peripheral pulses every hour.
- Observe for changes in mental status (could mean decreased cerebral perfusion).
- Maintain patient IV line to assure access for emergency medications.
- Ensure urinary output of at least 0.5-1.00 cc/kg/hour.
- When not in use, keep pacemaker at bedside or applied to patient for prophylactic uses (usually with pacing current turned off); manually initiate (turn on) pacing if need arises.

☐ EVALUATION CRITERIA/DESIRED OUTCOMES

The Patient

- Has cardiac electrical and mechanical activity that provides a viable blood pressure and pulse
- Has hemodynamic pressures and cardiac output within normal limits
- Has urinary output greater than 30 cc/hour
- Has improved level of consciousness
- Is paced within the normal current range (40-100 mA)

NURSING DIAGNOSIS #2

Impaired physical mobility related to enforced bedrest and positioning

Rationale: *The pacing electrodes and the cardiac monitor electrodes necessitate restricting the patient to bedrest. Position changes can necessitate the need for adjustment of current levels; therefore, the patient must remain relatively still and is restricted in gross movements of the torso.*

☐ GOAL

The patient will maintain the greatest possible mobility while maintaining proper electrode placement and lowest current settings for capture.

☐ IMPLEMENTATION

- Position for comfort in supine position with head of bed slightly elevated if vital signs permit.
- Explain need for mobility restrictions and enforced bedrest.
- Secure the electrodes to the chest wall to maximize good contact and minimize electrode displacement when patient movement occurs; apply tape if necessary over the complete electrode.
- Ensure electrode contact with skin when turning patient to maintain adequate pacing.
- Help the patient to maintain proper back

alignment with changes in position to prevent electrode displacement.

- Observe the QRS size, sensitivity and capture during and after position changes and adjust sensitivity and current if needed.
- Check bony prominences for reddened areas every 8 hours.
- Teach and encourage patient to perform active range-of-motion exercises every 4 hours if possible.

☐ EVALUATION CRITERIA/DESIRED OUTCOMES

The Patient

- Is free from complications associated with restricted movement
- Moves all extremities on command
- Has bilateral peripheral pulses

NURSING DIAGNOSIS #3

Impairment of skin integrity related to skin sensitivity to pacing electrodes, electrode adhesive material, and electrical pacing

Rationale: *Continuous external pacing causes capillary vasodilation and puts the patient at risk for skin impairment. The area under the electrode pads may be sensitive to the adhesive material. If the area has not been cleaned well of electrode paste, soap, lotion, powder, or cream prior to the application of the pads, good skin contact will be prevented and pain will be increased.*

☐ GOAL

The patient will maintain integrity of skin beneath anterior/posterior pacing electrodes.

☐ IMPLEMENTATION

- Check the position and condition of monitoring and pacing electrodes every 2-4 hours to be sure that they are securely attached.
- Change the pacing electrodes as needed, every 24-48 hours.
- Inspect the skin for breakdown when changing the electrodes.
- Use nonallergenic tape if taping the electrodes to the chest is indicated.
- Trim the hair directly under the adhesive with scissors if hair is preventing good contact; do not shave the skin as nicked areas can reduce skin impedance and cause severe pain with pacing.
- Wash the chest and back with soap and water gently before applying the pacing electrodes, if time allows; rinse and dry well; remove electrode paste, soap, powder, lotion and cream, which can alter skin resistance.
- Use no alcohol or benzoin under the electrodes, as this increases impedance and increases the voltage required to deliver current through the electrodes.
- Check diaphoretic patients more frequently; if ECG electrodes become detached, the pacemaker will interpret asystole and will initiate pacing.
- Turn the pace current or pace switch off while changing if the electrodes need to be changed.

☐ EVALUATION CRITERIA/DESIRED OUTCOMES

The Patient

- Maintains intact skin with minimal sensitivity beneath the electrodes

NURSING DIAGNOSIS #4

Alteration in comfort: pain related to skeletal muscle contraction and electrical skin stimulation during pacing

Rationale: *Skeletal muscle contractions that result when current passes through the chest wall can be uncomfortable or even painful. Descriptions range from sensations of a mild to severe thumping, or an intense burning or stinging pain. Physical observations during external pacing range from a mild pectoral twitching to a "hiccoughing" appearance of muscle contractions. The latter can be expected in all patients and the current should be adjusted to as comfortable a level as possible with the threshold maintained. The level of comfort is directly proportional to the level of current; every patient has an individual pain threshold. In thoracic surgery patients, or others with midline anterior chest incisions, placement of electrodes may require modification, thus increasing current needed to capture and increasing discomfort. Medication for pain or limited anesthesia may be indicated in these patients.*

GOAL

The patient will maintain a tolerable level of comfort during pacing.

IMPLEMENTATION

- Place electrodes to optimize capture and current levels.
- Encourage patient to verbalize tolerance to the muscle contractions to assist in selecting the correct mAs for capture.
- Increase the current slowly until capture is obtained.
- Increase current to 10 mAs above capture threshold to assure maintenance.
- Consider moving anterior pacing electrode to minimize threshold.
- Explain to patient/family using simple descriptions and terminology the realistic, expected sensations during pacing, sensations of "thumping," muscle contractions, appearance of "hiccoughing."
- Encourage patient to verbalize discomfort using a 0-10 scale; assess verbal/nonverbal cues of pain; note location, characteristics, onset, duration.
- Place the electrodes away from bone if possible because conduction through bone requires a more uncomfortable, higher voltage to produce a cardiac response.
- Administer analgesics as ordered; monitor effects on hemodynamic parameters.

EVALUATION CRITERIA/DESIRED OUTCOMES

The Patient

- Requests pain medication when needed
- Verbalizes pain relief
- Verbalizes the sensations to expect during pacing

NURSING DIAGNOSIS #5

a. **Anxiety** related to need for external pacemaker
b. **Fear** related to external pacemaker use
c. **Ineffective individual/family coping** related to need for life supportive device
d. **Knowledge deficit** regarding pacemaker function and indications

Rationale: *Information must be provided as to how the pacemaker functions. In emergency cases, when time cannot be taken to tell the patient what to expect, this can be accomplished if and when the acute phase resolves and mental status allows. The acute emergency and life-threatening situation causing a need for noninvasive pacing is likely to cause anxiety and fear for the patient and family. Anxiety/fear can be decreased with explanation of the procedure.*

GOAL

The patient will experience decreased anxiety and decreased fear; the patient/family will verbalize minimum knowledge of pacemaker purpose and function.

IMPLEMENTATION

- Assess for signs of anxiety (e.g., increased blood pressure, respiratory rate, irritability, crying, inability to concentrate, degree of stress).
- Assist to reduce anxiety level when emergency phase has resolved by reassuring patient that external pacemaker is a temporary device to be followed by further definitive and permanent therapy.
- Explain application of pacemaker to alert patients (or after application if mental status improves after perfusion improves) and their families.
- Explain function of pacemaker to patient/family including the expected skeletal muscle contractions and potential for discomfort.
- Explain to the patient/family the reasons for use (e.g., during cardioversion, instead of invasive pacing wire while a drug toxicity resolves); this may include brief overdrive pacing (pace rate setting above the patient's intrinsic rate) to obtain a capture threshold in order to establish pacing threshold.
- Administer medications such as diazepam (Valium) and oxazepam (Serax) as needed, when not contraindicated; evaluate effectiveness.
- Inform patient under what conditions pacing can be expected (i.e., what heart rate the pacer is set to initiate pacing) to alleviate fear or anxiety.
- Discuss the lack of risk of electrical shock to the patient or caretaker because of the very low energy levels used in pacing; alleviate

fears/anxiety of any similarity between external pacing and defibrillation.
- Provide emotional support at the bedside when pacing occurs, especially when rhythm has not necessitated pacing for long intervals.
- Encourage verbalization of fears, anxieties, concerns, and confrontation with death.
- Provide significant others with frequent updates on patient's condition and provide opportunities to be with the patient.
- Provide opportunity for questions.
- Encourage patient to repeat information to check for understanding.

☐ EVALUATION CRITERIA/DESIRED OUTCOMES

The Patient

- Verbalizes decreased anxiety
- Displays few physiologic/physical signs of anxiety

The Patient/family

- Describes pacemaker purpose and function in own words

The Patient with a Pacemaker: Temporary—Invasive

Definition/Discussion

A temporary pacemaker is an external electrical generator device that is attached to an electrode catheter. It is inserted through a large vein and advanced to the heart. This temporary device provides electrical stimulation to the atria and/or ventricles in order to produce consistent cardiac contraction until the sinus node resumes pacing or until a permanent pacemaker can be inserted.

Nursing Assessment

☐ PERTINENT HISTORY

Symptomatic bradycardia refractory to medications, complete heart block, prophylactic need for pacemaker post-open heart surgery, tachydysrhythmias (overdrive pacing), any dysrhythmia where there is a marked decreased or temporary absence of cardiac output; ECG demonstrating dysrhythmia, symptoms associated with dysrhythmia

☐ PHYSICAL FINDINGS

Lightheadedness, dizziness, forgetfulness, mental confusion, fainting, palpitations; fatigue, activity intolerance, seizures, cardiac arrest; heart murmurs and gallops; electrolyte imbalances, particularly potassium; patient may be asymptomatic

☐ PSYCHOSOCIAL CONCERNS/DEVELOPMENTAL FACTORS

Educational level, resource and support system, age, coping style

☐ PATIENT AND FAMILY KNOWLEDGE

Disease process and disease treatment, acceptance of treatment, level of knowledge, readiness and willingness to learn

Nursing Care

☐ LONG-TERM GOAL

The patient will maintain hemodynamic stability and proper pacemaker functioning during the acute phase of cardiac dysfunction until a permanent pacemaker can be implanted or until normal cardiac electrical stimulation is reestablished.

NURSING DIAGNOSIS #1

Alteration in cardiac output: decreased related to dysrhythmia secondary to impaired pacemaker function

Rationale: *Cardiac output is a product of heart rate and stroke volume. Pacemakers are needed when abnormalities of impulse formation or failures in the conduction system result in excessive slowing of the ventricular rate. In a pacemaker-dependent patient, an electrical impulse from an artificial pacemaker is used to provide the heart with an artificially stimu-*

lated rhythm so that the heart can contract and maintain cardiac output. Any disruption in that rhythm will decrease cardiac output and could cause death.

☐ GOAL

The patient will maintain adequate cardiac output with proper pacemaker function.

☐ IMPLEMENTATION

- Test pulse generator and battery before insertion of temporary pacemaker.
- Assess baseline information of pacemaker function (date and method of insertion), location of atrial/ventricular pacing leads, set rate, mA, threshold, sensitivity).
- Assess monitor pattern for percent paced rhythm, maintenance of preset rate, paced and nonpaced P or QRS configuration, pacemaker capture (pacemaker has initiated a QRS or caused ventricular contraction), pacemaker sensing (pacemaker senses patient's own electrical impulses and does not compete).
- Attach rhythm strip to chart at least every 4 hours.
- Check consistency between documented settings (rate, mA, and sensitivity) and those actually set on pacemaker generator.
- Observe for signs of battery failure (e.g., indicator lights not flashing sense/pace, battery test inoperable, loss of capture, failure to sense, loss of pacing spike, changes in preset discharge rate).
- Keep extra battery available; replace battery when low; document date of change.
- Observe for signs of pacemaker electrode displacement (e.g., change in P-QRS configuration, failure to capture or sense); notify physician if observed.
- Check generator-cable-pacing lead connections for fit and contact.
- Secure pacemaker generator to adjacent IV pole or to bed to prevent damage or disconnection.
- Observe for changes in pacemaker threshold (failure to capture, sense, pace).
- Monitor factors that alter pacemaker threshold
  - decreased threshold: myocardial ischemia, decreased postassium level, premature ventricular contractions, adrenergic drugs, hypoxemia
  - increased threshold: inflammation around catheter tip, poor contact with ventricular wall
- Monitor for dysrhythmias due to failure of pacemaker to capture or sense, premature ventricular contractions, and tachydysrhythmias.
- Have emergency equipment and drugs available (e.g., lidocaine, atropine, isoproterenol).
- If problem occurs because of failure to capture, increase stimulation (mA) threshold, prepare to support rhythm with drugs (e.g., atropine, isoproterenol, and inform physician of need to reposition.
- If problem occurs because of failure to sense, note where pacer spike falls in relation to T wave
  - if pacer spike falls on supernormal or vulnerable period of T wave and patient's own electrical rhythm is adequate, turn pacer off
  - if patient rhythm is insufficient without pacer, prepare for possible ventricular tachycardia or fibrillation and notify physician immediately
- Observe for signs of ventricular perforation and cardiac tamponade (e.g., decreased blood pressure, muffed heart sounds, pericardial friction rub, elevated venous pressure [increased central venous pressure, jugular venous distension], increased heart rate, paradoxical pulse greater than 10 mm Hg; dyspnea, cyanosis).

☐ EVALUATION CRITERIA/DESIRED OUTCOMES

The Patient

- Has blood pressure and arterial pulse within normal limits
- Is alert and oriented
- Has no threatening dysrhythmia

The Pacemaker

- has 100% sensing and 100% capture

NURSING DIAGNOSIS #2

a. **Anxiety** related to need for temporary pacemaker insertion

b. **Knowledge deficit** regarding procedure, pacemaker function

Rationale: *Inexperience may cause the patient to be unsure of what to expect from the pacemaker insertion procedure. Without correct information there may be misconceptions on how the pacemaker functions. Although the pacemaker is an identified threat, the patient experiences additional feelings of uneasiness due to unidentified and nonspecific threats to own well-being. Anxiety can be reduced by providing the patient with realistic information regarding the procedure and future expectations.*

GOAL

The patient will experience decreased anxiety; will verbalize at least minimum knowledge of pacemaker procedure and function.

IMPLEMENTATION

- Assess for indications of anxiety (e.g., increased heart rate, blood pressure, respiratory rate; irritability, anger, crying, nervousness; inability to concentrate, forgetfulness; degree of stress and effect on patient; patterns of coping).
- Diagnose level of anxiety; refer to *The Patient Experiencing Anxiety*, page 250.
- Assist to reduce present level of anxiety by encouraging questions and discussion of worries.
- Assess learning needs and readiness to learn.
- Assess personal factors that affect learning (e.g., physical condition, degree of anxiety, effect of dysrhythmia on mentation and concentration, degree of emergency for procedure, age, intelligence/education, past experience or knowledge, locus of control, support systems, cultural background).
- Individualize teaching plan.
- Explain purpose, procedure, and function of pacemaker to patient/family using concise descriptions and understandable terminology.
- Present realistic information; discuss prognosis; explain differences in temporary versus permanent pacemakers.
- Provide opportunity for questions and ask for feedback to evaluate understanding.
- Repeat information as needed.
- Reduce environmental distractions, which may interfere with learning.
- Provide ongoing explanation of care.

EVALUATION CRITERIA/DESIRED OUTCOMES

The Patient

- Verbalizes decreased feelings of anxiety
- Has no physical or psychologic manifestations of anxiety
- Asks appropriate questions; verbalizes understanding of purpose, procedure, function of pacemaker

NURSING DIAGNOSIS #3

a. **Alteration in comfort: pain** related to pacemaker insertion, position during insertion

b. **Fear** related to pacemaker insertion procedure

Rationale: *The insertion of a temporary pacemaker is usually done with local anesthesia using a percutaneous approach. There is some discomfort associated with infiltration of the local anesthetic and some pressure or pain with insertion of the catheter. The patient is often in the uncomfortable Trendelenburg's position. Sterile drapes may cover face, increasing discomfort. If the patient is unprepared for the procedure, fear of pain will intensify discomfort.*

GOAL

The patient will be as comfortable as possible during the pacemaker insertion.

IMPLEMENTATION

- Assess understanding and expectations of procedure.
- Assess factors that affect pain tolerance (e.g., culture, past experience with pain, degree of anxiety or fear, sleep deprivation, sensory overload, misconceptions regarding pain and procedure, previous pain tolerance, nurses'/

physicians' misconceptions of pain and pain tolerance; nurse-patient relationship); modify factors as possible (e.g., provide explanations, decrease unnecessary external stimuli).

- Present realistic expectations regarding discomfort of procedure.
- Assist to tolerate discomfort during procedure (e.g., premedicate and assess response to medication, provide encouragement and explain progress, hold hand, allow to express pain or emotions, use distraction techniques.
- Assist in aftermath of procedure by informing when procedure is over and encouraging discussion of experience; praise patient for endurance and cooperation.
- Notify physician if patient is hiccoughing.

☐ EVALUATION CRITERIA/DESIRED OUTCOMES

The Patient

- Verbalizes physical and psychologic comfort during/following procedure.
- Discusses fears and pain experience

NURSING DIAGNOSIS #4

Impaired physical mobility related to imposed restrictions on affected limb

Rationale: *The temporary pacemaker lead is passed through a central vein, usually the subclavian or jugular, with the polar tip positioned at the apex of the right ventricle. The catheter is sutured at the percutaneous insertion site but the polar tip simply rests against the ventricular wall. Motion of the affected shoulder or arm could dislodge the tip and the pacemaker will cease to sense or capture, losing effectiveness or causing life-threatening dysrhythmias.*

☐ GOAL

The patient will maintain the highest mobility possible while maintaining proper pacemaker function.

☐ IMPLEMENTATION

- Explain need and temporary nature of immobilization of extremity.
- Selectively minimize motion of extremity to prevent pacemaker wire dislodgment
  - *anticubital approach*: use padded armboard to immobilize arm; prevent abduction of arm by positioning with pillows or restraints if necessary; elevate with pillow to facilitate venous return, check pulses to determine adequacy of circulation
  - *femoral approach*: avoid outward rotation and flexion of hip
  - *jugular or subclavian approach*: prevent arm raising above shoulder; do not lift patient under arms; use extension cable to pulse generator for increased positioning range; use sling to immobilize shoulder
- Position extremity comfortably.
- Encourage to rest in bed for first 24-48 hours after insertion.
- Administer medication as needed for pain; evaluate effectiveness.
- Eliminate or reduce pressure points related to immobility; change position at least every hour; check orders for limitations on side-to-side turning or head elevation; assess armboard or sling for correct applications; monitor pressure areas; encourage patient to wiggle hands and feet; use sheepskins, egg-crate mattress, heel or elbow protectors as necessary.
- Encourage to use unaffected arm for self-care activities.
- Place self-care objects within reach of unaffected arm.
- Encourage to call for help when needed; place call bell within patient's reach.
- Increase limb mobility after temporary pacemaker is removed by assisting with range-of-motion exercises and encouraging use and exercise of extremity.

☐ EVALUATION CRITERIA/DESIRED OUTCOMES

The Patient

- Has no reddened or pressure sore areas
- Has warm, pink skin and strong pulses in involved extremity

The Pacemaker

- Is sensing and capturing appropriately

NURSING DIAGNOSIS #5

Potential for injury related to electrical microshock

Rationale: *An external pacemaker lead provides an alternative pathway for grounding electrical current. If a defective piece of electrical equipment is touched, the free current takes an alternative low-resistance pathway and a potentially lethal current passes through the patient's heart to the ground. The patient with a temporary pacemaker is particularly vulnerable. Not only is the patient connected to many electrical devices that could leak current, there is also an ideal low-resistant wire directing the free current to the myocardium. Microshock may be unnoticeable by the nurse but potentially fatal to the patient.*

☐ GOAL

The patient will remain hemodynamically stable in an electrically safe environment.

☐ INTERVENTIONS

- Cover the area of connection between the terminal pacer wires and the pacemaker generator with nonconductive material (if the generator is an older model); new models with rubber covered connections are safest.
- Report immediately to physician any deviation from expected function (e.g., inability to pace, unusual changes in the threshold, inability to sense, inaccurate rate).
- Wear rubber gloves if handling exposed wires.
- Use only appliances that have 3-wire prongs; never use an adaptor.
- Avoid extension cords unless they are redundant grounded.
- Do not use equipment with frayed wires or other signs of damage; if there is a question consult the electrician.
- Use nonelectric cardiac beds.
- Do not use any 100-volt appliances such as heating pads, radios, or electrical shavers.
- Avoid simultaneously touching electrical equipment and patient.
- Report immediately to physician any 60-cycle ECG noise or interference (indicates current leakage).
- Ensure that all electrical equipment in patient unit is checked to determine the amount of leakage current in accordance with biomedical-electrical safety guidelines.
- Have electrician check any equipment that has been dropped, wet, or otherwise damaged.
- Plug 2 or more line-powered machines into adjacent receptacles if used on the same patient.
- Notify the electrician if there is any question of electrical safety.

☐ EVALUATION CRITERIA/DESIRED OUTCOMES

The Patient

- Has no 60-cycle electrical interference on ECG
- Is maintained on a properly functioning pacemaker unit
- Has no threatening dysrhythmias

NURSING DIAGNOSIS #6

Potential for infection related to invasive procedure

Rationale: *There is a potential for infection with each invasive procedure. Temporary pacemakers are often inserted in the patient's hospital room under emergency conditions. In less than ideal conditions, poor aseptic practices of hospital staff contribute to potential infection.*

☐ GOAL

The patient will remain free from infection.

☐ IMPLEMENTATION

- Maintain sterile technique during insertion.
- Change dressings daily using sterile technique
  - cleanse insertion site with antiseptic solution and apply antiseptic ointment
  - apply dry sterile occlusive dressing
  - provide padding beneath wires to prevent pressure ulceration

- date dressing change
- note and report signs of infection (e.g., redness, swelling, drainage, warmth, tenderness, pain); catheter tip may be cultured on removal if signs of infection present

- Check vital signs every 4 hours.
- Notify physician of ECG abnormalities.

☐ EVALUATION CRITERIA/DESIRED OUTCOMES

The Patient

- Has normal body temperature
- Is free from insertion site redness, swelling, drainage, warmth, tenderness, pain

The Patient Experiencing Pain

Definition/Discussion

An unpleasant sensory and emotional experience resulting from the perception of noxious stimuli. Chronic pain is pain that continues for longer than six months.

Techniques to manage pain include

- *pharmacologic:* use of narcotic or non-narcotic analgesics administered orally, parenterally, rectally, or intrathecally
- *noninvasive:* applications of heat or cold, massage, topical anesthetics, hypnosis, relaxation, guided imagery, distraction
- *neurologic:* acupuncture, nerve block, cordotomies, transcutaneous electrical nerve stimulation (TENS).

Nursing Assessment

☐ PERTINENT HISTORY

Cause of pain; location (deep, superficial, referred); severity; duration, rhythmicity of episodes; quality; what time of day it is worse; precipitating, aggravating, alleviating factors; duration in weeks/months/years; fatigue, irritability; change in appetite or sleep patterns; decreased interest in living, recreational activities; rubbing of affected area; previous treatment; effect on activities of daily living (ADL); general health history

☐ PHYSICAL FINDINGS

Level of consciousness; changes in vital signs; diaphoresis; nausea and vomiting; muscle tension, weakness, spasms; changes in skin color; restlessness, agitation; change in facial expression (frown); apathy or withdrawal; crying, whimpering, moaning, screaming; clenching of fists or jaw

☐ PSYCHOSOCIAL CONCERNS/ DEVELOPMENTAL FACTORS

Attitude of family; concerns (e.g., diagnosis, prognosis, finances); perception of what will be helpful in management; amount of disruption; secondary gains; past experience with pain and coping efforts used, personality style, cultural influences or practices; meaning of pain, fears, perceptions regarding pain and pain relief; chronic pain: depression, guilt, hopelessness

☐ PATIENT AND FAMILY KNOWLEDGE

Cause of and ability to manage pain; strategies to tolerate chronic pain

Nursing Care

☐ LONG-TERM GOAL

The patient will be free from pain OR the patient will cope adaptively with chronic pain.

NURSING DIAGNOSIS #1

Alteration in comfort: pain related to injury, recent surgery, specific stimulus (specify)

Rationale: *Acute pain is of short duration; complete resolution is anticipated with treatment of the underlying etiology.*

☐ GOAL

The patient will experience reduction in or relief of pain.

☐ IMPLEMENTATION

- Assess the level of discomfort using a 0-10 point self-rating scale to obtain an objective measure of the pain.
- Encourage to talk about previous experience with pain.
- Attempt to understand the religious, cultural, and psychologic influences on this particular patient's reaction.
- Administer prescribed analgesics promptly PRN; know the time of onset and duration of effect of drug ordered.
- Utilize knowledge of patient's present reaction and tolerance to pain in addition to physician's orders to make your decisions about giving medication; do not withhold medication just because you feel the patient's pain is not real or should be adequately tolerated; remember that it is the patient who is feeling the pain; there is little fear of addiction to medication when given for acute pain over a short period of time.
- When giving pain medication, tell the patient about the medication and its expected effect; talk positively about it.
- Evaluate the effect of pain medication: did it eliminate or reduce the pain? If the latter only, consider changing medication as not all patients will respond in the same way to the same drug; consult with physician.
- Monitor for and take steps to prevent side effects of analgesics (e.g., respiratory depression, sedation, nausea, constipation).
- Medicate patient prior to participation in activities that will cause discomfort (e.g., coughing, turning, deep breathing).

☐ EVALUATION CRITERIA/DESIRED OUTCOMES

The Patient

- Rates pain less than 4 after pain medication
- Is free from side effects of drugs
- Demonstrates decreasing need for medication as days pass.

NURSING DIAGNOSIS #2

Alteration in comfort: chronic pain related to neurologic injury, metastatic cancer, altered body function

Rationale: *Chronic pain differs from acute pain in duration (over 6 months), physiologic indicators (the patient may exhibit none of the vital signs/behavioral responses to acute pain because of adaptation), and emotional reactions (e.g., anxiety, depression, withdrawal, anger or apathy, helplessness, hopelessness). The chronicity of the pain can make it much more difficult to manage.*

☐ GOAL

The patient will engage in ADL without preoccupation with pain; will achieve a satisfactory measure of pain control.

☐ IMPLEMENTATION

- Plan with patient the kinds and timing of activities that can reduce, eliminate, or minimize the suffering; educate regarding modification of activities (e.g., walk rather than jog).
- When patient is caring for self, allow as much time as needed to accomplish the task (patients in pain cannot tolerate being rushed); assist only when necessary.
- Provide opportunity for adequate rest as fatigue will increase perception of pain.
- Allow to talk intermittently, but not constantly, about the pain and suffering; finding the cause of the suffering often relieves or reduces it.
- Give positive feedback to efforts to share feelings and to cope with the suffering.
- Have friends/family/staff available when patient needs to see them.
- Ensure all staff is aware of the patient's usual response to pain; allow patient to participate in planning for management; ask what the patient thinks might be effective.
- Do not reinforce the focus on pain; instead begin to reward non-pain-focused behavior.
- Utilize activities and conversation (i.e., distraction) to help the patient focus on something other than the pain; find out what s/he likes to talk about, activities s/he enjoys.
- Hold patient care conferences to discuss responses to pain; plan approaches and write them in nursing care plan; be consistent in use of plan but be alert for new approaches.
- Take a few seconds and inwardly ask yourself, "What would I be like if I were suffering like this?"; identification of how we feel and respond increases our understanding of

the variety of ways other people respond to situations, particularly painful experiences.
- Facilitate family understanding of the suffering by giving careful explanations to them of how and why the patient responds as s/he does.
- Instruct in proper use of heat or cold applications when ordered by physician.
- Encourage regular exercise if tolerated.
- Teach body relaxation techniques (refer to *The Patient Experiencing Anxiety*, page 250) not only for pain reduction but also to use during periods of tension and anxiety; (tension and anxiety can increase the perception of and reaction to pain).
- Teach effective use of analgesics, side effects, efficacy; that pain should be managed, not endured.
- Help patient to be realistic in expectations of effects of medications; know that often pain medications can be reduced in frequency and amount as pain control is achieved or enhanced with other modalities.
- Consider with the physician the preventive approach if pain is expected to occur consistently; regular, rather than PRN pain medication may be more effective.
- Be alert to symptoms of depression (e.g., withdrawal, sad affect, suicidal ideation).
- Teach to use support systems and diversional therapy to cope with pain.
- Tell patient about outside resources such as pain clinics, reputable hypnotists, acupuncturists, family/individual psychotherapists.

☐ EVALUATION CRITERIA/DESIRED OUTCOMES

The Patient

- Describes events and conditions influencing the occurrence and level of pain
- Identifies a pattern of medication use, diversional and relaxation activities that assist in the reduction or elimination of pain
- Demonstrates use of relaxation techniques and distraction methods to manage pain
- Acknowledges utilization of outside resources for selected circumstances
- Requests information regarding noninvasive methods of pain relief

NURSING DIAGNOSIS #3

Fear related to pain, anticipation of pain, possible addiction

Rationale: *Fear about the return of pain can potentiate the patient's experience of it, making it more difficult to control. The patient may have specific fears concerning pain or may experience nonspecific anxiety and dread when pain occurs. When the patient's pain is not adequately relieved, a vicious cycle begins: unrelieved pain causes increased anxiety, which in turn increases the sensitivity to pain and diminishes the patient's confidence in the drug. Many patients will misuse analgesics because of unfounded fears of addiction.*

☐ GOAL

The patient will experience a lessening of fear and anxiety caused by pain; will employ adaptive coping mechanisms to keep the level of anxiety manageable.

☐ IMPLEMENTATION

- Assess for level of anxiety; refer to *The Patient Experiencing Anxiety*, page 250.
- Inform prior to tests or surgery when and where the pain can be expected to occur, possible severity, and how long it may last; instruct in measures to manage the pain; reassure that medication will be available.
- Be alert for denial of pain (e.g., saying everything is OK while grimacing, never complaining of pain or asking for medication).
- Encourage verbalization of past experiences, expectations, and perceptions of pain.
- Utilize pain-relief measures before pain becomes severe (they will be more effective).
- Encourage verbalization of feelings when pain is relieved to dissipate reactions to the stress; recognize that physiologic manifestations (e.g., shaking, chills, vomiting) may occur; attend to physical needs.
- Be supportive; the presence of the nurse is very effective in reducing fear and anxiety and encouraging development of trust.
- Reassure regarding addiction possibilities as necessary; encourage patient not to suffer because of an unfounded fear of becoming drug-dependant.

☐ EVALUATION CRITERIA/DESIRED OUTCOMES

The Patient

- States when feelings of fear and anxiety occur

- Verbalizes fears and concerns regarding the experience of pain
- Requests medication appropriately
- Acknowledges that addiction is unlikely

The Patient with Pancreatitis

Definition/Discussion

Pancreatitis is an inflammatory autodigestion of the pancreas caused by the enzymes it produces. Types of pancreatitis are

- *mild acute (interstitial)*: also known as acute pancreatic edema and characterized by an edematous swelling of the gland and enzyme leakage into the surrounding tissue and peritoneal cavity
- *acute hemorrhagic*: represents a more advanced form of interstitial pancreatitis; the tissue becomes necrotic with more widespread enzymatic digestion of the pancreas
- *necrotic hemorrhagic*: the most severe form of pancreatitis; can lead to pancreatic cysts or calculi or can be fatal

Nursing Assessment

☐ PERTINENT HISTORY

Medical and surgical history; alcoholism; bilary tract disease; abdominal trauma; viral infection (e.g., mumps); tumors; metabolic disorders (e.g., hypercalcemia or hyperlipidemia); drug use (e.g., oral contraceptives, corticosteroids or thiazide diuretics); family history of pancreatitis

☐ PHYSICAL FINDINGS

Severe, unremitting epigastric pain that may radiate to back or shoulder occurring after meals or after alcohol ingestion; elevated serum amylase and lipase; bulky, pale, foul-smelling stools (steatorrhea); nausea and vomiting; fever; diaphoresis; dehydration; abdominal distension; poorly defined abdominal mass; jaundice; mental confusion and agitation; respiratory distress; shock; coma

☐ PSYCHOSOCIAL CONCERNS/ DEVELOPMENTAL FACTORS

Sex (more common in men; women with biliary tract disease); age (40-50 years); alcohol abuse; usual coping mechanism, available support system; roles and responsibilities; occupation

☐ PATIENT AND FAMILY KNOWLEDGE

Disease process, necessary treatment and acceptance of realistic goals; level of knowledge; readiness and willingness to learn

Nursing Care

☐ LONG-TERM GOAL

The patient will resume activities of daily living experiencing minimum discomfort; the patient will recover within the limitations of the medical regimen, free from preventable complications.

NURSING DIAGNOSIS #1

Fluid volume deficit related to diaphoresis, nausea and vomiting

Rationale: *Nausea and vomiting, NG suctioning, NPO status, and decreased or restricted fluid intake all potentiate fluid deficit. Fever and diaphoresis also promote fluid loss. Third space fluid shifts associated with severe capillary leakage and blood loss also occur. Fluid losses promote electrolyte abnormalities.*

☐ GOAL

The patient will maintain an adequate fluid balance.

IMPLEMENTATION

- Record vital signs every 2-4 hours; note postural changes in blood pressure; assess apical rate and rhythm changes; observe ECG monitor.
- Monitor and record intake and output; include solution used to irrigate NG tube, amount of diaphoresis, and ice-chip intake.
- Monitor for signs of fluid alterations; monitor central venous pressure and other hemodynamic measures if appropriate.
- Keep Foley catheter patent; monitor urine output every 2 hours and maintain 30 cc/hour output; report oliguria promptly so that it can be corrected, thus preventing development of renal failure.
- Administer blood and plasma to keep circulating volume adequate.
- Infuse IV electrolytes (Na^+, K^+, Cl^-) to prevent electrolyte deficit.
- Assess for hyperglycemia with blood and urine glucose tests; administer insulin to control temporary pancreatic glucagon hypersecretion.
- Observe, document, and report signs of hypocalcemia (from calcium binding with fatty acids that are eliminated in stool); have IV calcium gluconate and IV magnesium readily available to facilitate metabolism of calcium.

EVALUATION CRITERIA/DESIRED OUTCOMES

The Patient

- Maintains adequate hydration
- Has balanced intake and output
- Has electrolytes within normal limits

NURSING DIAGNOSIS #2

Alteration in comfort: pain related to inflammatory process

Rationale: *Severe pain is the most frequently occurring problem with pancreatitis. The autodigestion of the pancreas by pancreatic enzymes and the blockage of the pancreatic duct causes inflammation, necrosis, and pain.*

GOAL

The patient will be comfortable.

IMPLEMENTATION

- Assess the level of discomfort using a 0-10 point self-rating scale as objective measure of the pain.
- Document and report patient's complaints of left shoulder pain caused by inflammation of the tail of the pancreas.
- Assist patient to assume a position of comfort such as a side-lying, knee-chest position with a pillow pressed against abdomen, or a sitting position with the trunk flexed.
- Administer medication in timely manner; document patient's response to pain medications; know that most opiate narcotics cause spasms of the sphincter of Oddi, so meperidine (Demerol) is usually the analgesic of choice.
- Teach patient if possible to use appropriate pain-relieving techniques of distraction, visual imagery, deep-breathing, and muscle-relaxation exercises; refer to *The Patient Experiencing Pain,* page 180.
- Reinforce drug effectiveness and reassure that the appropriate drug, dosage, and frequency are being employed.
- Explain all tests and treatments; encourage questions and help patient/family express fears and feelings.

EVALUATION CRITERIA/DESIRED OUTCOMES

The Patient

- Verbalizes relief of or decrease in pain
- Demonstrates use of alternate pain-relief measures

NURSING DIAGNOSIS #3

Alteration in nutrition: less than body requirements related to nausea, vomiting

Rationale: *The primary objective in treating the pain of pancreatitis is to decrease the pancreatic enzymes responsible for autodigestion of the organ. These enzymes, however, are essential to normal digestion and function in the breakdown of food into its basic components. The lack of these enzymes for normal digestion, decreased peristalsis, and the persistence of pain all contribute to stimulation of the nausea and vomiting reflex.*

GOAL

The patient will be adequately nourished.

IMPLEMENTATION

- Give antispasmodic and anticholinergic drugs to reduce gastric and pancreatic secretions.
- Keep patient NPO to decrease intestinal stimulus to pancreatic secretion.
- Maintain patient on bedrest to decrease body metabolism.
- Monitor IV rate carefully; refer to *The Patient Receiving Total Parenteral Nutrition,* page 229, if ordered.
- Care for nasogastric (NG) tube; record color, amount, and characteristics of drainage; reassure that tube relieves distension and contributes to decreased pancreatic secretions.
- Keep mouth and nares clean and lubricated with water-soluble lubricant to prevent dryness, irritation, and infection; provide oral hygiene every 4 hours.
- Administer antacids via NG tube to diminish gastric hyperacidity.
- Assure gag reflex.
- Begin oral feedings slowly after removal of NG tube; give water in small amounts progressing slowly to a liquid diet so symptoms do not recur; evaluate and record patient response/progress.
- Assess bowel sounds and passage of flatus; report diarrhea, which can alter electrolyte balance rapidly
- Administer replacement pancreatic enzymes with meals to correct enzyme deficit and to aid in digestion.
- Monitor blood glucose levels (administration of small doses of glucocorticoids may result in hyperglycemia).
- Weigh patient on admission and daily.

EVALUATION CRITERIA/DESIRED OUTCOMES

The Patient

- Is free from nausea, vomiting
- Participates in appropriate dietary regimen
- Will maintain weight within 1-2 kg of normal

NURSING DIAGNOSIS #4

Potential for infection related to immobility, inflammatory processes, fluid accumulation

Rationale: *The inflammatory process of pancreatitis predisposes patient to infection. Pseudocysts, fistulae, and abscesses are common complications and must be monitored for early treatment and resolution. Immobility and pain predispose the patient to respiratory complications.*

GOAL

The patient will be free from infection.

IMPLEMENTATION

- Monitor temperature every 4 hours and report developing or persistent elevations.
- Observe all drainage tube insertion sites every 8 hours for redness, swelling, leakage, warmth, or tenderness; use aseptic technique when caring for each tube and insertion site.
- Restrict visitors and staff who have upper respiratory tract infections from patient's room.
- Assess respirations; observe for signs of hypoxemia; position patient for optimal ventilation when acute pain subsides; assist with intermittent positive pressure breathing treatments; ensure effective coughing and deep breathing exercises every 2 hours to prevent respiratory infection.
- Administer antibiotics to control or prevent infection; assess effectiveness and document side effects.
- Auscultate lungs for adventitious sounds every 2-4 hours and as necessary; document and report abnormal breath sounds.
- Auscultate bowel sounds for peristalsis every 4 hours and as necessary; check for passage of flatus and observe for abdominal distension that may indicate an ileus, abscess, or pseudocyst.
- Observe for hyperglycemia that may indicate a pseudocyst or abscess.

EVALUATION CRITERIA/DESIRED OUTCOMES

The Patient

- Has temperature less than 99°F (37.2°C)
- Has lungs clear to auscultation
- Has active bowel sounds; no distension

NURSING DIAGNOSIS #5

Knowledge deficit regarding causes of pancreatitis, treatment, possible complications

Rationale: *Pancreatitis is a recurring disease that requires compliance with treatment regimen to decrease possible complications and/or further extension of the disease.*

☐ GOAL

The patient/family will be knowledgeable about disease process.

☐ IMPLEMENTATION

- Instruct patient or teach family about patient need to abstain completely from alcoholic beverages in order to prevent recurrent attacks of pancreatitis.
- Teach signs and symptoms of recurrence so treatment can be sought quickly.
- Teach family about excess use of coffee, spicy foods, and heavy meals; instruct to eat frequent small meals that are bland and low in fat to decrease stimulation of pancreatic secretions.
- Instruct regarding a high-protein, low-fat, moderate-to high-carbohydrate diet; teach to avoid substances that stimulate the pancreas (e.g., caffeine, alcohol, spices, nicotine).
- Refer patient/family to community self-help groups (e.g., Alcoholics Anonymous).

☐ EVALUATION CRITERIA/DESIRED OUTCOMES

The Patient/family

- Verbalizes understanding of diet
- Lists medications
- Lists signs and symptoms of recurrence

The Patient Requiring Peritoneal Dialysis

Definition/Discussion

Peritoneal dialysis is the diffusion of solute molecules through a semipermeable membrane (the peritoneum) from the side of higher concentration (the patient's blood) to that of lower concentration (the dialysate). Fluids pass through the semipermeable membrane by means of osmosis. The purpose is to remove toxic substances, body wastes, and fluids that the kidney normally excretes, and to maintain life until kidney function is restored, if possible.

Peritoneal dialysis (PD) is based on two principles

- *diffusion:* the random movement of molecules, ions, or small particles in solution or suspension toward a uniform concentration throughout the available volume
- *osmosis:* the diffusion of a solution through a semipermeable membrane

The dialysate is removed repetitively and replaced with fresh solution in order to maintain a high mean diffusion gradient between body fluids and dialysate.

Prior to dialysis, a catheter is inserted into the peritoneal cavity by a physician under strict aseptic technique (a signed operative permit is necessary). A Teflon catheter is used in intermittent PD and is removed following the PD treatment; for continuous PD, the catheter is made of silastic with a Dacron felt cuff (bacterial barrier) and has an average life of 9 months.

Dialysis is accomplished by repeating a 3-phase cycle. Each cycle includes

- *inflow:* the time it takes for the dialysate to flow into the peritoneal cavity by gravity (usually 10-15 minutes)
- *diffusion or dialysis:* the time that the dialysate is in contact with the peritoneal cavity (usually 30-40 minutes)
- *outflow:* the time it takes the dialysate to drain from the peritoneal cavity by gravity (usually 15-20 minutes)

Four common methods may be used

- *manual single-bottle method:* the catheter is attached to Y-tubing and prescribed fluid (usually 1-2 liter sterile dialyzing solution warmed to body temperature) is run in by gravity; the tubing is clamped just before the bottle or bag is empty (inflow phase); the dialysate remains in the peritoneal cavity until a degree of equilibrium between the dialysate and body fluids is achieved (diffusion or dialysis phase); the bottle or bag is lowered to the floor, the tubing unclamped, and the fluid drains out (outflow phase)
- *automatic PD system* (multiple cycler/reverse osmosis machine): this machine composes, sterilizes, and cycles the dialysate through the three phases; monitors and alarms are incorporated into the system. In either the manual or automatic method, the fluid exchange is repeated until blood chemistries are nearing normal, usually 36-48 hours (30-40 exchanges), and may be done as often as 3 times/week.
- *continuous ambulatory peritoneal dialysis (CAPD):* a prescribed amount of dialysate is connected to the *permanent* catheter and allowed to flow into the abdomen (inflow phase); the catheter is then clamped and the dialysate allowed to dwell for 4-5 hours (diffusion or dialysis phase). During this time the empty dialysate bag is folded and kept on the patient. After diffusion, the empty dialysate bag is lowered to a clean surface (usually a paper towel on the floor), unclamped, and the dialysate is allowed to flow out by gravity (outflow phase). The process is then repeated with new dialysate 3-5 cycles a day, 7 days a week. During the night cycle the dialysate is allowed to dwell 7-8 hours.
- *continuous cycling peritoneal dialysis (CCPD):* this method is basically a reversal of CAPD exchanges. CCPD does cycles during the

night with a simple cycling machine and the long dwell (diffusion or dialysis phase) during the day, which affords the patient much more personal freedom for day activity.

Peritoneal dialysis is superior to hemodialysis in that it requires a simple technique with no sophisticated equipment. However, it takes longer than hemodialysis and has increased risks for peritoneal and pulmonary infection and large albumin/protein loss. Peritoneal dialysis is contraindicated with bleeding or recent abdominal surgery.

Nursing Assessment

☐ PERTINENT HISTORY

Hyperkalemia, hypertension, hepatic coma, fluid overload, severe acidosis, severe edema, uremia, mental confusion, acute or chronic renal failure, drug poisoning, fatigue, headache, sleep difficulty; pruritus

☐ PHYSICAL FINDINGS

Congestive heart failure, pulmonary edema, hypotension/hypertension, rales, dyspnea; anorexia, metallic taste in mouth, ascites, uremic breath; oliguria, protein uria, increased urinary specific gravity and osmolality; anemia; short attention span, confusion, possible convulsions and coma; peripheral neuropathy (numbness, twitching, paresthesia); nystagmus; periorbital edema, rash, petechiae, ecchymosis; dryness, yellow bronzing, pallor of skin; uremic frost; resistance to infection; delayed wound healing; joint pain, loss of muscle mass; impotence, amenorrhea, infertility, decreased libido; increased BUN, increased creatinine, increased serum ammonia, increased uric acid, increased K^+, decreased Ca^{++}, increased phosphorus, increased Na^+ (may be decreased also), increased magnesium, increased albumin/casts in urine, increased levels of nephrotoxic drugs; acidosis, abnormal glucose tolerance; abnormal clotting times, decreased hemoglobin/hematocrit, decreased serum albumin levels, increased lipids; liver function test may be abnormal

☐ PSYCHOSOCIAL CONCERNS/ DEVELOPMENTAL FACTORS

Denial, anxiety, depression, personality changes, irritability; intermittent changes in memory/attention span (associated with elevated blood ammonia levels) may be particularly distressing to the patient; adaptation to body-image change, changed role in family, finances

☐ PATIENT AND FAMILY KNOWLEDGE

Disease and prognosis, support systems, treatment options, complications, home health maintenance regimen; level of knowledge, readiness and willingness to learn

Nursing Care

☐ LONG-TERM GOAL

The patient will adhere to prescribed regimen to aid recovery from the acute renal failure and to return to usual roles; OR the patient will adapt to the reality of long-term dialysis and will live within its accompanying limitations.

NURSING DIAGNOSIS #1

Anxiety related to fear of procedure

Rationale: *Lack of knowledge and not knowing what to expect leads to increased anxiety. Preprocedure explanation and question/answer periods have a calming effect on the patient and promote comfort. The nurse-patient relationship is also strengthened during this time.*

☐ GOAL

The patient will verbalize statements reflective of decreased anxiety.

☐ IMPLEMENTATION

- Explain each step of procedure; answer all questions as honestly as you can.
- Assess affect and mental status before dialysis; know that a dependence on the health team is established and that patient may respond with a variety of feelings; all can be considered adaptive except suicidal tendencies; refer to *The Patient with Chronic Renal Failure,* page 78.
- Recognize that questions about the procedure and necessary life-style changes are a sign of adaptation; when this occurs, it is important to provide information and to work with the patient to bring about changes.
- Plan care with patient, encouraging involvement as much as possible; if patient has been

dialyzed previously, ask what you can do to enhance comfort during this dialysis.

- Assess patient's support system, knowledge of procedure; provide as much information as patient requests and needs to know; speak in calm, reassuring tones; let patient know how long and at what times a nurse will be at patient's side.
- Emphasize that a variety of feelings and emotions are usual and expected in the adaptation process.
- Consult social worker, clergy, or mental health worker as needed.

☐ EVALUATION CRITERIA/DESIRED OUTCOMES

The Patient

- Verbalizes reduced anxiety about treatment

NURSING DIAGNOSIS #2

Alteration in comfort: pain related to dialysate in abdomen

Rationale: *The volume (3,000 cc) of dialysate may cause abdominal distension and create a feeling of pressure on abdominal organs. The dialysate may cause a chemical irritation; the peritoneal catheter may be malpositioned. Infection in the peritoneum will also cause pain.*

☐ GOAL

The patient will verbalize feelings of relative comfort during procedure.

☐ IMPLEMENTATION

- Assess for pain or discomfort during inflow and diffusion phases; have patient describe the timing and type of pain on a 0-10 point self-rating scale.
- Administer frequent back rubs, massage pressure areas, and change patient's position as needed; (during infusion, patient is usually supine with head slightly elevated to decrease discomfort of the abdominal organs pushing up against the diaphragm).
- Warm dialysate to core temperature before instilling into peritoneum.
- Check with physician to see if lidocaine can be ordered to be put in dialysate solution.
- Assure patient that feeling of fullness lessens after first few exchanges.
- Administer analgesic when indicated; monitor for effectiveness and side effects.
- Make certain that complete solution drainage is occurring.
- Notify physician for continuing pain.

☐ EVALUATION CRITERIA/DESIRED OUTCOMES

The Patient

- States absence of or decreasing discomfort during procedure
- Tolerates procedure comfortably

NURSING DIAGNOSIS #3

Potential for injury (bowel, bladder, vessel perforation) related to catheter insertion

Rationale: *The insertion site of the peritoneal catheter is 1-2 inches below the umbilicus and may perforate the bowel, bladder, or a blood vessel.*

☐ GOAL

The patient will remain free from or be promptly treated for any potential complications of peritoneal catheter insertion.

☐ IMPLEMENTATION

- Have patient void before catheter insertion; monitor for indications of bladder perforation (e.g., large amounts of urine output [urine + dialysate] with high glucose level, strong urge to urinate frequently).
- Be alert to signs of bowel perforation (e.g., fecal material in returning dialysate fluid, strong urge to have bowel movement; sudden decrease in blood pressure, tachycardia).
- Assess for vessel perforation by checking returning dialysate fluid for blood; the first few returns may have some blood because of rupture of superficial capillaries during catheter insertion, but then should be clear.
- Contact physician immediately should any of the above noted signs/symptoms be present.
- Monitor vital signs every 4-8 hours or as needed.

☐ EVALUATION CRITERIA/DESIRED OUTCOMES

The Patient

- Exhibits no signs of bowel, bladder or vessel perforation; dialysate solution is clear

---

NURSING DIAGNOSIS #4

a. **Fluid volume deficit** related to rapid removal of intravascular fluid

b. **Alteration in fluid volume: excess** related to fluid retention secondary to catheter problems (kinks, blockages)

Rationale: *Dialysate solutions are hypertonic (1.5% and 4.25% glucose), causing an osmotic gradient for fluid through the peritoneal membrane and may result in too rapid removal of fluid from the blood volume. Mechanical problems with catheter drainage may cause fluid retention and fluid overload.*

☐ GOAL

The patient will maintain fluid balance.

☐ IMPLEMENTATION

- Record baseline assessment of weight and vital signs; weigh after dialysis to check on fluid loss.
- Check vital signs when each outflow begins and ends.
- Do not administer antihypertensive medications during dialysis.
- Check urinary output hourly.
- If patient is slightly hypotensive, turn on side to decrease pressure on vena cava.
- Assess and record patient's hydration status prior to each dialysis by analyzing weight, skin turgor, thirst, mucous membrane moisture, intake and output, and edema; select tonicity of dialysate, as ordered, according to physician's or agency's protocol.
- Keep an accurate recording of patient's fluid exchange balance; for each exchange, record essential exchange times on flow sheet (time infusion started and ended, time outflow begins and ends, amount of solution infused and returned, computed balance—usually a plus or minus amount).
- Describe and record dialysate color and clarity; report any cloudy outflow to physician.
- If fluid does not drain in a steady stream, apply firm pressure to lower abdomen and ask patient to turn from side to side.
- Check with physician regarding amount of oral fluids permitted; accurately record intake and output.

☐ EVALUATION CRITERIA/DESIRED OUTCOMES

The Patient

- Remains in homeostasis as evidenced by normal vital signs and hydration status

---

NURSING DIAGNOSIS #5

Potential for infection related to possible contamination through direct access of peritoneal cavity, chemical irritation from dialysate solution

Rationale: *Infection is the major complication in peritoneal dialysis. There may be contamination during catheter insertion, during instillation of dialysate, or around catheter insertion site. Chemicals in the dialysate may also irritate the peritoneum significantly to start an infection leading to peritonitis (sterile peritonitis).*

☐ GOAL

The patient will remain free from peritonitis.

☐ IMPLEMENTATION

- Maintain strict aseptic technique at all times (e.g., dressing, peritoneal catheter care, skin care).
- Monitor continuously for signs of infection (e.g., increased temperature, increased white blood cell count, cloudy dialysate, persistent abdominal pain).
- Check site for redness and drainage.
- Administer antibiotics as ordered; monitor for effectiveness and toxicity.
- Observe for septic shock (e.g., tachycardia, decreased blood pressure, narrowing pulse pressure, tachypnea).

☐ EVALUATION CRITERIA/DESIRED OUTCOMES

The Patient

- Has a normal temperature
- Returns clear dialysate
- Is free from significant pain

NURSING DIAGNOSIS #6

Alteration in bowel elimination: constipation related to decreased peristalsis secondary to abdominal distention during dwell time

Rationale: *Peritoneal catheter and chemicals in dialysate may cause enough irritation to decrease or stop bowel activity.*

☐ GOAL

The patient will have normal bowel activity.

☐ IMPLEMENTATION

- Assess for bowel sounds, bowel movements, abdominal distension, increased nasogastric output prior to dialysis and during inflow and diffusion phases.
- Keep patient NPO if ileus is present.
- Have patient change positions and/or ambulate to decrease distension.
- If medications given to encourage peristalsis, evaluate effectiveness.

☐ EVALUATION CRITERIA/DESIRED OUTCOMES

The Patient

- Has normal bowel sounds, at least 3-4 bowel movements/week

NURSING DIAGNOSIS #7

Alteration in nutrition: less than body requirements related to excessive protein loss through dialysis outflow, anorexia secondary to abdominal distension, vomiting after too rapid instillation of dialysate

Rationale: *One of the disadvantages of peritoneal dialysis is the excessive protein loss through the semipermeable membrane. The presence of the dialysate in the peritoneal cavity may cause abdominal distension and feelings of fullness with resultant decreased appetite. Rapid instillation of dialysates, especially after meals, may cause vomiting with further loss of nutrients.*

☐ GOAL

The patient will maintain adequate nutrition.

☐ IMPLEMENTATION

- Monitor serum albumin levels daily or as ordered.
- Administer salt-poor albumin if prescribed.
- Provide protein supplements to diet.
- Plan meals to allow for approximately 2 hours absorption time prior to instillation of dialysate.
- Review foods allowed on diet; instruct as needed.

☐ EVALUATION CRITERIA/DESIRED OUTCOMES

The Patient

- Has normal serum albumin levels
- Maintains appetite and adequate nutritional intake
- Is free from vomiting

NURSING DIAGNOSIS #8

a. **Ineffective breathing patterns** related to pressure on diaphragm while dialysate fluid in abdomen
b. **Impaired gas exchange** related to ineffective breathing pattern
c. **Potential for infection** related to ineffective breathing pattern, impaired physical mobility

Rationale: *With 2,000 cc dialysate fluid in the abdomen, there may be sufficient pressure on the diaphragm to decrease inspiratory depth. Atelectasis/pneumonia may develop; the likelihood for these complications is increased by the necessity for limited mobility during dwell time.*

☐ GOAL

The patient will remain free from respiratory complications associated with peritoneal dialysis.

☐ IMPLEMENTATION

- Place patient in semi-Fowler's position.
- Turn and deep breathe every 2 hours.
- Have patient use inspirometer every hour while awake.

- Auscultate breath sounds every 2 hours.
- Check vital signs every 2 hours.
- Administer oxygen if appropriate.
- Note amount, color of respiratory secretions.
- Monitor chest films if indicated.

☐ EVALUATION CRITERIA/DESIRED OUTCOMES

The Patient

- Has no dyspnea
- Exhibits normal respiration and breath sounds
- Expectorates clear respiratory secretions easily

NURSING DIAGNOSIS #9

Knowledge deficit regarding treatment procedure, care of the catheter

Rationale: *Patient cooperation is needed to promote compliance and to prevent complications. Lack of understanding of treatment interferes with compliance.*

☐ GOAL

The patient will verbalize understanding of procedure and possible complications; the patient (with a permanent catheter) will demonstrate aseptic technique with catheter care.

☐ IMPLEMENTATION

- Instruct in all potential complications; give telephone number of physician and dialysis center, and explain when to call.
- If patient is on long-term dialysis, periodically review prescribed regimens to assess degree of compliance; praise all positive efforts and discuss areas for improvement.
- Teach aseptic catheter care and dialysis protocol to patient who goes home with indwelling peritoneal catheter; have patient return demonstration.
- Listen to patient's explanations, problems, and feelings; work out solutions with patient.

☐ EVALUATION CRITERIA/DESIRED OUTCOMES

The Patient

- States understanding of procedure and complications in own words
- Demonstrates proper catheter care

The Patient with Pneumonia

Definition/Discussion

Pneumonia is inflammation of the pulmonary air sacs with resultant filling of the alveoli with an exudate. Pneumonias are usually classified in terms of their etiology (either bacterial or nonbacterial [i.e., viral, fungal, chemical]) or structural distribution (*lobar pneumonia:* involvement of the entire lobe, *segmental or lobular pneumonia:* involvement of a portion of a lobe, or *bronchopneumonia:* involvement only of alveoli adjacent to the bronchi). Pneumonia is the fifth leading cause of death, especially in the very young and elderly. It is often seen coexisting with another disease, commonly alcoholism or influenza. When combined with the latter, it is the leading cause of death in infectious diseases. The causative organisms are around us all the time and are carried by droplet infection or contact with infected persons or carriers. Pneumonia generally occurs when body resistance is lowered, when a person is exposed to a large concentration of particularly virulent organisms, or by any bronchial obstruction associated with mucus formation. Every patient on bedrest is a potential candidate for hypostatic pneumonia.

Nursing Assessment

☐ PERTINENT HISTORY

Life-style patterns (e.g., smoking, nutrition, exercise); recent surgery; exposure to cold or dampness

☐ PHYSICAL FINDINGS

Shaking chills; fever (102°-104°F/39°-40°C); pleuritic chest pain; cough productive of greenish, purulent, blood-tinged sputum; rapid, shallow respirations; restricted mobility of the chest on affected side; nausea and vomiting; cyanotic nailbeds

☐ PSYCHOSOCIAL CONCERNS/ DEVELOPMENTAL FACTORS

Possible increased dependency or depression/ anxiety regarding disease-imposed changes upon usual role/life-style

☐ PATIENT AND FAMILY KNOWLEDGE

High-risk factors, strategies to reduce risks/recurrence, level of knowledge, readiness and willingness to learn

Nursing Care

☐ LONG-TERM GOAL

The patient will recover free from complications; will resume usual life roles in home, job, and community.

NURSING DIAGNOSIS #1

a. **Ineffective airway clearance** related to inflammation of respiratory passages, increased pulmonary secretions
b. **Impaired gas exchange** related to consolidation of lung tissue
c. **Ineffective breathing pattern** (shallow, rapid respirations) related to perceived "air hunger"

Rationale: *Ventilation is impaired because of secretions from exudate in the alveoli. Secretions need to be mobilized, loosened, and expectorated in order to provide an adequate gas exchange. Unless secretions are removed, the alveoli become/remain filled with exudate, causing consolidation of lung tissue and further interfering with gas exchange. In a hypoxic state, the individual becomes restless and anxious about the inability to obtain* *enough air and increases the rate of respiration to compensate. The increased rate, however, is likely to be ineffective in promoting oxygenation of body tissues as the respirations are shallow and inadequate gas exchange takes place.*

☐ GOAL

The patient will maintain a patent airway; will raise and expectorate pulmonary secretions; will regain adequate pulmonary ventilation.

☐ IMPLEMENTATION

- Monitor respiratory status every 2 hours; assess for increased rate/effort and abnormal breath sounds (inspiratory rales are present early in disease and should diminish as patient improves; increasing dullness indicates consolidation of lung tissue); notify physician of abnormal findings.
- Keep head of bed elevated; place patient on side with one pillow lengthwise to support entire back and to help expand chest.
- Turn every 1-2 hours; have patient cough and try to raise mucus at least every hour; splint chest with your hands to minimize pain; if unable to raise mucus, suction as needed; do cough routine one-half hour after giving pain medication; instruct to expectorate, not swallow mucus.
- Monitor arterial blood gases (ABGs) to assess oxygenation status.
- Administer oxygen as ordered; assist with intermittent positive pressure breathing and postural drainage as necessary; prevent smoking in room, even if patient not on oxygen.
- Monitor for indications of respiratory failure (e.g., depressed respiration, increased restlessness, confusion or abnormal ABGs); prepare for possible intubation and mechanical ventilation (refer to *The Patient Who is Ventilator-Dependent,* page 239).
- Explain cause of dyspnea and the expected outcome (should feel better in 24-72 hours).
- Check blood cultures and sputum cultures/sensitivity results; identify pathogen and check whether ordered antibiotic is sensitive to it; notify physician if discrepancy exists and obtain new antibiotic order.

☐ EVALUATION CRITERIA/DESIRED OUTCOMES

The Patient

- Has pink nailbeds and lips
- Expectorates secretions
- Breathes easily 20-30 times/minute

NURSING DIAGNOSIS #2

a. **Alteration in comfort: pain** related to pleuritic changes in chest
b. **Anxiety** related to physical effects of pneumonia

Rationale: *Patient comfort is important in order to enable the patient to participate fully in own care. Pleuritic chest pain can cause the patient to remain in one position, and not to take deep breaths or to cough. The physical effects associated with pneumonia (e.g., altered respiration, dyspnea, purulent or bloodtinged sputum) may be distressing to the patient/family.*

☐ GOAL

The patient will be free from pleuritic chest pain; will have adequate rest and sleep. The patient/family will have decreased level of anxiety.

☐ IMPLEMENTATION

- Monitor for expressed complaints of pain and behaviors (e.g., grimacing, splinting) indicative of pain (some patients may try to mask symptoms of pain); refer to *The Patient Experiencing Pain,* page 180.
- Assess the level of discomfort using a 0-10 point self-rating scale to obtain an objective measure.
- Give analgesics and sedatives as ordered; observe for depressed respirations; monitor for effectiveness.
- Plan and coordinate care with other disciplines to allow patient uninterrupted rest periods.
- Assess anxiety and fear (normally of choking, dying); assure patient you will be checking on him/her at least every 30 minutes to observe breathing.
- Know that abdomen and front shoulder pain often accompany early pneumonia; explain and reassure that they will subside.
- Explain that coughing up blood is common

after the first few days of unproductive coughing and does not mean worsening of condition.

☐ EVALUATION CRITERIA/DESIRED OUTCOMES

The Patient

- Expresses decreased/controlled pain
- Rests quietly

NURSING DIAGNOSIS #3

Fluid volume deficit related to fever

Rationale: *Increased metabolic demands from the disease process, fever, and diaphoresis can lead to dehydration.*

☐ GOAL

The patient will maintain a normal fluid balance.

☐ IMPLEMENTATION

- Monitor temperature, blood pressure and pulse at least every 4 hours; report increased temperature and pulse or decreased blood pressure to physician.
- Provide cooling measures (e.g., sponge baths, cooling blanket) for temperature over 102°F (39°C).
- Check linens for dampness (from perspirations) and change as necessary; protect patient from chilling.
- Give antibiotics on time in order to maintain blood levels; watch for sensitivity; report patient responses to physician.
- Record intake and output; assess for adequate urinary output, daily bowel movement.
- Monitor hydration status; insensible fluid loss will be high from fever, dyspnea, and diaphoresis; ensure high fluid intake within limits of patient's cardiac reserve (if no restrictions, 2-3 liters/day).
- Assess for indications of common complications associated with fluid volume deficit: abdominal distension (e.g., gaseous distension, tense abdomen, dull and diffuse pain) and paralytic ileus (e.g., depressed peristalsis, infrequent bowel sounds, vomiting after meals).
- Monitor for signs of other complications (e.g., pleural effusion, lung abscess, sustained hypotension and shock, meningitis, and congestive heart failure).
- Be aware that restlessness may precede delirium; withhold sedatives and check with physician; monitor patients with alcoholism or any chronic pulmonary problems carefully.
- Monitor laboratory results (e.g., BUN, hematocrit, electrolytes); report abnormal findings to physician.
- Refer to Table 1, *Common Fluid and Electrolyte Imbalances,* page 14, for additional interventions.

☐ EVALUATION CRITERIA/DESIRED OUTCOMES

The Patient

- Maintains adequate hydration
- Is afebrile
- Remains free from abdominal distension, constipation

The Patient with a Pneumothorax

Definition/Discussion

A pneumothorax is a life-threatening situation wherein air enters the pleural cavity causing a lung to collapse partially or completely on the affected side, resulting in a reduction in tidal volume and gas exchange. Medical treatment depends on the etiology, size, and duration of the pneumothorax. Small leaks (less than 20%) require no treatment beyond restricted activity, oxygen therapy, and cough suppression. Larger leaks require insertion of one or more chest tubes, which are then connected to a water-seal drainage system. Types of pneumothorax include

- *spontaneous*: the chest wall remains intact, but air enters the pleural cavity through a break in the surface of the lung (alveoli), thereby separating the two pleural layers
- *traumatic*: air entry results from an injury to the chest wall; *open pneumothorax* or penetrating injury (also called a sucking-chest wound) refers to wounds caused by stabbing, bullets, or other projectiles; *closed pneumothorax* or nonpenetrating injury can be caused by fractured ribs, electric shock, drowning, etc.
- *tension*: air enters the pleural cavity during inspiration and cannot escape with expiration (e.g., a persistent bronchopleural air leak); the increased intrathoracic pressure also affects the expansion of the unaffected lung. This is an emergency and requires immediate intervention (i.e., chest tubes) to prevent acute respiratory and circulatory impairment.

Medical treatment aims to establish a clear airway and ensure adequate alveolar ventilation to restore normal cardiopulmonary function as rapidly as possible. Diagnostic measures (chest x-ray, arterial blood gases [ABGs]) are delayed until the patient's condition becomes more stable. A spontaneous pneumothorax may resolve itself or, if patient has respiratory distress, a single chest tube will be inserted. To relieve a tension pneumothorax, a large-bore needle or dart may be inserted into the intercostal space until a chest tube can be inserted and connected to closed drainage.

Chest tube placement involves the insertion of one or more tubes through the chest wall and into the pleural space. Pleural chest tubes provide an outlet to evacuate air and/or fluid from the pleural space while preventing their return. A chest tube inserted for the removal of air will usually be inserted in the upper aspect of the anterior chest wall. A chest tube inserted to remove fluid will usually be inserted in the middle to lower aspect of the lateral chest wall. A chest tube may also be placed within the thoracic cavity to serve as a drain, as with mediastinal chest tubes that are commonly inserted following open heart surgery. Four types of drainage systems are available

- One-bottle system: commonly used in emergencies; the drainage goes directly into the bottle, which serves as both a collecting chamber and water seal; it is not recommended for the evacuation of fluid.
- Two-bottle system: provides an extra bottle for the separate collection of fluid directly from the patient. The drainage bottle is connected to the water-seal bottle, providing for release of air into the second bottle.
- Three-bottle system: provides separate bottles for collection of drainage, a water seal, and suction. Air from the pleural space passes through the collection and water seal bottles and is suctioned out. The fluid drainage remains in the collection bottle and does not interfere with the water-seal level.
- Disposable systems (e.g., Pleur-Evac, Thoradrain): contain all three chambers in one system; these function similarly to the three-bottle system.

Open chest wounds are immediately covered with an occlusive petrolatum gauze dressing. Seal-ing these open wounds can create a tension pneumothorax. If the patient's condition worsens, the dressing is removed.

Nursing Assessment

PERTINENT HISTORY

Recent accident or injury; life-style (e.g., alcohol or drug use, cigarette smoking); idiopathic (often young, tall, thin, healthy adult males), pathologic factors (carcinoma, pneumonia, tuberculosis, other infections, bronchitis, emphysema, asthma), iatrogenic effects (intermittent positive pressure breathing).

PHYSICAL FINDINGS

Severe, sharp, knife-like pain on affected side of chest; sudden shortness of breath worsening on exertion; diminished and delayed chest wall expansion; diminished or absent breath sounds, hyperresonant percussion on affected side; fall in blood pressure, weak rapid pulse, restlessness, diaphoresis, pallor, or cyanosis; decreased pO_2 and blood pH; decreased level of consciousness (symptoms depend on size of pneumothorax or extent of disease)

PSYCHOSOCIAL CONCERNS/ DEVELOPMENTAL FACTORS

Depression, increased dependency, altered roles; anxiety and fear of the unknown (unfamiliar hospital setting)

PATIENT AND FAMILY KNOWLEDGE

Possible cause, diagnostic and therapeutic measures; level of knowledge, readiness and willingness to learn

Nursing Care

LONG-TERM GOAL

The patient will achieve adequate lung reexpansion; the patient will return to a stable physical condition, adhering to a prescribed medical regimen designed to prevent recurrences.

NURSING DIAGNOSIS #1

a. **Ineffective breathing pattern** related to air in pleural cavity

b. **Impaired gas exchange** related to air in pleural cavity

Rationale: *Any pleural compromise can alter normal respiratory pattern and ventilation.*

GOAL

The patient will maintain effective pulmonary functioning.

IMPLEMENTATION

- Monitor for signs and symptoms of decreasing pulmonary function (e.g., dyspnea and other signs of respiratory distress, tachycardia, restlessness, anxiety, absent or decreased breath sounds on affected side, asymmetric chest movement [mediastinal shift], tracheal deviation, subcutaneous emphysema in neck and upper chest, sucking sound near open wound, cyanosis [late sign]); report significant findings to physician; prepare for possible intubation and mechanical ventilation (refer to *The Patient with Asthma,* page 32).
- Take vital signs every 30 minutes for 2 hours or until stable, then every 4 hours; report signs of shock, increasing respiratory distress, or exhaustion to physician.
- Place in a sitting position, supported by pillows to allow greater ventilatory efficiency; maintain a calm, unhurried manner to lessen anxiety.
- Monitor ABGs and observe for indications of hypoxia (e.g., confusion, drowsiness) and hypercapnia (e.g., elevated pCO_2); inform physician of patient status.
- Give oxygen via nasal catheter to relieve hypoxia and dyspnea (use with caution in patients with chronic obstructive pulmonary disease); if mechanical ventilation is used to ensure adequate alveolar ventilation, monitor settings and equipment carefully.
- Be prepared to assist with emergency measures at bedside if insertion of chest tubes cannot be done in surgery.
- Observe and note amount and type of chest drainage (should diminish steadily and change from sanguinous to serosanguinous to serous); record findings every 8-12 hours.
- Supervise regular deep-breathing and coughing exercises every 4 hours.
- Assist with removal of chest tube when no

longer needed; cleanse skin and apply dry, sterile, occlusive, petrolatum gauze dressing.

☐ EVALUATION CRITERIA/DESIRED OUTCOMES

The Patient

- Has regular respirations of 16-24/minute
- Maintains normal blood gases
- Shows no signs of respiratory distress

NURSING DIAGNOSIS #2

a. **Potential for infection** related to impaired skin integrity at chest tube insertion site, limited physical activity
b. **Impairment of skin integrity** related to limited physical activity

Rationale: *At the chest tube insertion site, the skin as a protective barrier is impaired, creating portal of entry for infectious organisms. Moreover, prescribed bedrest further increases the risk of infection as pulmonary secretions may pool and pneumonia develop. Additionally, decreased physical activity predisposes the patient to impaired skin integrity because of prolonged pressure over bony prominences.*

☐ GOAL

The patient will remain free from infection and impaired skin integrity.

☐ IMPLEMENTATION

- Monitor for signs of local (e.g., swelling, redness, warmth, tenderness to touch) and systemic (e.g., elevated temperature, decreased blood pressure, increased pulse and respirations) infection; review laboratory reports of cultures and sensitivities ordered.
- Inspect all skin surfaces every 8-12 hours, checking pressure points carefully; watch for signs of impaired circulation (e.g., pallor, delayed capillary refilling), pooling (e.g., redness, edema), or impaired tissue integrity (e.g., abrasions, ulcers); modify environment (e.g., use egg-crate or alternating pressure mattress, sheepskin, pillows/blankets for positioning).
- Maintain strict asepsis when assisting with insertion of chest tube and changing dressings; ensure that all connections are taped securely.
- Administer prophylactic antibiotics as ordered; monitor for effectiveness and toxicity; report patient responses to physician.
- Keep skin clean, dry, and pressure free over bony prominences; assist patient to modify position as needed to promote adequate circulation.
- Move arm on affected side, do range-of-motion exercises several times a day; increase as tolerated.
- Apply antiembolic stockings as ordered; remove for 15 minutes every 8 hours; inspect skin underneath before reapplying.

☐ EVALUATION CRITERIA/DESIRED OUTCOMES

The Patient

- Has no signs of local or systemic infection
- Maintains an intact, dry skin

NURSING DIAGNOSIS #3

a. **Anxiety** related to dyspnea, pain
b. **Knowledge deficit** regarding condition and treatment

Rationale: *Lack of knowledge about the disease process and treatment can provoke feelings of fear and anxiety. If these feelings go unrecognized the patient may experience an increase in severity of already preexisting symptoms. It is important to provide comfort and a low-stress environment for the patient; when comfort is promoted, pain and anxiety are reduced.*

☐ GOAL

The patient will verbalize and demonstrate a reduction in anxiety; will verbalize a decrease in dyspnea and pain.

☐ IMPLEMENTATION

- Plan 10-15 minutes daily to listen to patient/family concerns/feelings.
- Explain to patient/family the cause of dyspnea and pneumothorax and that reexpansion of lung usually occurs in 48-72 hours.
- Administer analgesics and sedatives as ordered PRN; evaluate effectiveness.
- Explain all procedures and treatment before carrying them out.
- Promote undisturbed rest to decrease meta-

bolic demands and thus decrease the dyspnea and anxiety.
- Assess specific learning needs and initiate individualized teaching plan.

☐ EVALUATION CRITERIA/DESIRED OUTCOMES

The Patient

- Expresses reduction of anxiety
- Has control of pain
- Verbalizes understanding of condition and treatment

NURSING DIAGNOSIS #4

Impaired gas exchange related to collapsed lung, mediastinal shift

Rationale: *Chest tubes may easily become nonfunctional if they are disconnected, kinked, or occluded by a fibrin clot. An air leak will cause an increased amount of bubbling in the water-seal chamber, which will not fluctuate if the tubing is obstructed. A continued air leak or persistent build up of fluid will result in alterations in intrapleural pressures.*

☐ GOAL

The patient will have easy, unlabored respirations of 20-30/minute; will have patent chest tube(s) with no obstruction.

☐ IMPLEMENTATION

- Make certain that all tubing is open and draining; check to see if water is fluctuating in the glass tube in drainage bottle.
- Milk the chest tube every 15 minutes immediately postoperatively until bleeding is stable or minimal, then at least 3 times daily or as needed; this will help push any clots or fibrin down the lumen, thus assuring patency.
- Check all connections for leaks; tape them securely.
- Check bubbling in water-seal chamber for presence of increased bubbling, suggestive of an air leak; if air leak detected/suspected, check for loose connections anywhere within the system: retape or reinforce taped connections; **do not clamp tube as this may put the patient at risk of tension pneumothorax;** notify physician; milk tubing, beginning close to insertion site and moving downward until the source is found; if disconnection is not evident and air leak is present, the bubbling will stop when tube is compressed below the air leak.
- Check insertion site if unable to find air leak in tubing: put gentle pressure on site; if bubbling stops, seal area with petrolatum gauze; know that the chest tube may be dislodged in the subcutaneous tissue and require reinsertion by physician.
- Replace drainage unit if leak cannot be found
Replace drainage unit if leak cannot be found
at site or in tubing; notify physician if problem is not resolved.
- Use proper safety precautions at all times
  - place bottles in a stand or other device to prevent them from being turned over or broken
  - ensure protection of collection unit during portable x-ray, when visitors present, etc.
  - clamp bottle tops or tape them securely, with a warning not to empty them (never empty bottles unless specifically ordered by the physician)
  - keep at least one clamp large enough to clamp chest tube attached to patient's bed sheet (on same side as tube); if bottle should break or fall over, clamp chest tube at once to prevent air from being sucked
at once to prevent air from being sucked
into pleural cavity; notify surgeon immediately and prepare another set-up
  - ensure chest bottles are kept below the level of the patient's chest if necessary to move patient's bed
  - never set bottles on the bed (water may run into patient's pleural cavity)
  - assist patient in ambulating to bathroom or transferring to a chair
- Explain that chest tubes usually stay in place for 48 hours, and that patient will have less discomfort in chest wall after removal.

☐ EVALUATION CRITERIA/DESIRED OUTCOMES

The Patient

- Breathes in a normal respiratory pattern
- Maintains integrity of water-seal drainage

The Patient with Pulmonary Edema

Definition/Discussion

Pulmonary edema exists when hydrostatic pressure in the pulmonary capillaries exceeds the intravascular osmotic pressure. This causes a life-threatening situation where fluid from congested lungs leaks through the capillary walls into the alveoli resulting in respiratory distress. Pulmonary edema is an extreme form of left-sided heart failure. A weakened left ventricle is unable to circulate sufficient blood to the body, while the right ventricle continues to pump blood into the lungs, resulting in lung congestion. Medical treatment aims at assisting respiratory function while correcting the underlying problem, congestive heart failure (CHF). Mechanical ventilation, hemodynamic monitoring, intra-aortic balloon pumping, or phlebotomy may be required, depending on the severity of the condition. Refer to *The Patient with Congestive Heart Failure,* page 88, and *The Patient with Cardiogenic Shock,* page 64.

Nursing Assessment

☐ PERTINENT HISTORY

Precipitating events leading to pulmonary edema (disease processes such as acute left ventricular failure, acute myocardial infarction, chronic CHF, mitral valve disease, central nervous system injuries, circulatory overload, hypertension)

☐ PHYSICAL FINDINGS

Severe dyspnea, tachypnea, orthopnea; frothy, pink-tinged sputum; bubbling rales; diaphoresis; tachycardia; anxiety; cyanosis, and cold, moist hands

☐ PSYCHOSOCIAL CONCERNS/ DEVELOPMENTAL FACTORS

Anxiety, fear of suffocation; most common in older adults with existing chronic diseases; lifestyle changes required to decrease risk of recurrence

☐ PATIENT AND FAMILY KNOWLEDGE

Current situation and prognosis; diet, medications, and activity needs related to precipitating causes; level of knowledge; readiness and willingness to learn

Nursing Care

☐ LONG-TERM GOAL

The patient will return to a stable physical condition, adhering to prescribed medical regimen designed to prevent recurrences; the patient will maintain adequate oxygenation and ventilation; hemodynamic stability will remain constant.

NURSING DIAGNOSIS #1

a. **Impaired gas exchange** related to accumulation of fluid in the alveoli
b. **Ineffective breathing pattern** related to hypoxia, anxiety
c. **Ineffective airway clearance** related to inability to cough up frothy secretions

Rationale: *Unless the effects of severe left-sided CHF are interrupted, the patient experiences increasing respiratory difficulty, possibly requiring intubation and mechanically assisted ventilation. The patient with acute pulmonary edema is literally drowning in the fluid accu-*

mulating in the lungs. The ventilation/perfusion ratio is drastically altered, with resultant hypoxia.

The hypoxic patient becomes anxious and attempts to hyperventilate in an unsuccessful effort to increase oxygen intake, as the effort required for breathing further compromises the ability of the damaged heart to supply an adequate cardiac output. The fatigued or intubated patient may be unable to cough forcefully enough to clear the airway of the increased secretions resulting from the pulmonary congestion.

☐ GOAL

The patient will be oxygenated adequately; will maintain a patent airway; will resume normal breathing patterns.

☐ IMPLEMENTATION

- Place in an upright sitting position, with feet and legs down to prevent further lung engorgement and to favor pooling of blood in dependent area of body.
- Administer oxygen in high concentration (unless patient has history of chronic obstructive pulmonary disease [COPD]) per mask or nasal cannula as ordered to relieve hypoxia and dyspnea (patients may tolerate mask poorly due to fear of suffocation).
- Auscultate lungs every 30 minutes or more frequently if indicated for presence of adventitious lung sounds (bubbling rales).
- Prepare for intubation/mechanically assisted ventilation, if indicated; refer to *The Patient with Asthma,* page 32.
- Monitor arterial blood gases for hypoxia and hypercapnea.
- Check blood pressure every 15-30 minutes or more frequently if indicated; hypotension may result as respiratory distress becomes evident (may result initially because of anxiety and activation of the sympathetic nervous system).
- Assess and record quality of pulse (full, bounding, weak, regular), respirations (shallow, rapid, slow), orthopnea, wheezing, cough (productive, dry), skin appearance (color, turgor, moistness) every 2-4 hours.
- Assess mental status for signs/symptoms of cerebral hypoxia (e.g., confusion, anxiety, restlessness, stupor, coma) every 8 hours or more frequently if condition deteriorates.
- Administer IV morphine sulfate as ordered by physician to control pain and decrease anxiety; monitor carefully for effectiveness, be alert to respiratory depression.
- Administer digoxin IV as ordered to improve left ventricular output; monitor for signs of toxicity; watch especially carefully if electrolyte imbalances present; report untoward effects to physician.
- Administer diuretics as ordered; keep accurate intake and output; watch for signs of hyponatremia or hypokalemia (refer to Table 1, *Common Fluid and Electrolyte Imbalances,* page 14) and administer replacement medications/fluids as ordered; record daily weight.
- Administer aminophylline IV as ordered to relieve bronchospasms; watch carefully for tachycardia, particularly if diuretics are being administered (possible cardiac dysrhythmias related to electrolyte imbalances); evaluate effectiveness; keep physician informed of patient's status.
- Apply rotating tourniquets as ordered to trap blood in the extremities
  - apply tourniquets to 3 extremities at one time for 15 minutes
  - rotate every 15 minutes, either clockwise or counterclockwise, but always in the same direction
  - record (diagram) direction and make it known to all care givers to avoid confusion or dangerous error
  - tourniquets should be tight enough to block venous return but not to cut off arterial circulation; check distal pulses after applying
  - to remove, continue rotating every 15 minutes removing one tourniquet each time until all are off (to remove all at once would overload the heart)
  - electric tourniquets may be used; if so, read operating instructions carefully; explain to patient that extremities will be swollen, mottled, and uncomfortable due to engorgement with venous blood, and that this will disappear after tourniquets are removed
- Prepare to assist with phlebotomy if indicated as a means of decreasing venous pressure and volume of circulatory blood; 200-500 cc is usually withdrawn by the physician (often results in dramatic improvement).

☐ EVALUATION CRITERIA/DESIRED OUTCOMES

The Patient

- Demonstrates a regular/normal respiratory pattern
- Has arterial blood gases within normal levels
- Has lungs clear to ascultation

> **NURSING DIAGNOSIS #2**
>
> **Anxiety** related to knowledge deficit regarding treatment modalities, fear of inability to breathe
>
> ***Rationale:*** *Many of the treatment modalities used to correct pulmonary edema (e.g., oxygen face mask, urinary catheter insertion, IVs, medications) can create or increase anxiety. The fear of suffocation can also increase anxiety level. The anxieties/fears of family members must be addressed as well as the patient's, as anxiety tends to have a "contagious" effect.*

☐ GOAL

The patient/family will express decreased feelings of anxiety.

☐ IMPLEMENTATION

- Stay with the patient, using physical touch as necessary to establish support and trust.
- Explain procedures/treatments including types of medications, how they work, and when relief of symptoms can be expected (usually within a few hours); share any signs of progress (e.g., favorable changes in respirations, pulse, output, blood gases).
- Maintain an ongoing assessment of anxiety level to determine whether it is induced by physical or psychologic factors; plan subsequent interventions to modify specific cause, if known.
- Administer morphine sulfate IV as ordered to relieve pain/anxiety; monitor for respiratory depression, expected relief; notify physician if pain persists or if respirations are depressed.
- Decrease environmental stimuli (e.g., audible alarms); realize that the patient may feel closed in and suffocated; open windows (if possible); use light bed covers.
- Provide comfort measures (e.g., positioning with pillows, mouth care, clean cloth to the face if the patient is diaphoretic).
- Review *The Patient Experiencing Anxiety*, page 250, for additional guidelines.

☐ EVALUATION CRITERIA/DESIRED OUTCOMES

The Patient/family

- States a feeling of reduced anxiety
- Verbalizes fears and feelings
- Demonstrates decreased fears of treatment as evidenced by cooperation in care

> **NURSING DIAGNOSIS #3**
>
> **Knowledge deficit** regarding illness, health maintenance plan
>
> ***Rationale:*** *In order to be able to comply with the discharge treatment regimen, the patient must first have a knowledge base regarding the disease process and the prescribed medical treatment. The patient must have sufficient knowledge to independently recognize warning signs and symptoms of pulmonary congestion should they recur.*

☐ GOAL

The patient will express understanding regarding the importance of compliance with the treatment of pulmonary edema during the acute phase; if discharged on medical regimen (e.g., for chronic CHF), will verbalize information necessary for compliance regarding activity, medications, diet, warning signs and symptoms of pulmonary edema.

☐ IMPLEMENTATION

- Institute teaching program for patient/family regarding the disease process, signs and symptoms, and treatment; provide literature together with drawings/audiovisual tools to enhance learning.
- Explain activity regulations and special diet instructions if ordered.
- Provide information regarding any prescribed discharge medications; have the patient identify the name and action, dosage, frequency, side effects of each medication prescribed.
- Provide a written list of medications, actions, and side effects to take home.

- Assess if patient/family know the warning signs and symptoms of pulmonary congestion (e.g., paroxysmal nocturnal dyspnea, cough, restlessness, anxiety) and how to seek medical help when these appear.
- Explain the need for limited amount of daily fluids (if ordered by physician), and to avoid ingestion of a large amount at one time; if on a sodium-restricted diet, explain and have patient select allowed foods and menus.
- Teach to weigh self daily to check on excess fluid retention (if applicable) and to report any excess.
- Teach to sleep with head of bed elevated approximately 10 inches and to avoid excessive, sudden exertion (if applicable).

☐ EVALUATION CRITERIA/DESIRED OUTCOMES

The Patient

- Expresses acceptance of need and value of following prescribed medical regimen
- Identifies restrictions on activity, diet
- Knows medication schedule, side effects, and when to call physician

The Patient with a Pulmonary Embolus

Definition/Discussion

Pulmonary embolism is an obstruction of the pulmonary artery or one of its branches by a blood clot, air, or foreign substance. Most emboli are thrombi, but may be air (from IV), fat (from fractures of large bones), tumors, or amniotic fluid. Approximately 38% of patients die within 2 hours of onset; with careful observation and intervention, the remainder recover. Clots usually disappear spontaneously in about 50% of those patients who survive 2-3 weeks.

Nursing Assessment

☐ PERTINENT HISTORY

Thrombus in the lower extremities; venous stasis resulting from conditions involving slow venous return to the heart (e.g., immobility, fractures, congestive heart failure, atrial fibrillation, hypercoagulability of blood, varicosities, phlebitis); heart disease, abdominal surgery, stroke, severe trauma, obesity, smoking, use of oral contraceptives; previous history of emboli; injury to wall of vein; subtle changes in temperature, pulse, respirations, blood pressure; sudden or gradual onset

☐ PHYSICAL FINDINGS

Pain, shortness of breath, tachypnea, tachycardia, cough, hemoptysis; with large embolus at bifurcation of pulmonary artery: sense of impending doom, sudden onset of substernal pain, diaphoresis, fever; with smaller embolus in terminal pulmonary arteries or arterioles: pleurisy-like pain, anxious expression, restlessness (symptoms reflect size of embolus and area involved)

☐ PSYCHOSOCIAL CONCERNS/ DEVELOPMENTAL FACTORS

Sudden onset leads to psychologic crisis with the fear/threat of dying; changes in life-style for those in high-risk groups (e.g., the obese, women who take birth control pills, smokers)

☐ PATIENT AND FAMILY KNOWLEDGE

Purpose of hospitalization or transfer to intensive care unit; rationale for therapy; posthospitalization regimen (measures to reduce risk factors and prevent recurrence); level of knowledge, readiness and willingness to learn

Nursing Care

☐ LONG-TERM GOAL

The patient will recover from the acute episode and will internalize a health-maintaining/alter life-style regimen designed to prevent future occurrences.

NURSING DIAGNOSIS #1

a. **Impaired gas exchange** related to intrapulmonary shunting, bronchoconstriction
b. **Ineffective breathing pattern** (hyperventilation) related to pain and anxiety
c. **Anxiety** related to knowledge deficit regarding condition, diagnostic procedures, treatment

Rationale: *When a pulmonary vessel is obstructed, inadequate perfusion distal to the embolus will result, decreasing the surface area for gaseous exchange. Pulmonary hypertension and right heart failure may develop. The* pO_2 *is decreased and the resulting hy-*

poxia causes severe dyspnea. The pCO_2 may be increased, decreased, or normal, depending upon whether or not the patient is hyperventilating and the extent of the embolism.

Bronchoconstriction can occur as a physiologic manifestation of anxiety, as a part of the sympathoadrenal response to pain (due to hypoxia and compounded by anxiety), or may result from the release of histamin or serotonin from the thrombus causing the embolus. The anxious patient in pain frequently hyperventilates in an unsuccessful attempt to increase the air supply, hoping to decrease the pain and feelings of air hunger.

The body attempts to compensate for the impaired pulmonary perfusion by intrapulmonary shunting to collateral vessels. Nursing measures aimed at promoting rest support this compensatory mechanism. Similarly, measures to relieve pain and decrease anxiety (and thus reverse hyperventilation and bronchoconstriction) will promote adequate gaseous exchange by increasing the air supply to the lungs and decreasing the cyclic hypoxic effects of pain and anxiety associated with pulmonary embolism.

When pulmonary embolism is suspected, the physician may order a lung scan, chest xray, ECG, arterial blood gases, bloodwork, and perhaps angiography, all to be done STAT. The patient/family may be worried and concerned about the number of studies, validating what they perceive as a very critical situation. IV fibrinolytic therapy with streptokinase may be used to dissolve the embolus. An embolectomy may be performed during angiography. Other surgical procedures that may be considered include vena caval plication (inserting a suture, clip, filter, or sieve to trap the thrombi while still permitting blood flow) and venous ligation. The patient/family will need information in order to provide informed consent for these procedures and to decrease their anxiety by increasing their understanding of the situation.

☐ GOAL

The patient will demonstrate an effective respiratory rate and experience improved gaseous exchange; will experience pain relief; will reduce anxiety.

☐ IMPLEMENTATION

- Maintain strict bedrest to decrease oxygen requirements of all body tissues; elevate head of bed to relieve shortness of breath; give oxygen as ordered; have intubation equipment ready for emergency use; watch for signs of respiratory insufficiency (e.g., dyspnea, tachypnea, sharp pleural pain, tachycardia, hyper/hypotension).
- Monitor blood gases for changes from baseline indicating improvement or worsening of condition; review x-ray reports for pleural effusion.
- Monitor vital signs every 5-15 minutes during acute episode, every 1-2 hours until stable, and every 4 hours afterwards; auscultate chest for rales/pleural rub every 2-4 hours or as needed; if central venous pressure (CVP) line and/or pulmonary artery pressure catheter are in place, monitor hemodynamic readings as ordered; report significant findings to physician.
- Administer IV analgesic (usually morphine sulfate) as prescribed and monitor for expected prompt relief; consult with physician about repeating dose if pain persists; question repeating medication if respirations are depressed—intubation may be required prior to administration of additional narcotic analgesic.
- Administer fibrinolytic agent, bronchodilator/sedative prescribed; monitor for desired and untoward effects.
- Explain all procedures prior to carrying them out; consult with physician regarding diagnostic tests, medical treatments, and surgical procedures planned.
- Emphasize how the patient can assist in controlling symptoms by remaining as calm as possible; refer to *The Patient Experiencing Anxiety*, page 250, for additional interventions.
- Stay with patient to ensure comfort and safety; ask to close eyes and visualize self breathing easily and comfortably; repeat as necessary; refer to *The Patient Experiencing Pain*, page 180, for additional interventions.
- Share signs of measurable progress with patient (e.g., improved or stabilized vital signs) as a way to decrease anxiety.

☐ EVALUATION CRITERIA/DESIRED OUTCOMES

The Patient

- Displays normal, unlabored respirations

- Has ABGs within normal limits
- Relates relief of pain
- Reports decreased anxiety

NURSING DIAGNOSIS #2

Fluid volume deficit related to inadequate oral fluid intake

Rationale: *During the acute episode, the patient in severe distress after a pulmonary embolism will not likely be able to maintain an oral intake sufficient to replace fluid losses, which are increased via diaphoresis and hyperventilation. The medical regimen (e.g., IV fluids, indwelling urinary catheter, intake and output monitoring) requires nursing implementation and evaluation. Treatment aims at avoiding fluid (and related electrolyte) imbalances, which would further compromise the patient's current status.*

☐ GOAL

The patient will maintain fluid balance.

☐ IMPLEMENTATION

- Monitor IVs and adjust rate as ordered; carefully inspect the area around the catheter insertion site for inflammation or bleeding every 4 hours.
- Monitor intake and output, CVP, and/or hemodynamic readings as needed; record measurements; report significant findings (e.g., abrupt changes from previous readings, excessive or diminished urinary output, elevated CVP) to physician.
- Encourage oral intake as tolerated.
- Assess for signs of dehydration (e.g., poor skin turgor, dry skin or mucous membranes, thirst, hypotension); report significant findings to physician.
- Monitor laboratory studies for abnormal electrolyte levels; assess for signs of imbalances, especially potassium (e.g., ECG changes, muscle aches, gastrointestinal (GI) irritability) and sodium (e.g., nausea, malaise, fatigue); record assessment and notify physician.
- Refer to Table 1, *Common Fluid and Electrolyte Imbalances*, page 14.

☐ EVALUATION CRITERIA/DESIRED OUTCOMES

The Patient

- Maintains a combined oral and IV fluid intake 100-300 cc greater than urinary output
- Has normal serum electrolyte levels
- Shows good skin turgor and moist mucous membranes

NURSING DIAGNOSIS #3

a. **Alteration in tissue perfusion: peripheral** related to restricted physical activity
b. **Impairment of skin integrity** related to restricted physical activity
c. **Potential for injury** (bleeding) related to side effects of anticoagulant/fibrinolytic therapy

Rationale: *The strict bedrest prescribed during the acute episode of pulmonary embolism predisposes the patient to complications related to immobility (e.g., impaired circulation, skin breakdown, risk of recurrent embolism). The physician may order anticoagulants to decrease the risk of thrombi and may also have ordered fibrinolytic agents to dissolve the occluding thrombus. Nursing measures to prevent complications of bedrest and quickly detect untoward effects of prescribed drug therapy are therefore high priorities in caring for patients with pulmonary embolism.*

☐ GOAL

The patient will maintain adequate peripheral circulation; will maintain intact skin surfaces; will be monitored closely for early signs of excessive bleeding.

☐ IMPLEMENTATION

- Assess peripheral circulation every 4-8 hours (palpable pulse, temperature, color, edema, pain); notify physician of signs of thrombophlebitis; check especially for Homan's sign (calf pain on dorsiflexion of foot indicative of deep vein thrombosis).
- Avoid use of knee gatch or pillow under knees when positioning patient; explain reason for avoiding rubbing or massaging legs (risk of dislodging thrombus).
- Consult with physician as to level of activity

permitted and use of active/passive range-of-motion (ROM) exercises; change position every 2 hours.
- Remove antiembolic stockings for 15 minutes every 8 hours; inspect skin underneath for signs of breakdown.
- Inspect all skin surfaces every 8 hours, carefully examining all pressure points and dependent areas; provide preventive skin care per unit or hospital protocol.
- As condition improves, encourage adequate nutritional and fluid intake to promote cellular nutrition and to ensure adequate circulating blood volume.
- Monitor for side effects of fibrinolytic/anticoagulant therapy (e.g., prolonged prothrombin and clotting times; nosebleed, petechiae, hematuria, GI or rectal bleeding).

☐ EVALUATION CRITERIA/DESIRED OUTCOMES

The Patient
- Has strong palpable pulses in all extremities
- Maintains intact skin surfaces, displays good skin color
- Shows no overt signs of bleeding
- Displays coagulation studies within acceptable limits

NURSING DIAGNOSIS #4

Knowledge deficit related to measures to prevent recurrence

Rationale: *To carry on with previous roles on an independent level, the patient needs information about post-hospitalization care (e.g., medications, exercise, indications for notifying physician) and methods of avoiding known risk factors of thrombophlebitis, the most common cause of pulmonary embolism.*

☐ GOAL

The patient/family will describe discharge regimen, including medications, precautionary measures to prevent venous stasis and bleeding, exercises, and signs/symptoms requiring medical follow-up.

☐ IMPLEMENTATION

- Teach about venous stasis and its relationship to embolus formation; instruct to avoid predisposing factors (e.g., sitting with legs crossed; massaging legs; immobility; pressure on popliteal areas; using tight straps/bands around thighs, knees, calves, or ankles).
- Explain vasoconstrictive effects of smoking; encourage patient's efforts towards stopping.
- Instruct to do full ROM exercises at least twice daily and to get up and ambulate for 5-10 minutes every 2 hours (except during the night), including when riding in an automobile or airplane.
- Ensure patient knows to wear elastic stockings (including wearing time) and to avoid wearing tight garters, girdles, or any other constrictive clothing.
- Instruct regarding medications; provide written list of medications including schedule, dosages, actions, and possible side effects to be reported to physician.
- Review with patient early signs of thrombophlebitis (e.g., stiffness, soreness, redness over affected area) and advise to notify physician if they occur.
- Provide helpful guidelines to avoid hazards that could cause bleeding while on anticoagulant therapy (e.g., use electric razor, soft bristle toothbrush; do not use power tools; avoid going barefoot; wear gloves while cleaning/gardening; use nonslip mat in shower/bathtub).
- Instruct patient to tell dentist or any other doctor that s/he is receiving anticoagulant medication.
- Structure teaching sessions to allow time for answering patient's/family's questions.

☐ EVALUATION CRITERIA/DESIRED OUTCOMES

The Patient/family
- Expresses accurate knowledge regarding exercise, drug/medical regimen, and precautionary measures to follow

The Patient with Pulmonary Emphysema

Definition/Discussion

Pulmonary emphysema is an irreversible condition of the lungs involving destruction of the alveoli with resultant chronic hyperexpansion of the lungs causing air to be trapped without gaseous exchange. It is one of three conditions (along with chronic bronchitis and asthma) that are collectively known as chronic obstructive pulmonary disease (COPD). It is usually the end result of a slowly developing process of chronic bronchial irritation (cigarette smoking and environmental, occupational pollutants) and infection leading to edema, mucus production, bronchospasm, constriction of the finer airways, and loss of lung elasticity. Occurs most frequently in persons over 45 years of age who have a history of smoking and/or inhalation of respiratory irritants; appears to be a genetic predisposition as well, which is associated with a deficiency of the plasma protein alpha-antitrypsin. COPD is a major cause of disability under Social Security and is the most common respiratory cause of death.

Nursing Assessment

☐ PERTINENT HISTORY

Long history of chronic cough, wheezing, and increasing shortness of breath; chronic respiratory infections; chronic fatigue; anorexia and weight loss; smoking; high-risk occupation (involving inhalation of known respiratory irritants); physical environment (living in a geographic area with known air pollution); family history

☐ PHYSICAL FINDINGS

Dyspnea with or without exertion; fatigue; increased thick pulmonary secretions with possible mucus plugs; diminished breath sounds from chronic obstruction (marked increase of airway resistance) of air exchange; tactile fremitus; decreased diaphragm excursion; hyperresonance on percussion; rigid barrel chest with ribs fixed at joints; forward bending posturing while breathing, using accessory muscles; retraction of the supraclavicular fossae on inspiration; with long-term disease, contraction of abdominal muscles on inspiration as well; pursed lips on expiration; cyanosis; with advanced disease digital clubbing, pulmonary hypertension leading to right-sided congestive heart failure (cor pulmonale), dependent edema, distended neck veins; hypoxia and increased carbon dioxide with acidosis in acute phases; chest x-rays indicate hyperinflation and presence of blebs; right axis deviation or atrial fibrillation; slowed expiratory flow rates, progressive reduction of vital capacity

☐ PSYCHOSOCIAL CONCERNS/ DEVELOPMENTAL FACTORS

Adaptation to changes in habits (smoking) and/or life-style (occupation, activity level, residence) to achieve control (not an easy or expected developmental task) necessitated by insidious onset, length of development of illness before diagnosis; increasing dependence upon others with disease progression further interfering with normal developmental tasks may predispose towards despair rather than maintenance of ego integrity

☐ PATIENT AND FAMILY KNOWLEDGE

Ways to delay progression of the disease, prevention and elimination of bronchial infections, reduction of bronchial secretions; guidelines for self-care, medications, exercise regimen, and use of ventilatory aids; signs of depression (frequently observed response in patients with a long history), possibly interfering with compliance with the planned regimen

Nursing Care

☐ LONG-TERM GOAL

The patient will carry out activities of daily living within limitations imposed by disease and treatment; the patient will make life-style changes to retard progression of the disease process.

NURSING DIAGNOSIS #1

a. **Ineffective airway clearance** related to excessive and tenacious mucus secretions
b. **Ineffective breathing pattern** related to tachypnea, rigidity of chest wall
c. **Impaired gas exchange** related to chronic tissue hypoxia

Rationale: *The patient with emphysema is often unable to cough forcefully enough to expel the copious, thick secretions produced; in times of distress, the air-hungry patient may increase the rate but not the depth of respirations, using all energy just to breathe, making respiration a muscular rather than a normal, involuntary act; interference with alveolar ventilation may occur due to chronic obstruction of the air flow in and out of the lungs, causing the patient to retain and tolerate higher levels of carbon dioxide and lower levels of serum oxygen (the long-term patient with emphysema breathes because of the "hypoxic drive" when circulating oxygen becomes too low rather than in response to elevated carbon dioxide levels as do most individuals).*

☐ GOAL

The patient will achieve maximum pulmonary function by demonstrating effective coughing and conserving energy; will demonstrate an effective respiratory rate with an increased air exchange in the lungs; will learn adaptive breathing patterns to decrease air hunger.

☐ IMPLEMENTATION

- Monitor for signs of acute respiratory insufficiency and possible failure (e.g., tachycardia and dysrhythmias; initial hypertension changing to hypotension; restlessness or agitation; impaired judgment; anxiety and confusion; headache, drowsiness, or dizziness; diaphoresis; reddening of skin, sclera, and conjuctiva; loss of consciousness); *apnea is a medical emergency;* stay with patient, initiate resuscitative measures or calmly reassure patient; call for help; endotracheal or tracheal intubation may be necessary to provide mechanical ventilation, which will permit rest of respiratory muscles and promote optimal gaseous exchange.
- Monitor oxygen therapy as ordered; carefully check flow rate (2-3 liters/minute to prevent overriding hypoxic drive) and ensure proper humidification to assist in liquefying secretions.
- If mechanical ventilation is required, ensure that equipment is functional (alarms, removal of excess moisture from tubing, intact system) and that settings are as ordered; assess patient's response to mechanical ventilation by observation, auscultation, and serial blood gases.
- Position in high-Fowler's with additional pillows as needed; to decrease energy expenditures, have patient sit on edge of bed or in a chair with arms folded in front, resting on pillows on top of overbed table or nightstand; or have patient sit in chair, spreading feet a shoulderwidth or more apart, leaning forward with elbows on knees and hands and forearms relaxed.
- Teach not to hold breath during an activity, but rather to inhale through nose beforehand and to slowly exhale while performing task.
- Demonstrate pursed-lip breathing while exhaling to prolong exhalation and more effectively remove residual air, thus enhancing subsequent inflow of air; advise normal rather than deep inhalation, encouraging a 1:2 inhalation:exhalation ratio.
- Assess need for suctioning (e.g., observed inability to expectorate; dyspnea; tachycardia; audible rales, diminished breath sounds, rhonchi; restlessness and agitation); maintaining sterile technique, gently suction as necessary to remove secretions; watch for signs of distress such as bloody aspirant, cardiac dysrhythmias (especially bradycardia due to accidental vagal nerve stimulation during deep suctioning), cyanosis or bronchospasm (if catheter is difficult to remove, disconnect from suctioning equipment and let catheter act as artificial airway, removing after spasm has ended); record amount and appearance of secretions (bronchoscopic re-

moval of mucus plugs by the physician may be indicated); obtain sputum specimens as ordered and monitor lab results.

- Encourage high fluid intake, 2,500-3,000 cc/day, to liquefy secretions and compensate for moisture loss through mouth breathing.
- Administer bronchodilators and expectorants as ordered; monitor carefully for side effects, toxicity, effectiveness.
- Monitor administration of intermittent positive pressure breathing, percussion/vibration of lower lobes, and postural drainage as ordered; consult with respiratory therapist to reinforce planned therapy.

☐ EVALUATION CRITERIA/DESIRED OUTCOMES

The Patient

- Exhibits improved respiratory functioning as evidenced by decreased respiratory rate, less dyspnea, fatigue, more normal breath sounds, and improved blood gases and pulmonary function studies
- Expectorates secretions adequately

NURSING DIAGNOSIS #2

Alteration in nutrition: less than body requirements related to anorexia, increased energy expenditures secondary to effort for breathing

Rationale: *Patients with COPD are often malnourished prior to hospitalization because of anorexia related to fatigue. Decreased nutritional intake further impairs lung function as it depresses the ventilatory response to hypoxia and hypercapnia, precipitating respiratory failure and prolonging recovery from failure. If sufficient protein and calories are not provided, the patient catabolizes muscles for fuel, contributing to atrophy of the respiratory muscles. It may be expected that nutritional support may improve respiratory muscle functioning and increase energy levels, thus decreasing the effort for breathing for the patient with emphysema. This diagnosis is especially relevant for ventilator-dependent patients, but is applicable to most patients with emphysema.*

☐ GOAL

The patient will ingest adequate oral intake; if that is not possible, will receive sufficient nutrients by alternate methods of feeding.

☐ IMPLEMENTATION

- Assess nutritional status: consider height, weight, body frame, ideal weight; condition of hair, skin, nails, and mouth.
- Carefully monitor daily weight, oral intake, and calorie count if indicated; assess prehospitalization dietary pattern, noting preferred foods; consult with dietician to plan acceptable diet.
- Encourage full consumption of prescribed diet; consider smaller, more frequent meals if easily fatigued; have family and friends bring in favorite foods; provide small, high-protein and high-calorie supplements between meals.
- Administer supplemental vitamins and minerals as ordered.
- Consult with physician about starting tube feedings if patient is unable to maintain oral intake to maintain or increase weight (hyperalimentation may also be considered but it is not the usual choice as it increases the risk for infection).
- If patient is ventilator-dependent, be aware of possible complications/implications and plan interventions to prevent their occurrence (e.g., infection secondary to aspiration may be precipitated by excessive filling of the stomach, malposition, or obstruction of feeding tube [check for placement and residual before feeding or every 8 hours if continuous feeding system in use and consider the use of food coloring or natural dye if a fistual is suspected]; frequent tracheal suctioning/postural drainage and chest physical therapy [turn off feedings for a short time before planned treatment if possible]; depletion of mineral stores [especially potassium, magnesium, phosphorus] secondary to diarrhea [alter strength or composition of feeding, provide mineral supplements]; and persistent gastric retention due to decreased gastric mobility [decrease rate of feeding]).

☐ EVALUATION CRITERIA/DESIRED OUTCOMES

The Patient

- Has observed/documented increased intake and weight gain or maintenance
- Expresses improved appetite

NURSING DIAGNOSIS #3

Potential for infection related to altered respiratory functioning, impaired nutritional state

Rationale: *The emphysematous lung does not fully contract on expiration, leaving secretions to pool in the alveoli and bronchioles, predisposing the patient to the development of respiratory infection. When the patient is malnourished as well, there are insufficient reserves to meet the increased metabolic requirements during respiratory distress. Infection further compromises lung function, creating a cyclic effect that if left untreated, may lead to respiratory failure and death.*

☐ GOAL

The patient will be free from infection.

☐ IMPLEMENTATION

- Monitor vital signs, watching for changes that might indicate the presence of infection (e.g., elevated temperature, tachycardia, hypotension).
- Observe and record amount and character of secretions expectorated or suctioned; send purulent secretions for culture and monitor lab results.
- Administer antibiotics, steroids, and antitussive-expectorants (coughing causes further damage to the lungs) as ordered, watching carefully for side effects, toxicity, and effectiveness.
- Use humidification as ordered; keep room free from known irritants.
- Encourage high fluid intake and good nutrition; offer supplements as needed or if indicated; monitor parenteral fluids.
- Encourage activity as tolerated, balancing with increased rest.
- Place in a private room, if possible, or at least away from any patient with a known infection.
- Caution visitors and staff who may have colds to wear a mask or not to enter the patient's room.
- Keep tissues handy at bedside, as well as a container for soiled tissues that can be removed and emptied at regular intervals.

☐ EVALUATION CRITERIA/DESIRED OUTCOMES

The Patient

- Maintains normal vital signs
- Expectorates clear or white-colored secretions

NURSING DIAGNOSIS #4

Activity intolerance related to dyspnea and fatigue

Rationale: *The patient with emphysema is frequently unable to perform even minimal self-care tasks without exertional dyspnea. Rehabilitation programs emphasizing physical conditioning have been demonstrated to improve activity tolerance and should be considered once the patient is past the acute exacerbation of the disease.*

☐ GOAL

The patient will spread out energy demands over the day and avoid becoming extremely fatigued; will develop a plan to conserve energy.

☐ IMPLEMENTATION

- Be aware that early morning and after meals are times when the patient is less likely to tolerate activity (in the morning energy is required to expectorate the secretions that have pooled during the night; after meals, especially the evening or main meal of the day, abdominal distension may interfere with diaphragmatic excursion and increase the effort of breathing); plan care and scheduled treatments accordingly.
- Review patient's usual patterns of activity and fatigue; attempt to schedule required activities at times when the patient usually has more energy.
- Plan care with the realization that patients with emphysema have a limited amount of energy, much of which is consumed with eating and talking and, in severe exacerbations, with breathing alone.
- Assist the patient in discovering own point of fatigue in order not to exceed it.
- Keep supplies close at hand within patient's easy reach.
- Schedule rest periods between treatments, meals, tests, visitors, etc., to prevent fatigue.
- Consult with physician and exercise physiol-

ogist about the advisability of prescribing an exercise/physical conditioning program to increase work capacity and exercise tolerance.

☐ EVALUATION CRITERIA/DESIRED OUTCOMES

The Patient

- Is free from periods of extreme fatigue
- Performs daily activities at own pace with minimal fatigue and dypsnea

NURSING DIAGNOSIS #5

Powerlessness related to perceived loss of control, chronic nature of emphysema

Rationale: *When acute episodes require hospitalization, the patient may express feeling overwhelmed by emphysema when, despite efforts at control, the disease is progressing. The long-term patient may exhibit depression because of this powerlessness, refusing to participate in decision making regarding care.*

☐ GOAL

The patient will be able to identify controllable aspects of emphysema; will participate in making decisions relating to treatment and daily activities.

☐ IMPLEMENTATION

- Identify specific causative factors of powerlessness, reviewing admission psychosocial assessment for individual patterns of coping and identified support systems.
- Observe family relationships to estimate the degree of support available and to identify situations in which the family member may require psychologic and emotional support as well (this is likely if the well family member has devoted life to caring for the sick person); include supportive persons in interventions; initiate referrals as appropriate.
- Allow the patient/family to express fears and concerns, listening attentively without minimizing feelings; offer suggestions without telling the person what to do; when possible, offer alternatives and encourage to choose a solution.
- Teach that emotional upsets and infection can increase symptoms; point out that by complying with the prescribed treatment regimen, s/he is controlling the disease process by avoiding situations that result in increased energy expenditures and further damage to lung tissue.
- Encourage attempts to decrease or stop any smoking, again pointing to the patient's ability to control symptoms by decreasing this source of irritation.
- Encourage to keep follow-up appointments, stressing their importance in maintaining control.
- Recognize financial and emotional strains of a chronic illness such as emphysema; initiate referrals to social service for follow-up care in the community after discharge.

☐ EVALUATION CRITERIA/DESIRED OUTCOMES

The Patient

- Identifies at least 2 aspects of regimen that s/he can control
- Increases participation in decision making regarding planned treatment

NURSING DIAGNOSIS #6

Anxiety related to uncertain prognosis, possible impending death

Rationale: *The patient with emphysema presents a physical appearance that suggests the anxiety commonly felt. Air hunger and the constant threat of not being able to breathe create a daily atmosphere of uncertainty where the patient may question, either overtly or covertly, whether or not this will be the time when recovery will not occur. Compounding this uncertainty is the reluctance of well-meaning family and friends to acknowledge the patient's anxiety, thereby denying the patient their support at a time it is most needed.*

☐ GOAL

The patient will experience emotional as well as physiologic comfort, expressing fears and concerns; the patient's family/supportive persons will assist patient to adjust to possible death/life-style changes.

☐ IMPLEMENTATION

- Assess for behavioral signs of anxiety (e.g., irritability, tenseness, nervousness, self-deprecation); recognize that common physiologic signs (e.g., increased pulse/respirations) are likely to be present because of the physical disease process, not because of anxiety.
- Explore expressed feelings about inability to breathe and fear of impending death, listening openly and giving the patient permission to discuss a subject that is a societal or cultural taboo.
- With the patient's permission, discuss these shared feelings with a supportive family member who has not been able to discuss the possibility of death with the patient; allow the family member to express concerns; offer gentle guidance to enable him/her to communicate these concerns with the patient without causing undue distress.
- Support adaptive coping mechanisms of both the patient/family; assist in planning strategies for more effective coping; initiate referrals to community agencies as appropriate.
- Refer to *The Patient Experiencing Anxiety,* page 250, for additional interventions.

☐ EVALUATION CRITERIA/DESIRED OUTCOMES

The Patient

- Expresses decreased anxiety and increased ability to adjust to prognosis
- Receives increased emotional support from family or supportive friends

NURSING DIAGNOSIS #7

Knowledge deficit regarding methods for delaying the progression of emphysema and maintaining optimal health level

Rationale: *Patient understanding of the disease process and methods of treatment can enhance compliance with the regimen and delay the progression of the predictable chronic course in emphysema. When the patient is in the end stage of the disease process, patient/family education is aimed at promoting comfort through symptom control.*

☐ GOAL

The patient/family will have sufficient information to promote control of the disease process and related symptoms.

☐ IMPLEMENTATION

- Instruct on methods of delaying the progression of emphysema through avoiding exposure to respiratory irritants (e.g., smoking, air pollution, pollens, allergens, extreme variations in temperature or humidity).
- Teach to protect self from respiratory infections by avoiding exposure to persons with known infection, avoiding crowds and poorly ventilated spaces, being immunized against influenza (if not allergic), taking prescribed prophylactic antimicrobials, practicing good oral hygiene, and promptly reporting to the physician/clinician any sign of respiratory infection (e.g., chest pain; change in color, character, or amount of sputum; increased difficulty breathing or talking; sore throat, fever, or chills).
- Discuss methods to remove secretions easily: maintaining an adequate fluid intake (8-10 glasses of fluid/day); humidification to loosen and mobilize secretions; avoiding self-medication, taking bronchodilators only as prescribed and avoiding over-the-counter medications that may suppress coughing and dry secretions; following postural drainage and breathing exercises as prescribed.
- Encourage maintenance of daily habits that promote healthy living: nutrition, vitamin/mineral supplements as directed (sodium may need to be restricted and potassium supplemented, particularly if the patient shows signs of right-sided heart failure), rest, physical activities as tolerated, use of community resources for physical, educational, and psychosocial support services.
- Plan methods for living within the physical limitations that emphysema imposes by avoiding activities that produce excessive shortness of breath, practicing relaxation techniques, using pursed-lip breathing, scheduling activities according to fatigue pattern, avoiding known stressors and energy-wasting activities, and considering such major life-style changes as retirement, occupational change, or moving to a smaller home or better climate.
- Review respiratory therapy aids to be used

after discharge or observe while the respiratory therapist gives instructions for use to reinforce teaching
  - have the patient practice assembling and disassembling equipment
  - review prescribed times for treatments and indications for use as needed
  - have the patient demonstrate ability to obtain the exact dosage of medication prescribed
  - have the patient practice controlled coughing after treatment to produce sputum (deep, slow diaphragmatic breathing, followed by breath-holding for a few seconds, then 2 short, forceful coughs with the mouth open, followed by a pause and quiet inhalation; (forceful inhalation may precipitate unproductive, energy-consuming cough and further damage the lung tissue)
  - encourage oral hygiene after treatment
  - tell to clean equipment daily
  - ensure that patient has a written list of instructions
- After consulting with physician and/or exercise physiologist, teach respiratory muscle-strengthening exercises
  - have patient in recumbent position with one hand on abdomen and other on upper chest
  - instruct to inhale through nose, raising abdomen against hand, then exhale while pursing lips, contracting the abdominal muscles, and moving abdomen inward without moving chest
  - have patient sit, with lighted candle 6 inches away; instruct to exhale slowly through pursed lips, attempting to make the flame flicker, not extinguish it; gradually, increase distance from candle by 2 inches/day to a maximum of 36 inches
  - have patient do return demonstrations
  - instruct to continue at home 3 times/day for 10-15 minutes each
- Encourage maintenance of body tone by regular exercise as tolerated; initiate referral to community service agencies or private exercise physiologist for specific programs if available.
- Follow a daily schedule of graded exercises (e.g., walking, riding stationary bicycle) using supplemental oxygen at prescribed low-flow rate if indicated; review signs of carbon dioxide narcosis (e.g., confusion, lethargy, change in depth of respirations); advise to discontinue oxygen immediately should these be present and to notify physician.
- Ensure that patient has a list of daily medications; review significant side effects to be reported; if steroids are prescribed, remind the patient that they may mask the signs of infection (by suppressing the inflammation response) and stress again the importance of protection from infection.

☐ EVALUATION CRITERIA/DESIRED OUTCOMES

The Patient

- Participates in planned regimen to promote control of disabling symptoms
- Demonstrates ability to provide self-care measures after discharge

The Patient Undergoing Renal Transplantation

Definition/Discussion

Renal transplantation entails removing a functioning kidney from a living related donor or from a cadaver and transplanting it into the right or left fossa of the recipient. Renal vessels are anastomosed to the recipient's iliac artery and vein. The ureter is transplanted into the bladder or anastomosed to recipient's ureter. Renal tranplantation is the treatment for end-stage renal disease (ESRD) and provides an alternative to dialysis with its increasing requirements, financial restraints, and needs for quality control. A successful renal transplant can allow a patient to return to an almost normal life. Most potential kidney recipients have a long waiting period because of a lack of suitable and available kidneys; 70% must await a cadaver transplant because they do not have a relative willing or able to donate a suitable organ.

Pre-op tissue typing ensures as histocompatible a transplant as possible. The highest degree of compatibility is with identical twins, then with a sibling, then parent, and, lastly, with a nonrelative. The transplant or allograft is a foreign body within the recipient that stimulates the antigen-antibody reaction, possibly leading to rejection. Types of rejection include

- *hyperacute rejection:* occurs on the operating room table
- *acute rejection:* occurs within the first year postoperatively
- *chronic rejection:* the rejection process continues despite repeated efforts to increase immunosuppression. A patient can survive several bouts of acute rejection, but once chronic rejection begins, it can become an insidious, irreversible process resulting in loss of the transplant. About 30%-40% of cadaver organs and 10%-20% of kidneys from live, related donors are rejected.

Pre-op management aims to put the patient in as normal a metabolic state as possible via dialysis and dietary measures. It also includes eliminating potential sources of post-op infection (e.g., extraction of carious teeth, removal of infected kidneys in those with chronic pyelonephritis or polycystic disease).

Nursing Assessment

☐ PERTINENT HISTORY

End-stage renal disease; history of chronic renal failure treated either by hemodialysis or continuous ambulatory peritoneal dialysis; age, presence of associated disease (e.g., coronary artery disease, malignancy, infectious or pulmonary disease)

☐ PHYSICAL FINDINGS

As for chronic renal failure (refer to *The Patient with Chronic Renal Failure,* page 78); normal lower urinary tract outflow; results of lab tests (e.g., BUN greater than 70 mg/dl; serum creatinine of 5 mg/dl; creatinine clearance of 15 ml/min), immunologic evaluation

☐ PSYCHOSOCIAL CONCERNS/ DEVELOPMENTAL FACTORS

Anxiety, fear about prognosis/possible rejection; possible body-image disturbance accepting donated kidney as part of self; donor anxiety regarding danger to own health, possible rejection)

☐ PATIENT AND FAMILY KNOWLEDGE

All options for treatment, risks/benefits of transplant versus continued dialysis, expectations of transplant, prescribed medications/side effects; level of knowledge, readiness and willingness to learn

Nursing Care

☐ LONG-TERM GOAL

The patient will adjust and adhere to a lifelong medical regimen imposed by the kidney transplant.

> **NURSING DIAGNOSIS #1**
>
> **Anxiety** related to fear of unknown, lack of understanding of procedure
>
> ***Rationale:*** *Lack of knowledge causes increased level of stress, discomfort, and anxiety.*

☐ GOAL

The patient will verbalize decreased anxiety and satisfactory knowledge of pre- and post-op instructions; will exhibit behavior consistent with decreased anxiety (e.g., uninterrupted sleep, decreased somatic complaints).

☐ IMPLEMENTATION

- Ask how it feels now to finally approach the reality of receiving a new kidney (usual feelings include euphoria, moderate apprehension, and anxiety, and fear of failure); share with patient that these feelings are commonly experienced by others in same situation, and are normal and expected; know that the patient needs you to help sort out, interpret, and suggest ways to cope with the many feelings, concerns, and questions.
- Assess current knowledge about the surgery and what patient wants and needs to know; usual questions revolve around potential for rejection of transplant, the shunt, the donor, the need for post-op dialysis, drugs, radiation, limited isolation, overview of surgical day, pain, and discomfort; teach as needed; have patient return demonstrate turning, deep breathing, effective coughing, use of pillow splint; be aware that these patients are usually much better informed than most surgical patients and tend to ask more questions; be honest; provide current information.
- Assess need to discuss potential post-op complications; be open, honest, and answer all questions.
- Reassure that a kidney can experience several bouts of acute rejection and still function.
- Reassure that feelings of euphoria and depression often result from taking steroids, and that these feelings will probably be short lived; help patient to express feelings to you/family, as a way of dealing with them.

☐ EVALUATION CRITERIA/DESIRED OUTCOMES

The Patient

- States decreased level of anxiety
- Indicates understanding of pre-op teaching

> **NURSING DIAGNOSIS #2**
>
> **Alteration in urinary elimination** (oliguria) related to kidney rejection
>
> ***Rationale:*** *Following transplant the body may attempt to reject the foreign protein by a severe antibody reaction that may impair renal functioning and cause symptoms of acute renal failure and rejection.*

☐ GOAL

The patient will have appropriate urinary output for post-op course; will experience no symptoms of rejection.

☐ IMPLEMENTATION

- Observe patient for signs of acute rejection of kidney transplant (fever, increased blood pressure, swollen tender kidney, decreased urine, proteinuria, weight gain, complaints of "getting the flu"); report significant findings.
- Explain any necessity for temporary post-op dialysis (especially with a cadaver kidney) until the transplant is functioning adequately (may be up to 7 weeks).
- Check shunt or fistula frequently for patency (high incidence of thrombosis postoperatively); refer to *The Patient Requiring Hemodialysis,* page 111.
- Observe patient for signs of hyperkalemia (may develop if massive blood transfusions are required or stored blood is administered); monitor serum potassium level at least every 4 hours; refer to Table 1, *Common Fluid and Electrolyte Imbalances,* page 14.
- Monitor acid-base balance; some base deficit

will be present but pH should not fall below 7.4; check with physician as to parameters for notification.

- Monitor kidney function tests (i.e., BUN, electrolytes, creatinine, urinalysis, renogram) and report significant findings.
- Administer immunosuppressive drugs as ordered, watch carefully for toxic effects, especially changes in white blood cell count, hemoglobin, hematocrit, liver studies, bleeding time, and lab tests indicative of extensive immunosuppressive activity (e.g., blastcell counts, antibody titers).

☐ EVALUATION CRITERIA/DESIRED OUTCOMES

The Patient

- Maintains urinary output between 30-300 cc/hour
- Has laboratory studies within physician or protocol designated limites
- Is free from rejection symptoms

NURSING DIAGNOSIS #3

a. **Alteration in tissue perfusion: renal** related to fluid volume imbalance (deficit or excess)

b. **Alteration in cardiac output: decreased** related to effects of electrolyte imbalance(s) associated with fluid imbalance

Rationale: *After receiving a donor kidney, the patient may be anuric, oliguric, or experience a massive diuresis. While there does not seem to be a cause-and-effect relationship, in all possible outcomes the implanted kidney may experience altered tissue perfusion (e.g., inadequate blood flow to the kidneys with fluid volume deficit, fluid overload with fluid volume excess); the ability of the implanted kidney to excrete fluid affects the circulating blood volume (e.g., with massive diuresis leading to fluid volume deficit and anuria predisposing the patient to fluid volume excess). Adequate tissue perfusion is necessary to decrease the possibility of rejection of the implanted kidney. Prompt recognition and implementation of measures to correct the underlying fluid imbalance and its associated electrolyte imbalances (which may cause cardiac dysrhythmias leading to a decreased cardiac output) are post-op nursing priorities.*

☐ GOAL

The patient will maintain fluid and electrolyte balance and cardiac output adequate to perfuse the implanted kidney.

☐ IMPLEMENTATION

- Monitor vital signs, peripheral pulses, and level of consciousness (LOC) every 1-4 hours; assess for signs of decreased cardiac output (e.g., dyspnea, decreased LOC, hypotension, pallor, peripheral edema).
- Record all fluid intake and measure urinary output every hour; report output of greater than 300 cc/hour or less than 30 cc/hour for 2 consecutive hours to physician; adjust fluid intake as ordered by physician or unit protocol.
- Keep indwelling catheter patent, irrigating only on physician order and using strict aseptic technique.
- Monitor serum electrolyte levels, hemoglobin and hematocrit as ordered; report significant findings.
- Monitor cardiac rhythm; treat any dysrhythmias per physician's order or hospital protocol; monitor patient's response to treatment.
- Refer to Table 1, *Common Fluid and Electrolyte Imbalances*, page 14, for care of specific imbalances.

☐ EVALUATION CRITERIA/DESIRED OUTCOMES

The Patient

- Has normal blood pressure, heart, respirations, and peripheral pulses
- Maintains urinary output of 30-300 cc/hour
- Remains alert and free from symptomatic dysrhythmias
- Has normal serum electrolyte, hemoglobin, and hematocrit values

NURSING DIAGNOSIS #4

Potential for infection related to administration of immunosuppressive drugs

Rationale: *Transplant patients are given medications to suppress the immune system to prevent rejection. Resultant immunosuppression may render any infection life threatening. Pa-*

tients with chronic renal failure are at particularly high risk because the disease had already decreased the effectiveness of their immune system. Detection of infection is difficult as the immunosuppressive drugs impair the usual inflammatory response that produces the common symptoms associated with infection (e.g., increased temperature, swelling, redness).

☐ GOAL

The patient will remain free from any infection.

☐ IMPLEMENTATION

- Limit contact with people outside the immediate family and hospital staff.
- Keep any infected persons away from patient.
- Use scrupulous hygiene measures; provide good oral hygiene every 4 hours or as needed.
- Provide early ambulation, if possible.
- Encourage good nutrition to prevent infection and enhance healing process.
- Maintain vascular access with aseptic technique.
- Discontinue indwelling urinary catheter as soon as possible.
- Assess very carefully for signs of any infection (e.g., slight increase in temperature, malaise, drainage, cloudy urine, frequency, lower back pain, cough).
- Obtain ordered specimens for culture and sensitivity studies promptly.
- Administer antibiotic therapy as ordered, carefully monitoring for expected and toxic effects, especially in drugs detoxified by the kidneys (e.g., gentamycin and tobramycin).

☐ EVALUATION CRITERIA/DESIRED OUTCOMES

The Patient

- Is free from nosocomial or iatrogenic infection
- Has negative bacterial cultures

NURSING DIAGNOSIS #5

a. **Alteration in nutrition: more than body requirements** related to stress, administration of steroids
b. **Fluid volume excess** related to elevated serum sodium level, associated water retention

Rationale: *Steroid therapy leads to excessive sodium and glucose being retained by the body. The stress of the operation also causes increased levels of cortisone to be released, resulting in hyperglycemia and hypernatremia. Excess sodium causes a retention of body water as the body attempts to dilute the solute excess.*

☐ GOAL

The patient will have normal blood glucose and serum sodium levels.

☐ IMPLEMENTATION

- Monitor blood glucose and sodium levels daily or as ordered.
- Check vital signs at least every 4 hours, especially for hypertension, tachycardia, and decreased respirations.
- Observe for signs of hyperglycemia (e.g., confusion, dry mucous membranes, increased blood sugar); initiate emergency measures as needed.
- Observe for signs of hypernatremia (e.g., thirst, anxiety, restlessness, dry skin and mucous membranes); report any significant findings.
- Administer medications as ordered: insulin for glucose excess, diuretics for sodium retention; monitor for effectiveness and toxicity; inform physician of patient responses.

☐ EVALUATION CRITERIA/DESIRED OUTCOMES

The Patient

- Has normal blood glucose and serum sodium levels
- Exhibits no signs of hyperglycemia or hypernatremia

The Patient with a Spinal Cord Injury

Definition/Discussion

A spinal cord injury is a fracture or displacement of one or more vertebrae causing damage to the spinal cord and nerve roots, with resulting neurologic deficit and altered sensory perception or paralysis, or both.

Nursing Assessment

☐ PERTINENT HISTORY

Trauma; tumor; level of injury; other medical problems (e.g., lung disorder, coagulation disorder, ulcer); medications; smoking; alcohol use

☐ PHYSICAL FINDINGS

Motor function (movement, strength, tone); sensory function; reflexes; respiratory status; symptoms of spinal shock (falling blood pressure, depression of all reflexes); absence of sweating below injury level; bladder and bowel function; symptoms of autonomic dysreflexia (headache, increased blood pressure, diaphoresis, flushing, pallor), skin integrity

☐ PSYCHOSOCIAL CONCERNS/ DEVELOPMENTAL FACTORS

Age, sex, life-style, occupation, usual role and responsibilities, available support systems, previous coping strategies, emotional reaction to injury

☐ PATIENT AND FAMILY KNOWLEDGE

Anatomy and physiology of spinal cord; treatment, prognosis/expected outcome; level of knowledge, readiness and willingness to learn

Nursing Care

☐ LONG-TERM GOAL

The patient will remain free from preventable complications; the patient will maintain maximal motor and sensory function; the patient will make successful adjustment to an altered style of living compatible with the injuries.

NURSING DIAGNOSIS #1

a. **Ineffective breathing pattern** related to muscle paralysis, spinal cord edema, fluid overload, impaired function of diaphragm
b. **Impaired gas exchange** related to muscle paralysis, spinal cord edema, fluid overload, impaired function of diaphragm
c. **Ineffective airway clearance** related to muscle paralysis, spinal cord edema, fluid overload, impaired function of diaphragm

Rationale: *Injury to C4 and above results in loss of innervation of the diaphragm, abdominal, and intercostal muscles. Injury below C4 leaves the diaphragm intact but the abdominal and intercostal muscles are impaired. Tidal volume and vital capacity are decreased resulting in an ineffective cough and retention of secretions that predispose the patient to pneumonia. Fluid overload can lead to pulmonary edema. If the patient develops an ileus as a result of decreased peristalsis, the extra abdominal pressure can further impair the functioning of the diaphragm. Immobility and flaccid paralysis of the lower extremities contribute to venous stasis and the development of thrombi that* *may travel to the lung and cause a ventilation/perfusion abnormality.*

GOAL

The patient will maintain adequate ventilation and be free from pulmonary complications.

IMPLEMENTATION

- Assess patient's ability to maintain a patent airway.
- Maintain a patent airway with proper positioning, suctioning, airway adjuncts; refer to *The Patient with a Tracheostomy*, page 236.
- Monitor respiratory rate, rhythm, and depth at least every 1-2 hours.
- Auscultate lung sounds every 2-4 hours to determine adequate aeration and detect adventitious sounds.
- Monitor serial vital capacity results; report decreasing volumes.
- Monitor arterial blood gas (ABG) values for acid-base abnormalities and decreased oxygen saturation.
- Monitor intake and output.
- Encourage coughing and deep breathing every 1-2 hours to mobilize secretions; perform postural drainage if needed; instruct in use of incentive spirometer if indicated.
- Utilize air mist/vaporizer to break up secretions and improve oxygenation; administer oxygen as ordered.
- Maintain ventilator function if necessary, refer to *The Patient Who is Ventilator Dependent*, page 239; when weaned, stay with patient, monitor ABGs, assess lung sounds and volumes.
- Administer heparin for actual/potential pulmonary embolus; monitor coagulation studies; report results.
- Apply antiembolic hose; remove every 8 hours to measure calf and thigh and assess skin integrity, circulation for potential deep vein thrombosis.

EVALUATION CRITERIA/DESIRED OUTCOMES

The Patient

- Maintains ABGs within normal limits
- Has clear bilateral breath sounds

NURSING DIAGNOSIS #2

Alteration in cardiac output: decreased related to spinal shock

Rationale: *Spinal shock is a state of transient depression of reflex activity below the level of injury. It happens immediately and may last from a few days to weeks or even months after injury. The result is a loss of vasomotor tone characterized by decreased blood pressure, bradycardia, loss of temperature control, sweating, and retention of urine and feces. Steroids and alignment are used to treat this disorder.*

GOAL

The patient will demonstrate cardiovascular stability.

IMPLEMENTATION

- Monitor vital signs (blood pressure and heart rate) every 2-4 hours (vasodilation and venous pooling lead to decreased cardiac output).
- Monitor temperature every 4 hours; keep patient warm but avoid overheating; prevent chilling especially at bathtime.
- Assess for presence/absence of rectal tone.
- Monitor urinary output and mentation to determine adequate perfusion to kidney and brain.
- Administer medications (steroids) and fluids as ordered and necessary to maintain normotensive state.
- Maintain proper body alignment with halo, traction, etc.

EVALUATION CRITERIA/DESIRED OUTCOMES

The Patient

- Maintains blood pressure and heart rate within normal limits
- Is afebrile

NURSING DIAGNOSIS #3

a. **Potential for injury** related to unstable vertebral column, stress, steroids
b. **Potential for infection** related to exogenous steroid administration

Rationale: Secondary injury to the spinal cord can occur as a result of inadequate stabilization of the vertebral column. A neurologic deficit not previously present may develop. An unexpected injury or illness can trigger the stress response and development of a gastrointestinal (GI) ulcer. The use of steroids to decrease spinal cord edema also contributes to GI bleeding and ulcer formation.

☐ GOAL

The patient will be free from further neurologic damage, GI bleeding, infection.

☐ IMPLEMENTATION

- Extend the neck and maintain in the position of extension to prevent further cord injury.
- Maintain hyperextension by use of Foster, Stryker frames and/or Crutchfield, Barton, or Vinki tongs as ordered.
- Apply and maintain traction weights; do not remove; ensure that they are free hanging.
- Report immediately any signs of motor or sensory loss indicative of further neurologic damage.
- Utilize sand bags on each side of head to prevent excess movement.
- Log roll patient until spine is considered stable.
- Assist with x-rays as ordered, maintaining proper alignment of head/neck.
- Utilize adequate help when lifting in order to maintain proper body alignment.
- Administer antacids and cimetidine (Tagamet) as ordered, if on steroids, to prevent potential GI bleeding.
- Assess for GI bleeding by testing pH and presence of blood in any emesis or nasogastric drainage; test stools for presence of blood.
- Ensure aseptic technique when caring for urethral catheter. Refer to Nursing Diagnosis #6.

☐ EVALUATION CRITERIA/DESIRED OUTCOMES

The Patient

- Has no further increase in neurologic deficit
- Is protected with stabilizing device
- Is free from GI bleeding
- Maintains correct alignment of spine and head
- Is free from signs and symptoms of infection

NURSING DIAGNOSIS #4

Impaired physical mobility related to spine instability and neurologic (motor/sensory) deficit

Rationale: An unstable spinal column requires immobilization to prevent further injury. The patient may be placed in a special bed (e.g., a Stryker frame) or in a regular bed with restricted activity and possibly a halo cast. Motor/sensory deficits resulting from the spinal injury will alter the ability to move.

☐ GOAL

The patient will be free from preventable complications of immobility (e.g., wrist or foot drop, contractures, external rotation of hip).

☐ IMPLEMENTATION

- Assess patient's motor and sensory functions daily to determine abilities and limitations.
- Utilize a firm mattress with a bedboard if patient is in a regular bed.
- Maintain patient in proper alignment at all times.
- Reposition or turn patient every 2 hours; log roll and support if patient is in a regular bed.
- Position feet against pillows or board to prevent footdrop.
- Apply and maintain orthopedic appliances, halos, collars, handsplints.
- Apply trochanter rolls from the crest of the ileum to the midthigh of both extremities to prevent external rotation of hip joints.
- Begin passive range-of-motion exercises within 48-72 hours of injury, 4-5 times daily.
- Consult physical/occupational therapist for exercises and appliances such as splints.

☐ EVALUATION CRITERIA/DESIRED OUTCOMES

The Patient

- Maintains flexibility of all joints
- Is free from of wrist or footdrop, contractures, hip rotation

NURSING DIAGNOSIS #5

Impairment of skin integrity related to immobility, sensory/motor deficits, circulatory impairment, traction pins, inadequate nutritional intake

Rationale: *Denervated areas break down faster and heal more slowly than those with normal nerve supply. Poor circulation resulting from venous stasis and decreased blood supply in the lower extremities can contribute to skin breakdown. Special beds as well as immobilization devices create additional potential pressure points. A patient in a halo will need attention to the areas where the pins pierce the skin. Adequate nutritional intake is necessary for maintaining skin integrity and healing.*

☐ GOAL

The patient's skin will remain intact.

☐ IMPLEMENTATION

- Assess patient's motor and sensory function, and peripheral circulation (pulses, color, temperature) to determine susceptibility to skin breakdown.
- Assess patient's skin (intactness, color) every 8 hours; palpate area under sheepskin pads of halo cast when patient is supine/prone.
- Position patient in anatomic alignment and use pads on bony prominences.
- Turn patient every 2 hours; use specialized equipment for turning (e.g., Stryker/Foster frame, CircOlectric/Roto-rest bed).
- Keep patient clean and dry as moist environment creates medium for breakdown; loosen lower straps of halo cast to reach otherwise inaccessible areas.
- Massage skin gently over bony prominences every 2 hours with a circular motion to promote circulation.
- Ensure adequate nutritional intake of foods and fluids.
- Provide high-protein formula feedings between meals to prevent hypoproteinemia.
- Keep heels off the bed.
- Keep linen free from wrinkles.
- Assess skin around pins of halo for erythema and drainage every 8 hours (some oozing and inflammation is expected the first few days).
- Provide ordered pin-site care every 4-8 hours with hydrogen peroxide, soap and water, or povidone-iodine solution.

☐ EVALUATION CRITERIA/DESIRED OUTCOMES

The Patient

- Has intact skin free from erythema
- Is free from infection at pin sites

NURSING DIAGNOSIS #6

a. **Alteration in patterns of urinary elimination** related to absence of volitional control/sensation

b. **Incontinence: total/functional** related to absence of volitional control/sensation

Rationale: *Impaired neural innervation predisposes the patient to the development of a urinary tract infection (UTI), reflux, stasis, or stone formation.*

☐ GOAL

The patient will establish a satisfactory pattern of urinary elimination free from retention or overflow; will be free from UTI or formation of urinary calculi.

☐ IMPLEMENTATION

- Monitor intake and output.
- Insert Foley catheter; begin aseptic intermittent catheterization as soon as possible to prevent complications associated with retention catheters (e.g., infection, atonic bladder).
- Assess odor, appearance, and amount of urine output to determine concentration, possible UTI.
- Ensure fluid intake of 2-3 liters/day if not contraindicated.
- Palpate bladder for distension gently and carefully as this procedure can trigger autonomic dysreflexia.
- Maintain acidity of urine by offering acid-ash diet; consult with dietician.
- Obtain urinalysis, culture and sensitivity samples as necessary.

- Monitor temperature every 8 hours as fever may indicate bladder infection.

☐ EVALUATION CRITERIA/DESIRED OUTCOMES

The Patient

- Maintains empty bladder without residual and distension
- Has clear, amber urine
- Has negative urine cultures

NURSING DIAGNOSIS #7

Alteration in bowel elimination: constipation, incontinence related to absence of sensation/volitional control, immobility

Rationale: *The patient with a spinal cord injury will be unable to feel an imminent bowel movement. Limited mobility during the acute phase contributes to potential constipation, as does the change in eating habits that comes with hospitalization.*

☐ GOAL

The patient will establish a satisfactory pattern of evacuation without dependence on laxatives.

☐ IMPLEMENTATION

- Determine patient's previous pattern of elimination.
- Auscultate bowel sounds and palpate abdomen for distension every 8 hours.
- Assess and record number and character of bowel movements.
- Provide for privacy during period of elimination.
- Encourage fluids and foods high in fiber and roughage when able; consult with dietician.
- Encourage patient to avoid gas-forming foods and liquids.
- Administer suppositories and/or institute manual extraction of stool every other day.
- Administer laxatives when necessary and evaluate effectiveness.
- Insert a rectal tube to relieve abdominal distension.

☐ EVALUATION CRITERIA/DESIRED OUTCOMES

The Patient

- Is free from impaction or constipation
- Passes soft, formed stools every other day
- Is continent of stool

NURSING DIAGNOSIS #8

a. **Grieving** related to body changes
b. **Ineffective individual coping** related to inability to deal with severity of injury
c. **Disturbance of self-concept: body image, personal identity, self esteem** related to loss of body function, physical changes, dependence
d. **Powerlessness** related to loss of ability to walk and/or limited use of arms/hands
e. **Fear** related to unknown prognosis
f. **Ineffective family coping** related to inability to deal with severity of injury

Rationale: *Insult to the spinal cord is often sudden and unexpected. The individual's lifestyle is significantly altered, and as a result of physical losses and hospitalization the patient is in a dependent position even for the most basic needs such as eating and personal hygiene. The patient's ability to deal with the injury depends on age, personality, relationship with the health care providers, and information provided about the extent of the injury and prognosis.*

☐ GOAL

The patient/family will effectively adapt to an altered appearance and abilities; will participate in care within limitations of illness.

☐ IMPLEMENTATION

- Orient patient/family to extent, nature, and probable outcome of the injury.
- Offer realistic hope.
- Allow patient to grieve in own way.
- Provide simple, concrete explanations.
- Assess patient's/family's ongoing understanding of information provided; clarify misconceptions, false hopes; gently return to reality.
- Permit family involvement in patient care as much as possible within unit restriction
- Encourage verbalization of fears, loss of independence, and loss of control of body functions.

- Allow choices and decision-making opportunities when possible.
- Allow patient to participate in care within limitations of illness.
- Decrease stress in the environment by providing for continuity of care, privacy, adequate rest periods, limited or extended visitation if requested.
- Consult social services, counseling, spiritual care as needed.
- Reinforce positive gains and abilities.
- Refer to *The Patient Experiencing Grief and Loss*, page 272, and *The Patient Experiencing a Body-Image Disturbance*, page 253.
- Provide patient with information about support groups when appropriate.

☐ EVALUATION CRITERIA/DESIRED OUTCOMES

The Patient/family

- Participates in care as able
- Increases independence gradually
- Verbalizes accurate understanding of situation, concerns
- Utilizes family for support

NURSING DIAGNOSIS #9

Knowledge deficit regarding disease process/treatment, prognosis/outcomes

Rationale: *The need for immediate stabilization may result in the patient/family having insufficient time to accept information concerning the injury, its treatment and prognosis, or being overwhelmed with more information than they can comprehend. Denial and anxiety are normal as the patient seeks to integrate and understand the situation.*

☐ GOAL

The patient/family will demonstrate adequate knowledge of spinal cord injury.

☐ IMPLEMENTATION

- Introduce new information slowly allowing patient time to comprehend situation.
- Inform patient/family of progress, prognosis, plan of care.
- Encourage verbalization and questions if possible.
- Teach reasons for treatment measures, why patient is experiencing certain signs and symptoms.
- Explain rehabilitation options; assist with decision making regarding appropriate rehabilitation plans.

☐ EVALUATION CRITERIA/DESIRED OUTCOMES

The Patient

- Verbalizes understanding of current situation
- Initiates discussion of rehabilitation options

The Patient Undergoing a Thoracotomy

Definition/Discussion

A thoracotomy is an incision into the chest wall. It may be done to remove an entire lung (pneumonectomy), a lobe (lobectomy), or a segment of a lobe. Patients with decreased pulmonary function are at greater risk postoperatively than those with adequate pulmonary function. Pre-op preparation is vitally important to post-op recovery.

Nursing Assessment

☐ **PERTINENT HISTORY**

Nature of illness, cardiovascular status, chest x-ray, pulmonary function, ECG, history of smoking, allergies, respiratory distress, activity tolerance, occupational history

☐ **PHYSICAL FINDINGS**

Auscultation, inspection, ability to cough, fluid intake, nutritional status, pain, hemoptysis

☐ **PSYCHOSOCIAL CONCERNS/ DEVELOPMENTAL FACTORS**

Known/possible malignancy: overlying concerns for long-range prognosis; nonmalignancy: patient attitudes are generally more optimistic, with less apprehension

☐ **PATIENT AND FAMILY KNOWLEDGE**

Pre-op diagnostic studies and preparation; post-op expectations/routines; purpose of thoracotomy; prognosis for recovery from underlying condition; posthospital regimen

Nursing Care

☐ **LONG-TERM GOAL**

The patient will recover from the surgery free from preventable complications; the patient will have optimum gas exchange.

NURSING DIAGNOSIS #1

Anxiety related to anticipated surgical procedure, post-op prognosis, expectations for recovery

Rationale: *Patient participation is crucial to the success of the procedure. Thorough pre-op teaching is helpful in decreasing patient and family anxiety by promoting feelings of control through knowledge of procedure and post-op routines.*

☐ **GOAL**

The patient/family will experience decreased anxiety.

☐ **IMPLEMENTATION**

- Plan to spend at least fifteen minutes daily with patient/family to listen to their concerns/feelings; validate that other patients/ families may have expressed similar feelings.
- Encourage questions about proposed surgery and prognosis; reinforce what physician has instructed; correct misunderstandings; provide additional information as requested or required.
- Teach to deep breathe and cough forcefully; provide with an opportunity to cough with splinting support; instruct in use of blow

bottles or inspirometers and provide time for practice.

- Explain that pain medication will be provided as necessary before activities are attempted.
- Explain purpose and use of assistive devices (if necessary) for turning and sitting up in bed.
- Teach arm exercises to be used postoperatively.
- Explain rationale for all activities to promote patient/family cooperation.
- Refer to *The Patient Experiencing Anxiety*, page 250, for additional interventions as needed.

☐ EVALUATION CRITERIA/DESIRED OUTCOMES

The Patient/family

- Verbalize decreased levels of anxiety
- Discuss post-op expectations

The Patient

- Returns demonstration of post-op activities

NURSING DIAGNOSIS #2

a. **Impaired gas exchange** related to effects of thoracotomy
b. **Ineffective airway clearance** related to inability to expel secretions
c. **Ineffective breathing pattern** related to anxiety/fear of suffocation

Rationale: *When the pleural space is entered surgically, the lung collapses; respiratory function is then carried out by the remaining lung. Overall ventilation, perfusion, and diffusion capabilities are greatly decreased while demands on the unoperated lung are greatly increased. The patient may remain intubated during the immediate post-op period or have an ineffective cough and will require suctioning to remove secretions. Feelings about not being able to breathe may trigger rapid, shallow respirations that further impair gas exchange and increase the metabolic requirements and therefore interfere with healing.*

☐ GOAL

The patient will have optimum respiratory functioning during the post-op period.

☐ IMPLEMENTATION

- Provide care in a calm, assured manner to decrease patient/family anxiety; limit visitors if you assess that increased respiratory distress or fatigue results when visitors are present.
- Elevate had of bed 30°-45° when blood pressure is stabilized.
- Assess rate and quality of respirations every hour; report and record diminished sounds, rales, rhonchi.
- Monitor arterial blood gases (ABGs); inform physician of patient status; implement orders for oxygen/mechanical ventilatory assistance.
- Observe for signs of respiratory distress (e.g., increased dyspnea, restlessness, tachycardia, cyanosis, increased pain); report significant findings to physician; initiate measures (e.g., suction if patient is unable to raise sputum by deep breathing and coughing, and medicate to control pain) to correct precipitating factor if known; prepare for possible reintubation and mechanical ventilation as ordered (refer to *The Patient who is Ventilator-Dependent*, page 239).
- Observe for dysrhythmias, especially tachycardia and PVCs that may be initiated by hypoxia; inform physician; administer antidysrhythmics as ordered; monitor for effectiveness and toxicity.
- Clarify with physician exact orders for positioning and activity (e.g., dangling); turning is usually done from back to either side after lobectomy or segmental resection; after pneumonectomy, extreme lateral positions are avoided although brief periods with patient turned slightly to operated side may be permitted.
- Turn patient at least every two hours; encourage to cough and deep breathe before repositioning; splint incisional site with pillows; ask patient to demonstrate activities practiced preoperatively; provide reinforcement (e.g., praise for correct efforts; reinstruction of incorrect or insufficient actions).
- Refer to *The Patient with a Pneumothorax*, page 197, for specific additional interventions as required.

☐ EVALUATION CRITERIA/DESIRED OUTCOMES

The Patient

- Has respiratory rate and rhythm and ABGs within acceptable limits

- Has chest clear to auscultation and percussion
- Reexpands lung on operated side (except in pneumonectomy)
- Is free from dysrhythmias

NURSING DIAGNOSIS #3

Alteration in fluid volume: excess related to decreased lung area for receiving unoxygenated blood from the heart

Rationale: *Depending on the exact surgery, the pulmonary vascular vessels may be decreased as much as from 50% with pneumonectomy to a relatively small amount with segmental resection.*

☐ GOAL

The patient will maintain fluid balance.

☐ IMPLEMENTATION

- Regulate IV flow carefully and maintain prescribed oral fluid restriction to guard against fluid overload; measure urinary output every 1-2 hours; assess for fluid balance; refer to Table 1, *Common Fluid and Electrolyte Imbalances,* page 14.
- Observe hemodynamic catheter pressures to monitor fluid levels; adjust fluid intake according physician's order; report patient response to physician.
- Observe for other signs of fluid excess (e.g., increased dyspnea, rales, rhonchi, pallor, cyanosis, frothy sputum, tachycardia, neck vein distention at 45° elevation, increased blood pressure); report significant findings to physician; refer to *The Patient with Pulmonary Edema,* page 201, for specific interventions.

☐ EVALUATION CRITERIA/DESIRED OUTCOMES

The Patient

- Is free from signs of fluid overload
- Has hemodynamic pressures within acceptable limits

NURSING DIAGNOSIS #4

Alteration in comfort: pain related to surgical procedure

Rationale: *The thoracic cage is never at rest. Therefore, the constant motion of inspiration/respiration will cause considerable incisional pain. In addition, the patient is required to deep breathe (expand the site) and forcefully cough (place pressure on the site) to prevent atelectasis.*

☐ GOAL

The patient will be comfortable and have pain controlled.

☐ IMPLEMENTATION

- Assess discomfort using a 0-10 point self rating scale to obtain an objective measure.
- Administer pain medications 20-30 minutes before patient is asked to sit up, turn, deep breathe, or cough.
- Avoid overmedication so that respiratory rate and depth are not decreased.
- Splint operative side during activity.
- Include patient as much as possible in planning activity/sleep/rest schedule.
- Promote arm exercises on operative side as soon as feasible.

☐ EVALUATION CRITERIA/DESIRED OUTCOMES

The Patient

- Verbalizes relief from or control of thoracic pain
- Tolerates prescribed level of activity with minimal discomfort

The Patient Receiving Total Parenteral Nutrition

Definition/Discussion

Total parenteral nutrition (TPN), sometimes called hyperalimentation, is the infusion of hypertonic solutions of dextrose, nitrogen, and additives (vitamins, minerals, electrolytes, essential trace elements) directly into the blood stream through an indwelling venous catheter in order to restore/maintain normal body composition and nutrition in individuals who are unable to meet their needs via the gastrointestinal (GI) tract. TPN is usually administered via an established central venous line or a right atrial catheter. Hypertonic solutions need to be infused directly into a central vein with high blood flow. Less concentrated solutions may be given via a peripheral vein.

Nursing Assessment

☐ **PERTINENT HISTORY**

Health problem that interferes with normal nutrition (e.g., Crohn's disease, chemotherapy, surgical manipulation of GI tract); anticipated duration of treatment (short-term during acute illness or lifelong); previous parenteral nutrition experiences; other chronic illnesses that may affect treatment (e.g., diabetes mellitus, renal disease requiring protein and calcium restrictions, cardiac disease requiring sodium restriction)

☐ **PHYSICAL FINDINGS**

Height and weight; muscle mass; serum proteins, electrolytes, minerals; fluid status (skin turgor, edema, diaphoresis); ability to ingest oral foods; method of elimination (usual urinary and GI patterns, ostomies, abnormal losses via vomiting); presence of wounds or fistulas that increase nutritional requirements for tissue repair and growth; anticipated caloric and nitrogen needs; established venous access

☐ **PSYCHOSOCIAL CONCERNS/ DEVELOPMENTAL FACTORS**

Age; sex; usual coping mechanisms; stage of grief response to loss of normal body functioning; changes in role, family dynamics, daily activities, and employment; mental stability, personal resources to perform home parenteral nutrition

☐ **PATIENT AND FAMILY KNOWLEDGE**

Level of knowledge; patient acceptance of health problem necessitating parenteral nutrition; understanding of purpose and mechanics of parenteral nutrition, patient role, and problems to report; readiness and willingness to learn

Nursing Care

☐ **LONG-TERM GOAL**

The patient will receive total parenteral nutrition infusion free from preventable complications.

NURSING DIAGNOSIS #1

Alteration in nutrition: less than body requirements related to inability to absorb nutrients via GI tract, inability to ingest sufficient nutrients

Rationale: *Pathophysiology making GI absorption of nutrients a problem for the patient will vary depending on specific health problem. Regardless of the specific situation, a person needs enough protein for tissue repair and growth, enough calories for energy (both carbohydrate and fat sources), and enough electrolyte, vitamins, minerals, and trace elements* *for normal body functioning. The specific health problem determines exact amount of nutrients needed. General guidelines for daily parenteral nutrition (for adults) are: amino acids—1-1.5 gm/kg; glucose and lipids—25 cal/kg + 10%-30%; sodium—50-120 mmol; potassium—80-120 mEq.*

☐ GOAL

The patient will receive adequate nutrition to restore/maintain health.

☐ IMPLEMENTATION

- Assist with assessment of nutrition needs by
  - measuring height and daily weight
  - accurately recording foods eaten
  - collecting ordered laboratory studies
  - observing fluid status via intake and output (include unusual losses such as vomiting, diarrhea, ostomies, and wounds)
  - performing a daily physical assessment
- Administer using an electronic infusion pump to accurately control rate.
- If solution infuses too slowly do not increase rate to catch up; if solution infuses ahead of schedule, infuse 20% dextrose in water to keep system open until time to resume TPN.
- Monitor blood sugar according to method ordered (e.g., Accucheck, serum glucose) closely during this interim and when TPN is resumed (there may be decreased blood sugar when TPN is not infusing because 20% dextrose is usually a less concentrated glucose solution and it will be infusing at a slower rate).
- Administer intralipids as ordered using an electronic infusion pump (intralipids may be given via a peripheral vein because these solutions are isotonic; they are occasionally piggybacked into TPN solution, sometimes given simultaneously via a second intravenous access site, and sometimes given while TPN is turned off).
  - do not use an IV filter because particles are too large to pass through filter
  - take baseline vital signs and repeat every 10 minutes during first 30 minutes of infusion to monitor for side effects (chills, fever, flushing, diaphoresis, allergic reactions, chest and back pain, nausea and vomiting, headache, vertigo, pressure over the eyes)
  - discontinue infusion if side effects occur
- Monitor patient for hyper/hypoglycemia refer to Nursing Diagnosis #2.

☐ EVALUATION CRITERIA/DESIRED OUTCOMES

The Patient

- Receives infusions on time, free from side effects
- Maintains ideal body weight
- Heals existing wounds
- Is free from electrolyte imbalance or excess/deficit of vitamins and minerals

NURSING DIAGNOSIS #2

a. **Potential for injury** (air embolism, glucose imbalance, impaired catheter integrity) related to infusion of TPN via a central line
b. **Potential for infection** related to central line,TPN

Rationale: *Patients receiving TPN are frequently malnourished and at risk for infection. Hypertonic glucose solution is an excellent culture medium for bacteria and yeast. Poor aseptic technique may result in contamination of catheter or solution. In addition, TPN bypasses the normal defenses of the GI tract. Disconnection of IV tubing attached to a central line without proper clamping may result in air embolism. Inconsistent rate of infusion and inadequate or overdosage of insulin to cover glucose load may lead to hyper/hypoglycemia. Improper clamping or inadequate heparinization of catheter may result in breaks in catheter integrity. Any of these problems may result in breaks and interruption of needed nutrition and can cause serious, even life-threatening problems for the patient.*

☐ GOAL

The patient will be free from complications associated with parenteral nutrition.

☐ IMPLEMENTATION

- Use strict aseptic technique when handling catheter; follow established hospital protocol; refer to Table 3, *Right Atrial Catheter Care*, page 121.

- Check temperature every 4-6 hours and report elevations above 100°F (37.8°C).
- Culture any purulent drainage from any part of body; perform routine blood and urine cultures as ordered.
- Refrigerate TPN solution (which has been prepared by pharmacist under laminar flow hood) until 1 hour before administration to retard the growth of yeast that grows easily in high dextrose solution; inspect solution for turbidity, precipitates, or cracks in the bottle before administration.
- Administer solution via IV tubing with 0.22 micron in-line filter to remove impurities; do not allow solution to hang for more than 12 hours.
- Tape all catheter connections securely to avoid inadvertent disconnections; instruct patient to bear down and/or hold breath when changing IV tubing to avoid air embolism; if patient becomes short of breath with chest pain, coughing, or cyanosis, clamp catheter and position on left side to keep air from going into pulmonary circulation, left heart, and into arterial circulation; report immediately.
- Check fingerstick blood sugar or urine sugar/acetone every 4 hours during therapy; administer insulin coverage as ordered; observe for manifestations of hypoglycemia (sweating, pallor, palpitations, nausea, headache, hunger, shakiness, blurred vision) or hyperglycemia (nausea, weakness, thirst, headache, polyuria).
- Flush catheter with heparin solution between infusions if treatment is intermittent rather than continuous; clamp catheter with specially designed toothless nontraumatic clamp between infusions; clamp tubing at a different place each time to prevent clot formation within catheter and breaks in catheter.

☐ EVALUATION CRITERIA/DESIRED OUTCOMES

The Patient

- Is afebrile
- Has no redness, swelling, or discharge at catheter insertion site
- Maintains negative urine and blood cultures
- Is free from shortness of breath, chest pain
- Maintains serum glucose between 80-120 mg%; urine sugar less than 3+

NURSING DIAGNOSIS #3

a. **Alteration in health maintenance** (need for parenteral nutrition) related to digestive dysfunction
b. **Social isolation** related to fear of being different
c. **Grieving** related to lost body function and inability to eat normally
d. **Ineffective individual coping** related to altered health status

Rationale: *Eating is both a time to meet the body's need for nutrition and a time for social interaction. The person who is unable to eat normally due to dysfunction of the digestive system may experience a grief process over the loss. This may progress normally with development of alternative behaviors to deal with the loss or may develop into ineffective coping behaviors. The patient may feel so abnormal that s/he avoids social contact with others. Whatever the response, the patient will need to adjust to a new method of health maintenance regarding diet.*

☐ GOAL

The patient will develop effective coping behaviors to deal with a new method of nutritional support.

☐ IMPLEMENTATION

- Be an empathic and supportive listener during the patient's stages of grief (patient may be in shock; may be mistrustful of an artificial method of nutritional support); use open-ended, leading statements to facilitate expressions of feelings.
- Assess for fluid and electrolyte balance, sepsis, protein imbalance if patient demonstrates delirium; if no metabolic cause or evidence of substance abuse, consult psychologic professionals; refer patient as necessary.
- Assess for signs of depression and hopelessness; provide support and clarify facts as needed.
- Educate patient regarding the treatments and long-term needs; assist in the resumption of normal social contacts.
- If family is overprotective, work with members to encourage patient progress toward an independent life-style.

- Encourage patient to participate in meals; patients can often tolerate small amounts of clear liquids and can schedule this during usual mealtimes.
- Encourage resumption of normal work and leisure activities
  - most patients infuse their solutions at night and are able to conceal catheter beneath clothing during the day
  - contact sports are not allowed due to possibility of damage to the catheter
  - if swimming, cover dressing with plastic wrap and change dressing right after swimming
  - travel is possible with planning
  - sexual activity is also possible with good communication and planning in terms of how to avoid catheter displacement
- Ensure patient has address of a national organization such as Lifeline Foundation, Inc. (2 Osprey Rd., Sharon, Maine 02067) in order to obtain support and ideas for adaptation to condition (local health care centers may also have support groups available).

☐ EVALUATION CRITERIA/DESIRED OUTCOMES

The Patient

- Progresses normally through grief response
- Utilizes effective coping behaviors to deal with alteration in diet
- Participates in family meals and social situations that include food
- Resumes preillness work and leisure activities, making changes as needed to protect catheter
- Expresses feelings to staff and family

NURSING DIAGNOSIS #4

Knowledge deficit regarding new method of nutritional support

Rationale: *The patient/family who understands health problems and treatment will be better able to participate in therapy. They will be willing to ask questions, avoid many problems (e.g., sleep pattern disturbances, sexual dysfunction, noncompliance with treatment), and know how to recognize and deal with complications.*

☐ GOAL

The patient will verbalize need for parenteral nutrition; will cooperate with treatment.

☐ IMPLEMENTATION

- Explain treatments as patient is interested; keep explanations brief; including
  - need to keep head turned away from insertion site during dressing changes to maintain asepsis
  - that TPN is a method of supplying complete nutritional need
  - importance of not turning suddenly or pulling at dressings to avoid dislodging the catheter
- Teach patient how to monitor blood/urine glucose at home and administer insulin as needed.
- Teach to weigh every other day to detect fluid retention and assess nutritional status.
- Assess patient's usual routine and help incorporate TPN into usual work and social schedule.
- Include family members in the instruction.
- Refer patient/family to support groups appropriate to their needs, as necessary.

☐ EVALUATION CRITERIA/DESIRED OUTCOMES

The Patient

- Explains reasons for TPN
- Asks questions and discusses concerns freely

Table 4 Guidelines for Right Atrial Catheter Care

A right atrial catheter is an indwelling catheter made of polymeric silicone rubber that can be left in place for several months. The catheter is positioned in the right atrium, tunnels through the subcutaneous tissue of the chest, and exists between the nipple and the sterum. Two incisions are made, one below the right clavicle (entrance site) and the second between the right nipple and the sternum (exit site). A tunnel is made with long forceps through the subcutaneous tissue between the upper and lower incisions. The catheter is pulled through the tunnel and inserted into the selected vein. The catheter may enter the vein by cutdown or a percutaneous stick; in the latter case, there would only be one incision at the exit site. The catheter is then advanced into the right atrium. A dacron cuff lies about midway between the entrance and exit sites to help anchor the catheter in place and also act as a protective barrier to prevent ascending infection.

The single, double, or multiple lumen catheters are used to administer TPN, to administer blood/blood products, and medications and to draw venous blood samples. Multilumen catheters have the same uses as the double-lumen catheter with the advantage of an additional fluid access line. The proximal lumen (18 gauge, color-coded white, and the longest lumen externally) is for blood samples, medications, and blood administration. The middle lumen (18-gauge, color-coded blue, and of middle length externally) is used for TPN or medications (the latter only if TPN is not used and is not expected to be used). The distal lumen (16-gauge with the shortest external length) is used to monitor CVP or to administer blood, high volumes of fluids, coloids, or medications.

The catheters are inserted by a surgical procedure that lasts about one hour. Diazepam (Valium) may be given when local anesthesia is used. General anesthesia may be indicated, particularly for small children who have difficulty lying still. Right atrial catheter care includes changing the dressings and injection cap, irrigating, drawing blood samples, administering IV push medications and repairing catheter damage. Each institution has specific policies for these procedures. Use the following guidelines, but follow the procedures that your institution has outlined.

- Apply pressure dressings at the entrance and exit sites for the first 24 hours; observe dressings for drainage; the sites may produce serosanguinous drainage for several days (especially if patient is thrombocytopenic), but this should becontrolled with pressure dressings; if bleeding continues, notify physician; expect some bruising and tenderness along the tunnel.
- Keep a flow sheet of intake and output including the blood sample volume withdrawn at the bedside.
- Assess for signs of venous thrombosis (e.g., tenderness and edema of the shoulder, neck, and arm, usually on the side of the catheter), unexplained difficulty infusing IV fluids, edema or subcutaneous fluid along the tunnel, or leakage around the catheter at least every 4 hours.
- Prevent thrombosis by irrigating catheter as ordered with heparinized saline (usually twice/day when not in use) and after drawing each blood sample; know that the frequency of irrigation and concentration of heparin used varies among hospitals and patients depending on the RAC and the patients vulnerability to the effects of heparin; check product information literature for the specific volume the catheter holds.

Irrigation

- Gather supplies
  - povidone-iodine or alcohol swabs
  - 10 cc syringe
  - 1 inch, 21-25 gauge needles
  - heparinized saline (usually 100 units heparin/cc saline; follow hospital policy for heparin concentration and irrigation volume)
- Wash hands; clamp catheter over protective tape if not already clamped.
- Cleanse top of heparinized-saline bottle with alcohol or povidone-iodine swab and allow to air dry.
- Prepare syringe with appropriate amount of heparinized saline.
- Cleanse injection cap with alcohol or povidone-iodine swab and allow to air dry.
- Insert needle, unclamp catheter, and inject heparinized saline.
- Clamp catheter while infusing the last 0.5 cc of solution to prevent backflow of blood.
- Leave clamp in place if IV fluids are not to follow; loop the catheter and tape to chest dressing.
- Document type and amount of irrigation solution used and ease of flow into catheter.

Blood Sampling

- Draw as ordered through a single lumen catheter or through the proximal lumen (white) of a multilumen catheter; irrigate using procedure outline above; attach a sterile injection cap securely or reconnect the IV after withdrawing desired blood sample; document amount of blood drawn and patient's response to procedure.
- Ask the patient what usually facilitates blood withdrawal if you have difficulty withdrawing blood (catheter may be lodged against the wall of the atrium) or have patient try one or a combination of the following to facilitate obtaining desired blood sample:
  - –change position (roll to side, sit upright, lie flat, etc.)
  - –take a deep breath
  - –perform Valsalva's maneuver (unless contraindicated because of change of bradycardia)
  - –raise one or both arms overhead, or lower arms

IV Administration

- Infuse IV at 30 cc/hour or more; flush catheter with normal saline (or dextrose if appropriate) before and after administering any medications not compatible with IV solution; double check that IV is restarted after drawing blood or giving medication; ensure that electronic pumps are not inadvertently turned off.
- Teach patient to help keep tubing unkinked.
- Prevent air embolism by taping all connections securely; remove air bubbles from IV tubing and syringes; clamp catheter before changing injection cap or tubing.

Injection Cap

- Know that when the right atrial catheter is not connected to continuous IVs (or one of the lumens is not connected), the lumens are capped like a heparin lock, enabling the patient to move around freely while maintaining a closed, sterile system; because the cap may be punctured several times a day, change it at least every third day and each time a blood sample is taken.
- Inspect the cap integrity every shift.
- Change cap as required.
  - –gather supplies (irrigation supplies, new injection cap)
  - –wash hands
  - –clamp catheter over protective tape and prepare supplies
  - –put on sterile gloves
  - –cleanse cap-connection site with povidone-iodine swab and allow to air dry
  - –remove old cap and replace with new cap, twisting securely but without force
  - –unclamp catheter and irrigate if needed (see irrigation procedure)
  - –tape cap-catheter junction securely, folding ends of tape onto itself (creating tabs to facilitate tape removal)
  - –wrap the catheter end in sterile gauze and tape to chest

Catheter damage

- Prevent catheter damage
  - –use toothless clamps (e.g., bulldog or rubber-tipped hemostats) on catheter
  - –keep clamp attached to patient's chest dressing, clothing, or on tape tabs around catheter at all times for emergency use
  - –do not use scissors to remove old dressings or tape
  - –use 1 inch needles for irrigation and medication administration
  - –clamp only over protective tape and rotate clamp sites daily
- Clamp catheter close to the patient's chest immediately if catheter leaks or is damaged.
- Cut off the damaged portion of the catheter with sterile scissors or scalpel (as long as more than 4 cm of catheter remains intact).
- Insert a 2 inch angiocath (using the appropriate gauge for the lumen) into the catheter end and remove the stylus.
- Follow the irrigation procedure and replace the injection cap or reconnect the IV fluids.
- Tape connections securely.
- Obtain a repair kit and repair catheter per directions.
- Document procedure and patient's response.

Dressing Changes

- Check hospital protocol regarding dressing change procedures; use aseptic technique at all times; assess entrance and exit sites for signs of infection at each dressing change; report minor temperature elevations since neutropenic patients have a poor immune response.
- Gather supplies
  - –clean gloves
  - –bag for contaminated supplies
  - –sterile towel and gloves
  - –hydrogen peroxide (H_2O_2)
  - –sterile bowl
  - –3 povidone-iodine swabsticks
  - –3 cotton-tip swabs
  - –alcohol swab
  - –povidone-iodine or antibiotic ointment
  - –2 × 2 inch gauze
  - –2 isolation masks
  - –transparent dressing
- Place patient in supine position with equipment on bedside or overbed table.
- Mask self and patient; turn patient's head away from dressing site; wash hands and put on gloves.
- Remove and bag old dressing; loosen the dressing with an antibacterial soap if the tape removal is painful (this has not been shown to increase infection rate).
- Inspect entrance and exit sites for indication of infection (e.g., redness, ecchymosis, swelling, exudate).
- Remove gloves and wash hands; prepare sterile field, open sterile supplies onto field; pour H_2O_2 into sterile bowl, open alcohol swab; put on sterile gloves
- Cleanse a 3-4 inch area around the exit site with a circular motion using one povidone-iodine swabstick at a time; move each swabstick from the inner to the outer aspect of the circle; allow to air dry; if skin is sensitive, substitute hexachlorophene for povidone-iodine.
- Cleanse the area with H_2O_2 on cotton tip swabs using the same procedure; allow to air dry; clean catheter with alcohol swab, moving from chest outward; allow to air dry.
- Apply a small amount of povidone-iodine ointment to the exit site and cover with sterile 2 × 2 inch gauze; apply an occlusive transparent waterproof dressing that allows the skin to breathe; use tincture of benzoin on skin if susceptible to breakdown.
- Permit patient to shower (with physician's order) with the dressing in place; redress site after shower as needed.
- Change tubing every 24-48 hours (depending on hospital policy).
- Monitor for any systemic manifestations of infection (e.g., fever, tachycardia, tachypnea, hypotension) every 4 hours; report significant findings.
- Administer antibiotics as ordered; monitor for effectiveness and toxic effects.

The Patient with a Tracheostomy

Definition/Discussion

A tracheostomy is the surgical creation of an opening (stoma) into the trachea. It is performed to circumvent upper airway obstruction, to facilitate removal of tracheobronchial secretions, to optimize mechanical ventilation, or to enhance ventilation for any patient with decreased chest muscle capability. The tracheostomy may be temporary or permanent.

Nursing Assessment

☐ PERTINENT HISTORY

Reason for tracheostomy, date of procedure, temporary or permanent; oral fluids/foods status

☐ PHYSICAL FINDINGS

Color; vital signs with emphasis on respirations, breath sounds; condition of skin around stoma; humidification, cuff (inflated/deflated), closed/open system

☐ PSYCHOSOCIAL CONCERNS/ DEVELOPMENTAL FACTORS

Inability to communicate verbally, fear of asphyxia, change in body image

☐ PATIENT AND FAMILY KNOWLEDGE

Hygiene regimen to be followed after discharge; purpose of tracheostomy, permanent or temporary; indications for contacting physician after discharge; level of knowledge; readiness and willingness to learn

Nursing Care

☐ LONG-TERM GOAL

The patient will maintain optimum ventilation; the patient will care for own stoma, incorporating changes necessary to accommodate this alteration in life-style.

NURSING DIAGNOSIS #1

Ineffective airway clearance related to inability to expel excess secretions

Rationale: *This artificial opening into the tracheobronchial tree bypasses the glottis and the expulsive forcefulness of the cough is reduced. The upper airway passages are also bypassed so that humidification and warming are decreased.*

☐ GOAL

The patient will maintain a patent airway.

☐ IMPLEMENTATION

- Auscultate chest; record respiratory rate and characteristics every 4 hours.
- Suction every 2-4 hours or as needed; record color, consistency, and amount of secretions.
- Observe for restlessness, anxiety, stridor, tachycardia, cyanosis; monitor blood gases if ordered, especially pCO_2.
- Assess for tactile fremitus.
- Turn, cough, and deep breathe every 2 hours.
- Provide humidification.
- Ensure fluid intake of 2,000 cc/day unless contraindicated.

- Elevate head of bed or place patient in semi-Fowler's position.
- Keep obstructive materials such as sheets or cotton away from stoma.
- Tape obturator to head of bed; maintain an extra tracheostomy tube/hemostat at bedside.
- Provide tracheostomy care every 8 hours or as necessary; keep ties securely knotted; never remove old ties until new ones are in place or unless a second person holds the flange in place.
- Inflate cuff during and for 30 minutes after each feeding.
- Flex neck and thrust chin downward to facilitate swallowing of food/fluids.

☐ EVALUATION CRITERIA/DESIRED OUTCOMES

The Patient

- Breathes easily with a respiration rate between 8 and 20
- Demonstrates clear breath sounds upon auscultation
- Takes food and fluids without choking

NURSING DIAGNOSIS #2

Potential for infection related to altered pattern of ventilation, ineffective airway clearance

Rationale: *With the body's first line of defense (an intact skin as a protective barrier) compromised and the upper airway passages no longer functional, there is an access route for infectious organisms to enter the respiratory tract. If the patient is unable to expel excess secretions, the likelihood of infection increases as the accumulated secretions provide a medium for the growth of organisms.*

☐ GOAL

The patient will remain free from infection.

☐ IMPLEMENTATION

- Inspect skin around stoma for signs of inflammation (e.g., redness, swelling, warmth, increased tenderness) every 2-4 hours during first few days postoperatively, then at least every 8-12 hours; recognize that some incisional inflammation is expected during the early post-op period; report unexpected changes in appearance (e.g., exacerbation of signs of inflammation or drainage around stoma).
- Use sterile technique in suctioning and in performing tracheostomy care.
- Change external dressing and ties when wet or soiled.
- Administer prophylactic antibiotics if prescribed, carefully monitoring for effectiveness (afebrile, normal pulse and respiratory rate, white blood count within normal limits, negative sputum cultures) and toxicity (abnormal hematologic, renal, liver function studies).
- Assess for other etiologic factors (e.g., impaired nutritional status, immunosuppression, environment, existing disease processes) that might contribute to the development of infection; initiate measures to modify these factors.

☐ EVALUATION CRITERIA/DESIRED OUTCOMES

The Patient

- Has clean, dry skin around the stoma
- Maintains temperature within normal limits
- Expectorates clear respiratory secretions
- Exhibits normal laboratory studies

NURSING DIAGNOSIS #3

Impaired communication: verbal related to effects of tracheostomy

Rationale: *The artificially created opening bypasses the larynx, making phonation impossible.*

☐ GOAL

The patient will establish an effective method of communication.

☐ IMPLEMENTATION

- Provide pad/pencil or erasable slate for writing.
- Arrange signals for bells or buzzer.
- Work out an alternative method of communication for common needs (e.g., tongue clicks, eye blinks, finger taps).

☐ EVALUATION CRITERIA/DESIRED OUTCOMES

The Patient

- Communicates needs and wants effectively with minimal frustration

NURSING DIAGNOSIS #4

Anxiety related to weaning process

Rationale: *Some patients will need a tracheostomy for a limited period of time. It is likely that the patient will display some anxiety about getting enough air when the decision is made to start weaning. In addition, the patient with a chronic respiratory condition may be concerned that the weaning will be unsuccessful. The return to normal ventilation pathways can be achieved by a planned progressive set of actions.*

☐ GOAL

The patient/family will express decreased anxiety; the patient will ventilate through the nose, pharynx, larynx, and trachea.

☐ IMPLEMENTATION

- Explain the process to the patient/family carefully, showing a fenestrated tracheostomy tube.
- Begin by suctioning the tracheostomy thoroughly.
- Deflate the cuff; remove inner cannula; clean and store in hydrogen peroxide solution.
- Insert the plug in outer cannula for 5-10 minutes; monitor the patient constantly for any sign of respiratory distress.
- Do not leave patient unattended while tube is plugged.
- At the end of 10 minutes, remove plug; rinse inner cannula in saline solution and reinsert.
- Gradually (over a period of several days) increase the time the outer cannula is plugged.
- Decrease the size of, remove the tube as ordered by the physician; cover stoma site with light dressing until edges are closed.

☐ EVALUATION CRITERIA/DESIRED OUTCOMES

The Patient/family

- Expresses decreased anxiety about weaning process

The Patient

- Breathes through normal passages

NURSING DIAGNOSIS #5

Knowledge deficit related to tracheostomy care

Rationale: *The tracheostomy requires constant care in order to provide the patient with adequate ventilation.*

☐ GOAL

The patient/family will suction the airway and provide routine care; will know how to proceed if the outer tube should become displaced; will take caution with environmental factors that might lead to aspiration of foreign particles.

☐ IMPLEMENTATION

- Implement teaching plan for tracheostomy care with adequate time for practice and mastery of skill before discharge.
- Encourage the patient to increase amount of self-care while still in the hospital.
- Review physician's instructions as to what to do should the outer tube become displaced.
- Advise to avoid swimming; showers may be taken if the spray is directed below the stoma and if a water-deflective mask can cover it.
- Suggest using a porous covering for the stoma to filter out dust/foreign objects.
- Encourage wearing a Medic-Alert bracelet to advise of tracheostomy.

☐ EVALUATION CRITERIA/DESIRED OUTCOMES

The Patient/family

- Demonstrates the procedure for suctioning and routine care with minimal anxiety
- Describes the process for reinserting the outer cannula and avoiding aspiration

The Patient

- Wears a Medic-Alert bracelet upon discharge

The Patient Who Is Ventilator Dependent

Definition/Discussion

When the patient is unable to maintain safe levels of carbon dioxide and/or oxygen by spontaneous breathing, mechanical ventilation may be used to artificially substitute for the bellows action of the thoracic cage. This artificial mode can maintain automatic ventilation for prolonged periods of time. There are 3 major categories of commonly used ventilators: external body ventilators, pressure-cycled ventilators, and volume-cycled ventilators.

Nursing Assessment

☐ PERTINENT HISTORY

Respiratory insufficiency/failure resulting in alteration of the ventilation/perfusion ratio secondary to pulmonary diseases, neuromuscular diseases, central nervous system depression/injury/disease, musculoskeletal diseases, chest trauma, thoracic malformation, severe cardiac or renal diseases

☐ PHYSICAL FINDINGS

Tachypnea, hyperventilation, dyspnea, wheezes, rhonchi; hypoxemia (on room air, PaO_2 below 50), hypercapnea (room air $PaCO_2$ above 50); vital capacity less than 15 ml/kg body weight, inspiratory force of less than −25 cm H_2O; nasal flaring, use of accessory muscles for respiration, intercostal and sternal retractions; dusky skin color due to cyanosis, especially of lips and nailbeds; alteration in sensorium (e.g., restlessness, agitation, confusion, decreased level of consciousness), headache; diaphoresis; tachycardia and other dysrhythmias, abnormal serum electrolytes (particularly potassium and sodium), alterations in extracellular fluid balance

☐ PSYCHOSOCIAL CONCERNS/ DEVELOPMENTAL FACTORS

Fear of inability to control breathing or not being able to communicate, onset of acute episode (history of chronic illness versus unanticipated respiratory distress), previous coping strategies of patient/family/support system, prognosis and implications of projected lifestyle changes

☐ PATIENT AND FAMILY KNOWLEDGE

Causative factors, including pathology of respiratory system; explanations of machinery used and diagnostic studies performed; prognosis and rehabilitative strategies, readiness and willingness to learn

Nursing Care

☐ LONG-TERM GOAL

The patient will receive mechanical ventilatory assistance until such time as s/he is capable of maintaining normal spontaneous respirations.

NURSING DIAGNOSIS #1

a. **Ineffective breathing pattern** related to bronchospasm, mucosal edema, hypoxemia, hypercapnea
b. **Ineffective airway clearance** related to bronchospasm, inability to expectorate excessive or thick secretions, mucosal edema
c. **Impaired gas exchange** related to hyperinflation of alveoli, ventilation/perfusion mismatch

Rationale: *Respiratory failure is caused by any condition that results in alterations in the ven-*

tilation/perfusion ratio. The patient may become hypoxic and compensatory mechanisms (e.g., hyperventilation, tachypnea) may be manifested. While these mechanisms may be effective for a short period of time, they are fatiguing and soon are no longer compensatory. The lungs can then no longer maintain gaseous exchange adequate to provide oxygen to all body tissues. Depending upon the specific causative factor, the patient may also have secretions or alterations in the respiratory anatomy (mucosal edema) or physiology (bronchospasm) that can interfere with the patency of the airway. Mechanical ventilation, when properly regulated, should result in resolution of ineffective breathing patterns and impaired gas exchange. However, the patient who is ventilator dependent is frequently unable to maintain a clear airway without being suctioned.

☐ GOAL

The patient will maintain optimal ventilation with mechanical assistance; will maintain a clear airway; will resume normal breathing patterns when mechanical assistance is no longer necessary.

☐ IMPLEMENTATION

- Monitor respiratory status every 1-2 hours or as necessary; *do not depend solely on digital readouts of ventilator*; auscultate and document breath sounds; inspect and record chest movements/use of accessory muscles; note character and rate of spontaneous respirations.
- Verify that endotracheal or tracheal tube is secured in place and that ventilator settings (tidal volume, oxygen percentage [FiO_2], respiratory rate, airway pressures [high airway pressure limit is usually 20 cm H_2O above peak pressure selected; low limit is 5-10 cm H_2O below peak pressure], sensitivity and mode) and cuff pressures (if applicable) are as ordered; record every 8 hours or whenever changes are made.
- Ensure delivered air is humidified; check water level in reservoir at least every 8 hours; validate patency of all tubing; remove pooled liquids, reconnect tubing securely.
- Check ventilator alarm system every 8 hours; ensure alarm indicator is in the "ON" position at all times.
- Monitor patient's response to mechanical ventilation; check and record vital signs, skin color, level of consciousness every 2-4 hours or as ordered; report changes in status to physician.
- Troubleshoot alarm conditions; disconnect patient from mechanical ventilator and manually ventilate with resuscitation bag if necessary to ensure proper ventilation.
- Suction every 2 hours or as necessary; monitor for bradycardia (may be caused by stimulation of the vagus nerve while suctioning) or other dysthythmias; record amount and character of secretions.
- Avoid having suctioning catheter in place for longer than 12-15 seconds at a time; reconnect ventilator tubing between insertions of suctioning catheter; consult with physician or unit protocols regarding increasing the percentage of oxygen received or "sighing" the patient (providing a longer, deeper breath manually with a resuscitation bag or mechanically by adjusting the ventilator setting) before or after suctioning.
- Monitor arterial blood gases as ordered; report changes to physician.
- Watch for signs of "fighting" the ventilator; may be related to pain, fear, hypoxia, or blocked airway; initiate appropriate action to correct situation (e.g., suction, medicate with analgesics or sedatives as ordered, offer brief explanations to decrease fear); note results of nursing action; report changes in status to physician.
- Watch very carefully if pancuronium bromide (Pavulon) (which paralyzes respiratory muscles) is prescribed to correct "fighting or bucking the ventilator"; patient is completely dependent upon ventilator and will be unable to breathe should the tubing become disconnected or the ventilator malfunction in any way.

☐ EVALUATION CRITERIA/DESIRED OUTCOMES

The Patient

- Maintains normal baseline arterial blood gases
- Maintains a patent airway
- Has clear breath sounds, normal heart rate and skin color
- Maintains normal baseline respiratory rate af-

ter mechanical ventilation is no longer necessary

NURSING DIAGNOSIS #2

Potential for infection related to inability to expel accumulated secretions

Rationale: *With the upper airway passages no longer functional, natural barriers to airborne infectious agents are bypassed, providing a route of transmission into the lower respiratory tract. Accumulated secretions provide a medium for the growth of these organisms. Frequent suctioning, while necessary to maintain airway clearance and promote gaseous exchange, does increase the risks of infection as the closed system used for mechanical ventilation is disrupted, allowing for the possible entry of infectious organisms.*

☐ GOAL

The patient will remain free from infection while intubated.

☐ IMPLEMENTATION

- Use sterile technique when suctioning and performing tracheostomy care (refer to *The Patient with a Tracheostomy*, page 236); when possible, use suctioning catheters that attach to ventilatory tubing to decrease the incidence of disrupting the closed system.
- Assess and record characteristics of secretions obtained during suctioning (appearance, odor, amount); obtain specimens for culture as ordered; monitor results and report findings to physician.
- Turn patient side-to-side every 2 hours; recheck tubing after turning to ensure patency and that excess moisture is drained rather than allowed to pool in tubing.
- Monitor for systemic signs of pulmonary infection (e.g., elevated temperature and heart rate, decreased blood pressure) every 2-4 hours or as ordered; obtain blood cultures for elevated temperature as ordered by physician; report significant findings.
- Administer prescribed antibiotics, checking culture and sensitivity reports and monitoring for desired and toxic effects; report significant findings to physician.
- Assess for other etiologic factors (e.g., impaired nutritional status or existing disease states) that might further increase the risk of infection; monitor serum proteins and report decreased levels or disruption of albumin/globulin ratio to physician.

☐ EVALUATION CRITERIA/DESIRED OUTCOMES

The Patient

- Remains afebrile
- Has clear secretions
- Exhibits normal flora on cultured sputum

NURSING DIAGNOSIS #3

Alteration in nutrition: less than body requirements related to increased metabolic demands secondary to illness

Rationale: *Illness states resulting in respiratory insufficiency/failure requiring mechanical ventilation place increased metabolic demands on the patient. Patients with chronic illnesses (e.g., chronic obstructive pulmonary disease or neuromuscular disorders) may also have had impaired nutritional status because of fatigue and/or decreased appetite prior to mechanical ventilation. If infection is present, the metabolic demands further increase. Ensuring adequate nutritional intake is a priority nursing responsibility when caring for ventilator-dependent patients.*

☐ GOAL

The patient will maintain/regain nutritional balance.

☐ IMPLEMENTATION

- Assess for signs of nutritional imbalance at least every 8 hours; monitor skin turgor, inspect oral mucous membranes, check laboratory studies (especially serum proteins and electrolytes) as ordered; report significant findings to physician.
- Provide prescribed nourishment (usually via enteral or parenteral feedings); accurately monitor rate of tube feeding or total parenteral nutrition (TPN) and note expected and unexpected responses; consult unit protocols for specific procedures.
- Encourage patients with tracheostomy tubes in place to eat slowly; ensure that cuff is in-

flated while patient is eating and for 15-30 minutes afterwards (patients requiring continuous mechanical ventilation will always have the tracheal cuff inflated but those being weaned from ventilator may have cuff deflated).
- Provide oral care at least every 8 hours.
- Assess for presence of bowel sounds every 8 hours; if absent, hold feeding while contacting physician.
- Check stool for presence of occult/overt bleeding (patients requiring mechanical ventilation and feeding tubes are at increased risk for developing stress ulcers); report abnormal findings to physician.
- Refer to *The Patient Receiving Total Parenteral Nutrition*, page 229, as needed.
- Weigh daily or every other day as prescribed; report losses of more than 3 pounds.

☐ EVALUATION CRITERIA/DESIRED OUTCOMES

The Patient
- Has normal serum proteins and electrolytes
- Maintains/regains body weight
- Has intact mucous membranes and normal skin turgor

NURSING DIAGNOSIS #4

Impaired verbal communication related to intubation

Rationale: *The endotracheal tube passes between the vocal cords, preventing speech. The tracheostomy is an artificial opening that bypasses the larynx, making phonation impossible. The patient's hands may be restrained to prevent injury caused by pulling on the tubing; therefore, communication with the hands may also not be possible.*

☐ GOAL

The patient will establish and maintain an effective method of communication while intubated.

☐ IMPLEMENTATION

- Ask yes/no questions to which patient can nod/shake head in response.
- Provide alternative communication means (e.g., pencil/paper, magic slate, alphabet board) for patients who do not require arm restraints.
- Have nursing call light accessible, especially if patient is restrained; arrange for signals if patient desires to use that method for communicating.
- Suggest other methods of communication for patients unable to use hands (e.g., eye blinks, tongue clicks, or finger taps); record method chosen on care plan and share with other staff members and visitors.
- Be alert to changes in facial expression or indications that patient is attempting to extubate self; remain with patient; convey acceptance and understanding by remaining calm while stating what you perceive the patient is trying to express.

☐ EVALUATION CRITERIA/DESIRED OUTCOMES

The Patient
- Conveys desired information to caregiver and visitors
- Indicates that messages are understood

NURSING DIAGNOSIS #5

a. **Anxiety** related to dependence upon mechanical ventilator
b. **Fear** related to feelings of suffocation

Rationale: *When the patient is unable to breathe spontaneously, s/he is frequently very anxious and may, in fact, be afraid of dying because of this inability. It is imperative that nurses act to resolve these diagnoses as the manifestations of fear and anxiety (e.g., restlessness, irritability, "fighting" the ventilator) further compromise the patient's ability to maintain adequate ventilation. Family members may also share these anxieties/fears. Helping family members is a priority as their approach to the patient can be beneficial if they are calm and confident or detrimental if agitated and worried.*

☐ GOAL

The patient/family will experience decreased anxiety and/or relief from fear.

IMPLEMENTATION

- Provide explanations for all nursing actions, even if treatment/procedure was previously explained.
- Explain functions of equipment in use at bedside and used for diagnostic procedures; plan time for answering family's questions and include patient in explanations.
- Respond quickly to patient's signals for help; remain with agitated patient; quietly provide reassurance and explanations of what is happening at the time; consider holding patient's hand or lightly massaging forearm or face.
- Encourage physical closeness of family; be alert for interactions that seem to have a calming effect and encourage situations likely to produce these interactions; limit visitation that seems stressful to patient.
- Medicate with prescribed bronchodilators, analgesics, sedatives, and hypnotics; observe for desired and untoward effects; report patient responses to physician.
- Collaborate with discharge planner, social worker, and/or nursing staff to promote adjustment to new area when transfer to another unit is planned.

EVALUATION CRITERIA/DESIRED OUTCOMES

The Patient/family

- States that anxiety and/or fear has decreased
- Expresses understanding of equipment and procedures

Section II

Nursing Care for Selected Psychosocial Problems

The Patient Manifesting Anger

Definition/Discussion

Anger is a strong feeling of displeasure, usually of antagonism, excited by a real or supposed injury; a learned means of avoiding anxiety that arises in response to interpersonal threat; and a normal response to loss (refer to *The Patient Experiencing Grief and Loss,* page 272). *Aggression* is a forceful, attacking action that may be physical, verbal, or symbolic. It is unrealistic and directed outwardly toward the environment or inwardly toward the self. *Violence* is any physical behavior that is destructive to self, others, or property.

Nursing Assessment

☐ **PERTINENT HISTORY**

Previous acute or chronic episodes/outbursts of angry or aggressive behavior; behavioral manifestations of anger (abusive language, frequent negative verbalizations regarding care givers and peers, refusal to conform to hospital routine, acting out, dysfunctional dependent or independent behaviors)

☐ **PHYSICAL FINDINGS**

Physical illness, trauma, organic disorder, inadequate nutrition, refusal of treatments, neglect in self-care

☐ **PSYCHOSOCIAL CONCERNS/ DEVELOPMENTAL FACTORS**

Ineffective patterns of communication, inadequate or underdeveloped socialization skills, dysfunctional family relationships, dependency, chronic or acute anxiety, feelings of inadequacy, history of emotional difficulties, hostility towards self or others, fear, depression

☐ **PATIENT AND FAMILY KNOWLEDGE**

Ability to recognize behaviors of anxiety and feelings of powerlessness, ability to assess family interactions; socialization skills and interpersonal relationships of family, readiness and willingness to learn

Nursing Care

☐ **LONG-TERM GOAL**

The patient will verbally identify causative internal and external stressors; the patient will use realistic and assertive behavior to express displeasure and anger.

NURSING DIAGNOSIS #1

Ineffective individual coping related to anxiety

Rationale: *Ineffective individual coping is manifested when the individual experiences an inability to manage either internal or external stressors adequately related to inadequate resources. Anxiety is a feeling aroused by a vague nonspecific threat. The individual experiences feelings of discomfort and uneasiness, activating the autonomic nervous system. The feelings may be expressed through angry outbursts, hostility, and acting-out behavior, either overt (e.g., fighting, hitting, verbal attack) or covert (e.g., somatizing, depression, suicide).*

☐ **GOAL**

The patient will eliminate the physically harmful and attacking expressions of anger; will express anger assertively rather than aggressively; will identify and use effective coping mechanisms to manage own anxiety.

☐ IMPLEMENTATION

- Assess level of anxiety and remove excess stimulation.
- Tell the patient you will prevent any further expression of anger that is physically harmful in nature.
- Find physical outlets for anger that are acceptable (e.g., hitting punching bag, using batakas).
- Spend time with the patient; ask what the anger is about and if patient refuses to answer, just sit with him/her while s/he is silent.
- Praise any efforts to put the anger/feelings of anxiety into words and to share the causes with you.
- Be aware that this anger is usually not meant for you personally, so do not respond defensively.
- Assist in making connections between feelings of frustration and subsequent behavior.
- Assist in reevaluation of the perceived threat and the anxiety produced.
- Have patient analyze consequences of behavior.
- Set limits on irrational or manipulative demands; state those limits clearly with consequences if limits are violated.
- Assist to develop alternative adaptive coping mechanisms for dealing with anger (e.g., discussion, one-to-one communication, physical exercise).
- Provide positive feedback when patient utilizes adaptive coping mechanisms.

☐ EVALUATION CRITERIA/DESIRED OUTCOMES

The Patient

- Verbalizes when feeling anxious or frustrated
- Describes the difference between the conversational expression of anger and physically harmful/forceful behavior
- Uses a minimum of one alternative adaptive coping mechanism when angry
- Acknowledges the limits set on manipulative or demanding behavior

NURSING DIAGNOSIS #2

Powerlessness related to hospitalization

Rationale: *Powerlessness is a subjective state in which the individual perceives a lack of personal control over events or situations that are occurring to and about him/her. Anger may be seen as a response to feelings of powerlessness and an attempt by the individual to regain control.*

☐ GOAL

The patient will discuss situations that provoke angry feelings; will verbalize both positive and negative feelings related to angry outbursts; will identify factors that contribute to a sense of powerlessness; will identify factors that s/he can control.

☐ IMPLEMENTATION

- Invite to participate in own care and discuss feelings about the hospitalization.
- Assess knowledge of hospitalization and illness.
- Assess present ability to control behavior and to make decisions.
- Determine the patient's feelings of powerlessness before beginning teaching.
- Explain all procedures, rules, and options.
- Keep informed about condition, treatments, and results.
- Provide opportunities for the patient to control decisions by offering alternatives and increase decision-making opportunities as patient progresses.
- Involve in own care on a continuing basis; ask to do specific tasks while you do others; discuss the results of this shared responsibility with the patient.
- Inform patients of scheduled tests/procedures to eliminate unpredictability of events.
- Provide specific times each shift for communication and interaction.
- Be sensitive to the factors that contribute to feelings of helplessness (e.g., strange environment, unknown outcomes, pain), and allow patient to discuss concerns and feelings.
- Direct conversation towards those aspects of the illness for which patient has the most negative feelings; use open-ended questions.
- Spend time with family explaining patient's

need to have the opportunity to express both positive and negative feelings about what is happening.
- Praise the efforts of others to accept the conversational expressions by the patient of negative feelings.
- Praise staff/family efforts to support the patient and to understand the behavior without personalizing it.

☐ EVALUATION CRITERIA/DESIRED OUTCOMES

The Patient/family

- Verbalizes behavior or demands that trigger the physically harmful aspects of patient's anger
- Shares both positive and negative feelings about an individual experience
- Participates in decision-making for self/family
- Experiences a sense of control and power

NURSING DIAGNOSIS #3

Knowledge deficit regarding use of adaptive coping mechanisms to deal with manifestations of anger

Rationale: *Giving information to the patient helps decrease feelings of anxiety and powerlessness, thus reducing angry outbursts as a means of expressing these feelings. Patients who express anger in nonadaptive ways usually have not learned alternative methods of dealing with anger.*

☐ GOAL

The patient/family will use adaptive coping mechanisms in dealing with angry feelings.

☐ IMPLEMENTATION

- Discuss with patient adaptive ways that patient has developed for dealing with feelings of anger, anxiety, powerlessness.
- Identify anger-producing situations with patient; use role playing to practice alternative methods of expressing anger.
- Help patient to plan ways to maintain self-care after discharge; help set personal goals.
- Discuss available community resources and support groups; supply list of such groups as needed.

☐ EVALUATION CRITERIA/DESIRED OUTCOMES

The Patient

- Identifies and expresses angry feelings in adaptive way
- States feelings and behaviors of anxiety, powerlessness that should be reported to the physician/therapist/clinic
- Knows and identifies community resources and support groups

The Patient/Family Experiencing Anxiety

Definition/Discussion

Anxiety is the uncomfortable feeling of tension or dread that is unconnected to a specific stimulus; it can be vague or intense. It occurs as a reaction to some unconscious threat to biologic integrity and/or self-concept. Anxiety can be assessed according to level.

- *Mild:* increased alterness and motivation and ability to cope with daily problems
- *Moderate:* decreased perception of the environment with selective inattention; decreased ability to think clearly
- *Severe:* drastically reduced perceptual field; can focus on only one detail at a time
- *Panic:* inability to integrate environment with the self; cannot function; physical activity is disorganized or the patient may be "frozen"

Nursing Assessment

☐ PERTINENT HISTORY

Recent environmental or family changes, school changes, change in life-style; family stability; employment stability; losses, absence of supportive relationships, confusion of values/beliefs; previously experienced anxiety and coping methods; financial status, health status

☐ PHYSICAL FINDINGS

Increased vital signs; muscle tension, sweating, headaches, dizziness, tremors, sweaty palms, flushing, fatigue; GI discomfort, hyperventilation, somnolence or insomnia; crying, irritability, dry mouth, capillary dilation; inability to concentrate or understand explanations

☐ PSYCHOSOCIAL CONCERNS/ DEVELOPMENTAL VARIATIONS

Age, sex, degree of perceived disruption, patterns of dependency, usual coping patterns of family, socialization pattern (e.g., values, belief systems, culture), occupation, usual roles and responsibilities

☐ PATIENT AND FAMILY KNOWLEDGE

Identifiable cause(s)/agreement about causes and management, involvement of community agencies, level of knowledge, readiness and willingness to learn

Nursing Care

☐ LONG-TERM GOAL

The patient will be able to cope effectively with anxiety and use it as a motivation for change.

> NURSING DIAGNOSIS #1
>
> **Ineffective individual/family coping** related to anxiety
>
> ***Rationale:*** *Anxiety of more than a mild level will impair the individual's ability to cope.*

☐ GOAL

The patient/family will be able to cope with the anxiety and reduce it at least one level.

☐ IMPLEMENTATION

- Determine level of anxiety patient/family is experiencing and use interventions appropriate to that level
  - mild: does not require any intervention
  - moderate
    - spend 5-10 minutes with the individual at least three times daily; show interest and support

* determine cause if possible, since anxiety may decrease if it can be explained
* focus on the immediate problem; stay in the "here and now"
* do not give more information than the individual can handle
* be clear and concise in communication and with explanations; repeat if needed
* attend to physical comforts and needs
* do not make demands of the individual
* do not confront individual or argue regarding unrealistic perceptions
* encourage coping mechanisms such as verbalization
* allow to cry
* teach relaxation exercises

Guide patient through a relaxation exercise to experience its usefulness. Begin relaxation with deep breathing. Use guided imagery to induce relaxation (e.g., "Take another deep breath and let all the tension release. With each breath you become more relaxed. Now, imagine yourself in a peaceful, quiet setting [garden, beach, etc.]). Refer to cassettes, books, and classes on learning and practicing relaxation techniques.

Practice diaphragmatic breathing, with patient

- sit or recline in a comfortable position with legs uncrossed
- place on hand on the chest and the other hand on the diaphragm, approximately 2 inches below the bottom center of the breastbone
- inhale so the diaphragm expands and the hand covering the diaphragm moves out while the other hand remains almost still
- as you exhale, the diaphragm relaxes and the hand covering it moves inward
- as you exhale, the diaphragm relaxes and the hand covering it moves inward
  * do not allow your own personal anxieties be perceived by the individual
- severe
  * use previously stated interventions as applicable
  * decrease environmental stimulation; refer to *The Patient Experiencing Sensory Alteration*, page 275
  * if individual is hyperventilating, encourage to take slow deep breaths and ask to focus on how body feels on expiration; breathe with individual to provide support
  * use only brief, simple communications
  * structure activities into concrete tasks that do not require concentration
  * attend to somatic complaints
  * consider use of a minor tranquilizer if ordered
  * stay with individual until anxiety is lessened
- panic
  * remain with individual; demonstrate competence
  * use physical touch judiciously; some individuals are comforted by touch and some are threatened by it
  * remain calm; reassure that control will be maintained
  * use firm, professional manner
  * use a small room or separate area to provide privacy and security to family
  * direct individual's energy into motor activities; repetitive actions are helpful in concentrating attention; continue close observation
  * administer medication if ordered (imipramine [Tofranil] is often used to treat panic attacks); evaluate effectiveness

☐ EVALUATION CRITERIA/DESIRED OUTCOMES

The Patient/family

- States anxiety is decreased to a tolerable level
- Channels energy into goal-directed activity
- States willingness to learn new ways to cope with anxiety

NURSING DIAGNOSIS #2

Sleep pattern disturbance related to anxiety

Rationale: *Physiologic disturbances caused by anxiety may be reflected in a disturbance in sleep patterns.*

☐ GOAL

The patient will achieve a sleep/rest pattern appropriate to individual needs.

☐ IMPLEMENTATION

- Determine type of sleep disturbance patient is experiencing.
- Ask what the patient/family perceives are the reasons for the patient's disturbed sleep pattern.

- Encourage verbalization of problems causing anxiety if able.
- Provide measures appropriate to reduce insomnia, if indicated and appropriate
  - quiet, secure environment
  - relaxation techniques
  - night light
  - decreased number of unnecessary distractions
  - structured bedtime routine (e.g., personal hygiene, music)
  - maximum measures for comfort of bed, clothing, etc.
- Provide daytime stimulation and a regular schedule that discourages napping and dozing if increased somnolence is exhibited.

☐ EVALUATION CRITERIA/DESIRED OUTCOMES

The Patient

- Identifies disturbances in sleep patterns
- Utilizes measures to achieve appropriate rest and sleep without medication

NURSING DIAGNOSIS #3

Knowledge deficit regarding recognition and effective management of anxiety

Rationale: *The individual can use anxiety as a motivating rather than a destructive force if it is recognized and successful coping mechanisms developed.*

☐ GOAL

The patient will be able to identify sources of own anxiety; will employ effective measures to manage own anxiety.

☐ IMPLEMENTATION

- Be aware of the impact of anxiety on ability to learn
  - mild: learning can occur at this level
  - moderate: learning can occur but it must be directed
  - severe: inability to learn at this level
  - panic: unable to learn
- Help patient identify those tensions and environmental factors that create a feeling of anxiety; attempt to identify precipitating factors or situations.
- Include the patient in decisions about care in order to encourage patient responsibility.
- Give careful explanations of what will occur; encourage questions and verbalization of any concerns that patient may have.
- Encourage supportive family members to be patient since the patient may not respond to them as before; involve them in prevention or management as much as possible.
- Encourage establishment of regular physical activity as tolerated.
- Praise staff and family members who are able to maintain an environment for the patient that allows an understanding of and control over the anxiety.
- Teach assertive techniques to assist in keeping anxiety manageable.
- Provide information regarding community supports available for socialization, services, information, or support.

☐ EVALUATION CRITERIA/DESIRED OUTCOMES

The Patient/family

- Can list environmental factors that elicit anxiety
- Can discuss ways of keeping responses to anxiety at a mild or moderate level and successfully cope with it
- States willingness to learn ways to cope with anxiety
- Can verbalize ways to cope with severe anxiety if it occurs

The Patient Experiencing a Body-Image Disturbance

Definition/Discussion

Body image is a person's image or concept of their own body. It is formed from internal development as well as from environmental experiences including input from others, societal views, cultural practices, and previous experience with persons whose bodies have changed.

A body-image disturbance reflects the inability of an individual to perceive and/or adapt to an alteration in structure, function, or appearance of a part of or the entire body.

Nursing Assessment

☐ **PERTINENT HISTORY**

Surgeries, illness, trauma causing change in body form; rapidity of change; permanent or temporary refusal to participate in care; denial of change(s)

☐ **PHYSICAL FINDINGS**

Loss of body part and/or its function; neurologic, metabolic, or toxic disorders; progressively deforming disorders; acute dismemberment; disability or handicap; visibility of change; withdrawal, apathy, crying, agitation

☐ **PSYCHOSOCIAL CONCERNS/ DEVELOPMENTAL FACTORS**

Previous experience with someone with altered physical appearance, cultural practices, coping patterns, personality style, dependency patterns; depression, shame

☐ **PATIENT AND FAMILY KNOWLEDGE**

Possibility of rehabilitation or repair, degree of change in life-style and functional significance, value placed on alteration, perception of what change means, available community agencies, level of knowledge, readiness and willingness to learn

Nursing Care

☐ **LONG-TERM GOAL**

The patient will acknowledge and integrate body change(s) into adaptive and realistic management of own life.

> NURSING DIAGNOSIS #1
>
> **Disturbance in self-concept: body image** related to altered body structure or function
>
> ***Rationale:*** *A real or perceived change in body image results in a need to modify one's self-concept. Certain areas of the body have greater value and meaning to an individual; threats to these areas cause more disruption and require more adjustment.*

☐ **GOAL**

The patient will acknowledge and begin to accept body change(s).

☐ **IMPLEMENTATION**

- Provide openings to enable patient to express feelings by validating your observations and feelings (e.g., "You look down in the dumps. How are things going for you today?" or "You seem upset/sad. Are you?); be a good listener and accept what patient verbalizes; remember not to take anger or hostility personally (this may be the only way possible for the patient to handle these feelings).

- Focus on the patient's feelings and deal with the presenting behavior (e.g., do not challenge patient's denial that a body change has actually occurred).
- Determine what the body-image change means to the patient and what effect the patient thinks it will have on life; if you think these perceptions are unrealistic, do not challenge them but continue to provide opportunities for patient to share these perceptions and feelings with you.
- Include in nursing care plan patient's own perception of meaning of body change, the objectives, and nursing actions; share plan with all care givers, including family.
- Be accepting of patient's body changes; if patient is repulsed or ashamed of physical changes, s/he will be watching the faces of others for negative signs; assist the family to accept changes also and to avoid reinforcement of the patient's negative feelings.
- Provide basic needs for patient; very dependent behaviors may be exhibited at this time.
- Let the patient know that the feelings and concerns that are being experienced are normal and that you are there to listen as well as to help cope with the changes.

☐ EVALUATION CRITERIA/DESIRED OUTCOMES

The Patient

- States that a change in the body has occurred
- Begins verbalization of feelings regarding the change
- Exhibits fewer negative reactions to staff and environment
- Shows occasional interest in self-care

NURSING DIAGNOSIS #2

Grieving related to loss or alteration in body form, function

Rationale: *Resolution of a loss through successful management of the grief process will allow the patient to progress effectively toward adjustment to changes in body structure and function.*

☐ GOAL

The patient will acknowledge, express, and resolve grief related to change(s) in body form or function.

☐ IMPLEMENTATION

- Recognize individual responses to grief; these are determined by ego strengths, perception and meaning of loss, previous experiences, and present support systems; refer to *The Patient Experiencing Grief and Loss,* page 272.
- Know that the nurse's personal feelings toward loss must be recognized before the nurse can accept those of others.
- Be empathetic and understanding; educate family/patient regarding normal grief reactions to permit more realistic expectations.
- Encourage verbalization of feelings toward the loss of the body part or function, the pleasures provided, and the needs it fulfilled in the past in order to promote acceptance and to lessen denial.
- Allow patient to cry.
- Be alert for signs of depression (e.g., isolation or withdrawal, inability to grieve, fatigue, anorexia).
- Do not encourage fantasizing or false hopes regarding reversal of change in body form or function.
- Know that resolution of loss is accomplished a little at a time; be realistic about time required to achieve resolution.
- Involve family in the grieving process.

☐ EVALUATION CRITERIA/DESIRED OUTCOMES

The Patient

- Verbalizes sadness and feelings of loss; identifies this as part of the normal grieving process
- States what the change in body image means
- Begins to regard the future in a positive way
- Is able to cry
- Begins to share feelings of loss with family

NURSING DIAGNOSIS #3

Knowledge deficit regarding adaptation to alteration in body image

Rationale: *When changes in one's body occur, new coping mechanisms and changes in*

life-style may be required for successful adjustment.

GOAL

The patient will accept the alteration in body image and successfully adapt to required changes in life-style.

IMPLEMENTATION

- Give positive reinforcement for efforts to adapt; patient behavior will indicate when acceptance of body alterations has begun (e.g., may ask questions; will start to look at the incision, dressings, etc.).
- Accept, but do not support, expressions of denial.
- If a prosthesis will be used, assist patient in choice by providing information and arranging for a visit by a member of an ostomy club, Reach to Recovery, or other appropriate group; let patient determine time of visit, but try to arrange it as soon as possible.
- Involve in self-care activities; begin slowly and add new activities one at a time; reinforce any efforts to participate.
- Assist to adjust to awareness of the extent of the loss since there is frequently a lag between initial alteration and realistic perception.
- Tell family how they can help by listening, supporting reality, allowing expressions of anger, denial, and not challenging them, permitting patient to cry and giving positive reinforcement for all efforts to cope/adapt; praise the family for participation in efforts to assist.
- Hold a team conference, including family if you wish, and share information on grief and loss (see page 272) and crisis intervention (see page 256) with each other; discuss what parts of these concepts apply at this time; revise the care plan as necessary.
- Refer for employment counseling if change in occupation is required.
- Refer for continued contact with community support group, home health nurse, and appropriate community agencies.

EVALUATION CRITERIA/DESIRED OUTCOMES

The Patient

- Accepts continued support and positive input from family
- Utilizes community resources such as Reach to Recovery, ostomy club, to provide ongoing support, reassurance, and assistance in recovery
- Resumes predisturbance activities

The Patient Requiring Crisis Intervention

Definition/Discussion

Crisis intervention refers to those approaches used to restore a patient to a state of emotional equilibrium, from one of disequilibrium (the crisis state), that is equal to or better than the functioning at the precrisis level.

Nursing Assessment

☐ **PERTINENT HISTORY**

Recent illness or loss; stresses of the past year; transitions; trauma, catastrophic illness or accident; marriage, job, family stability; decreased ability to carry out activities of daily living (ADL); current threatening event

☐ **PHYSICAL FINDINGS**

Altered vital signs, anxiety (severe to panic), decreased concentration, somatic complaints, agitation, tension, neglect in self-care

☐ **PSYCHOSOCIAL CONCERNS/ DEVELOPMENTAL FACTORS**

Normal coping methods, supportive nuclear or dysfunctional family history, ego strengths, dependency patterns, apathy, distorted perceptions, regression to lower levels of functioning

☐ **PATIENT AND FAMILY KNOWLEDGE**

Previous experiences; perception of the problem, severity of disruption; internal and outside support or agencies; ability to decrease anxiety; socialization, interpersonal, and communication skills

Nursing Care

☐ **LONG-TERM GOAL**

The patient will achieve adaptive resolution of the crisis; the patient will return to usual job/roles with a realistic perception of what has occurred and with adequate coping mechanisms.

NURSING DIAGNOSIS #1

Ineffective individual coping related to perceived inability to deal with problem, distorted perception of the problem

Rationale: *Usual coping mechanisms may not be able to prevent increased stress when a threatening event occurs. The individual may have a distorted perception of the problem and may feel unable to deal with it. The inability to manage the stress situation results in disequilibrium.*

☐ **GOAL**

The patient will state perception of stressful situation and develop coping mechanisms effective in the crisis state.

☐ **IMPLEMENTATION**

- Ask to identify feelings regarding the stressful event and what patient perceives the problem to be; remember perception is what is important and patient's may differ from yours.
- Allow to respond at length and in detail to your questions; do not challenge any statements; try to determine exactly what is most threatening; listen and encourage patient to keep talking.

- Determine the real/anticipated patient loss/losses involved; assess behavior in light of the grief and mourning process; see *The Patient Experiencing Grief and Loss*, page 272.
- Determine the usual ways patient copes with a problem and how successful these methods are.
- Encourage verbalization about supportive individuals or agencies and whether or not they would be of value in the present situation.
- Ask what you could do to make patient feel better right now; if at all possible, provide it.
- Provide basic needs; patient may be very dependent in ADL; allow this dependency to occur for the immediate time.
- Help patient to gradually increase independence in ADL: involve in self-care, slowly at first, then gradually add more activities.
- Provide opportunities for patient to make decisions about daily care (to give some control over own life); praise patient for making decisions, for coping with current stress, for helping self to feel better.
- Ask for patient's ideas on what can be done next to improve the situation; incorporate your ideas with patient's to give a sense of control.
- When behavior indicates that patient is beginning to adapt or cope (e.g., begins to ask questions, focus on reality), support and reinforce reality; share with patient how you see it; ask patient to clarify or validate your perceptions.
- Incorporate into the nursing care plan suggestions for new methods of coping with the crisis state; enlist the cooperation of staff in assisting the patient with these.

☐ EVALUATION CRITERIA/DESIRED OUTCOMES

The Patient

- Appraises situation realistically
- Verbalizes feelings regarding the threatening event
- Identifies usual methods of coping with problems
- States need for new ways to handle the disequilibrium
- Identifies at least two effective strategies

NURSING DIAGNOSIS #2

Anxiety related to feelings of being overwhelmed by threatening event

Rationale: *Situations perceived as threatening produce increased anxiety that can result in inability to manage situation, which leads to feeling overwhelmed.*

☐ GOAL

The patient will identify causes of threat; will achieve skill in managing the anxiety.

☐ IMPLEMENTATION

- Refer to *The Patient Experiencing Anxiety*, page 250.
- Ask what the patient is feeling at this time (e.g., scared, anxious, panicky) and what occurred to cause these feelings (e.g., new diagnosis, new roommate, new equipment).
- Encourage verbalization of feelings of anxiety and discern those that are the most threatening; listen actively and with empathy.
- Make any environmental changes that are possible to decrease the impact of the threat (e.g., change room, allow family to stay for additional support).
- Share information regarding tests, procedures, etc.; tell what to expect and how orders are carried out.
- Enlist the help of other personnel in planning for care that will decrease anxiety; share your perceptions and information with them.
- Teach simple relaxation techniques (e.g., deep breathing) to use whenever needed to keep anxiety from increasing.
- When leaving room, tell patient when you will be back; return at the appointed time.

☐ EVALUATION CRITERIA/DESIRED OUTCOMES

The Patient

- Verbalizes causes of threat and describes threatening event
- Can make realistic requests to keep anxiety manageable
- Uses relaxation techniques
- Requests staff assistance appropriately

NURSING DIAGNOSIS #3

Grieving related to an actual or perceived loss

Rationale: *An individual's grief is affected by many factors, including personality, previous losses, intimacy of relationship, and personal resources. Unresolved grief is a pathologic response of prolonged denial of the loss or a profound psychotic response that leads to problems in coping. Dysfunctional grieving is evidenced by loss of self-esteem, depression, excessively strong dependency needs, and ambivalent feelings for the lost person or object. Such unresolved grief leaves the individual susceptible to further psychologic trauma that can in turn lead to crisis, depression, and suicide.*

☐ GOAL

The patient will describe loss and the meaning of the loss; will express and share grief with family; will resolve the loss in an adaptive manner.

☐ IMPLEMENTATION

- Review *The Patient Experiencing Grief and Loss*, page 272.
- Assess for any contributing/causative factors that may delay the grief work.
- Listen to patient, encourage expression of feelings (e.g., fear, despair, anger, sadness).
- Develop a relationship of trust through one-to-one interactions.
- Give support and reassurance by accepting patient's feelings and experiences.
- Explore what it is that makes patient feel hopeless, worthless, that life is not worth living.
- Provide support for the patient/family members by discussing feelings and coping mechanisms.
- Encourage patient/family to share grief and provide support for each other.
- Discuss new coping mechanisms; encourage to practice them.
- Involve patient in the decision making process.

☐ EVALUATION CRITERIA/DESIRED OUTCOMES

The Patient

- Expresses feelings
- Shares feelings and concerns with family members
- Participates in decision making for the future

NURSING DIAGNOSIS #4

Alteration in family process related to situational or pathophysiologic stressor

Rationale: *When the normally supportive and adaptively functioning family experiences a stressor, the family's previously effective functioning ability may be challenged. Common factors that contribute to an alteration in family process include illness of a family member, trauma, loss of a family member or valued object, gain of a new family member, disaster, economic crisis, change in family roles, conflict, psychiatric illness, and social deviance. When the patient's/family's usual problem-solving methods are inadequate to resolve the situation, a crisis may occur. The patient/family in response to crisis will either return to precrisis functioning, develop a higher level of functioning, or develop an ineffective (lower) form of functioning.*

☐ GOAL

The patient/family will return to the precrisis level of functioning; will verbalize feelings to nurse and to each other on a regular basis; will participate in care of family members; will maintain a functional system of mutual support for each other.

☐ IMPLEMENTATION

- Assess patient/family patterns of interaction and coping.
- Help patient/family members identify feelings of stress, past and current methods of coping, strengths and weaknesses.
- Encourage to share thoughts and feelings with each other, to interact and communicate daily.
- Encourage verbalization of guilt, anger, hostility, blame, and to recognize own feelings in patient/family members.
- Help patient/family to make realistic appraisal of the situation.
- Urge to list choices, available resources.
- Assist to reorganize roles as needed at home and to set priorities to maintain family integrity and to reduce stress.

☐ EVALUATION CRITERIA/DESIRED OUTCOMES

The Patient/family

- Share feelings and concerns

- Participate in care appropriately
- Set priorities and implement adaptive coping strategies
- Reorganize home roles as needed
- Avoid crisis or return to precrisis level of functioning

> **NURSING DIAGNOSIS #5**
>
> **Knowledge deficit** related to utilization of support systems, problem-solving techniques needed to avert a crisis state
>
> ***Rationale:*** *A crisis will not develop if situational supports are sufficient, perception of the problem is realistic, and effective coping solutions are available.*

☐ GOAL

The patient will identify available support; will develop alternative coping to solve current problem.

☐ IMPLEMENTATION

- Continue to give as much information as needed about hospitalization, treatment therapy, etc.; ask for feedback to ensure understanding.
- Teach to brainstorm alternate solutions to current problem, to look at the pros and cons of each one; do not tell patient what to do, but ask if one of the solutions could possibly work.
- Check the effectiveness of patient's new coping options by asking what actions patient would take if confronted with a situation similar to the one just experienced; reinforce positive adaptation and coping and teach as necessary.
- Refer to outside support or agency to correct family or individual dysfunction once crisis is resolved.

☐ EVALUATION CRITERIA/DESIRED OUTCOMES

The Patient/family

- Has a realistic expectation of what occurred
- Has adequate situational supports in the form of family, friends, job
- States at least 3 options available to use to cope with stress
- Has name of a community resource to go to if another threatening situation occurs

The Patient Experiencing Depression

Definition/Discussion

Depression is an alteration in mood, usually related to a loss, characterized by sadness, pessimism, despondence, hopelessness, and emptiness. It can also be related to internalization of anger or aggressive feelings.

Nursing Assessment

☐ **PERTINENT HISTORY**

Recent or unresolved loss; crises; suicidal ideation; cultural or social isolation; changes in location, status, employment, home, body, school, health, abilities, finances; alcohol or substance abuse; anhedonia, withdrawal; sleep disturbances

☐ **PHYSICAL FINDINGS**

Psychomotor retardation, crying, anorexia or overeating, apathy, decreased concentration, anxiety, fatigue, sad expression, poor eye contact

☐ **PSYCHOSOCIAL CONCERNS/ DEVELOPMENTAL FACTORS**

Personality, normal coping patterns, self-esteem, introjection of anger, feelings of failure, familial pattern of depression or dependency, importance of real or perceived loss, degree of disruption perceived; adolescents: acting-out, problem behaviors; elderly: sensory-perceptual changes

☐ **PATIENT AND FAMILY KNOWLEDGE**

Dynamics of depression, community resources, treatment plan, readiness and willingness to learn

Nursing Care

☐ **LONG-TERM GOAL**

The patient will be able to acknowledge and resolve the loss; the patient will resume management of own life and plan for the future.

NURSING DIAGNOSIS #1

Ineffective individual coping related to feelings of depression associated with loss, failure

Rationale: *Feelings of depression associated with loss or failure prevent the individual from effective role performance.*

☐ **GOAL**

The patient will express feelings; will develop skills to effectively manage readjustment.

☐ **IMPLEMENTATION**

- Make frequent, intermittent contact with the patient, both verbal and nonverbal.
- Give attention consistently, even when the patient is unwilling/unable to converse with you; this approach will establish you as an interested, caring person; be aware that depressed patients usually feel alone and worthless; a belief that someone is interested in and cares about them is the most helpful intervention.
- Involve in self-care and activities of daily living (ADL); start with one activity and gradually add others; prevent withdrawal by encouraging social interactions; recognize patient's efforts.
- Explore how patient feels about listening to

others' feelings (often people who have problems tolerating their own feelings tend to feel overwhelmed with those of others).
- Use open-ended questions to elicit expression of feelings, (e.g., "You look sad today. What is it that makes you feel this way?"); acknowledge and reinforce any expression of feelings.
- Do not tell patient the feeling of depression is not as bad as it is perceived to be; this approach only serves to reinforce the feeling that no one understands.
- Ensure that staff knows not not to chastize the patient when feelings of sadness are evident; allow the patient to cry.
- Praise for any involvement in self-care or other activities; encourage staff/family to praise patient for these efforts; structure schedule to provide adequate and enjoyable activities.
- Help patient do things for self and explain that activity usually helps people to feel better.
- Assist staff in their efforts to draw out the patient; direct them to pay as much attention as possible.
- Monitor physical needs and encourage patient to maintain good hygiene and grooming.
- Provide sufficient nourishment; allow favorite foods and choice of diet when possible.
- Assess sleep and activity pattern; provide adequate rest and a regular bedtime routine that promotes sleep without medications; limit daytime sleeping; encourage morning activities as patient will usually feel best then.
- Encourage participation in regular exercise program if possible.
- Help patient focus on meaning of loss, somatic symptoms, depressed feeling tone (e.g., "You've had a hard time lately and you're learning to deal with your feelings." "You've lost functioning and you're going through grief and mourning.")
- Reinforce reality and realistic expectations.
- Identify problem areas and work out alternatives with patient; take care to consider individual preferences and needs.
- Assess areas in which patient is making own decisions and give positive reinforcement to self-enhancing ones; assist with decision making when profoundly depressed; as depression lifts, expect patient to make own decisions with support.

☐ EVALUATION CRITERIA

The Patient

- Identifies events/loss that led to feeling depressed
- Demonstrates increasing self-direction in self-care and activities
- Has stable physical condition
- Participates actively in unit activities
- Participates in regular exercise

NURSING DIAGNOSIS #2

Disturbance in self-concept: self-esteem related to lack of appreciation for own value and abilities

Rationale: *The characteristic present in all depressions is lowered self-esteem. Attention to improving self-esteem will assist in lifting depression.*

☐ GOAL

The patient will experience an increase in self-esteem.

☐ IMPLEMENTATION

- Approach the patient in accepting, respectful way; keep promises and agreements to demonstrate caring.
- Recognize patient's prior abilities and display a positive attitude toward recovery; do not reassure but ask patient to describe feelings.
- Offer alternative statements to ruminative or self-deprecatory remarks but do not argue with the patient.
- Determine interests and activities that were enjoyed previously and try to incorporate these into the care plan.
- Ask patient to describe positive thoughts and write them down; suggest that when negative thoughts occur, producing feelings of helplessness, that the patient state "I will stop thinking about that."
- Begin with small tasks and activities where success will be possible and give honest praise for accomplishments; increase requirements as patient improves; provide recognition consistently.
- Encourage verbal interaction and communication with staff and other patients to pre-

vent isolation; role play situations of potential concern to the patient.
- Encourage increasing decision making in as many areas as possible; ask for participation in planning for own care.
- Support any evidence of motivation or initiative and praise efforts and progress.
- Assist in reevaluation of goals and expectations and recognize efforts being made to adjust; continue to focus on positive aspects and strengths.
- Encourage attendance and participation in group therapy, occupational therapy, and recreational activities.
- Convey an attitude of confidence in the abilities of the patient.

☐ EVALUATION CRITERIA

The Patient

- Identifies successful aspects of life
- Demonstrates adequate communication skills; makes few self-deprecatory remarks
- Participates in therapies and plan for care

NURSING DIAGNOSIS #3

Knowledge deficit regarding behaviors of depression, responses to loss, treatment plan, need for support system

Rationale: *Often new supports and adjustments in life-style are necessary to cope with changes that preciptated the depression. Patients can learn new coping strategies and problem solving.*

☐ GOAL

The patient will adapt to changes, utilize support systems, and plan constructively for the future.

☐ IMPLEMENTATION

- Assist to understand behaviors that usually occur with depression and how the resolution of a loss may be accomplished; refer to *The Patient Experiencing Grief and Loss*, page 272.
- Encourage development of techniques to help in management of life changes and alterations of mood.
- Teach assertive techniques and their appropriate application.
- Instruct regarding prescribed medication: actions, side effects, compliance, how to obtain refills.
- Educate regarding symptoms of recurring depression so early assistance can be obtained.
- Encourage evaluation of environmental situation and assist with changes if indicated; involve the social worker in areas indicated.
- Encourage continuation of social contacts and discuss the importance of their maintenance.
- Inform patient/family regarding self-help or informational groups for outpatient assistance (e.g., Reach-to-Recovery, spouse groups.)
- Tell about local mental health center, crisis and suicide prevention centers.
- Inform regarding benefits of continuing individual, family, or group therapy; ensure understanding of indicated referrals; arrange for follow-up appointment prior to discharge.

☐ EVALUATION CRITERIA/DESIRED OUTCOMES

The Patient

- Understands need to monitor follow-up care
- States understanding of causes of depression
- Has plans for alterations in life-style
- Describes correct use of medications
- States optimism and a constructive plan for the future

The Patient who is Dying/Terminal

Definition/Discussion

The process of dying is the final stage of life and involves the patient, family, friends, and all members of the health care team. Although death is a universal experience, the feelings and attitudes each person has regarding death are unique and affect the way his/her life is lived and terminated. People will usually face death in a manner similar to how they dealt with other crisis situations throughout life.

Kübler-Ross has identified 5 psychological stages of grieving that are usually experienced when an individual is facing death.

1. *Denial* is an adaptive coping mechanism to delay the pain and shock until the patient is better able to deal with the reality. Patients go in and out of denial throughout the grieving process as a protection against the anguish and despair of the situation. "Oh, no. This can't be true. I don't believe it!" demonstrates denial.
2. *Anger and rage* are felt regarding the unfairness of the diagnosis. The question asked during this stage is "Why me?". These feelings are projected onto family and care givers who are able to continue with life and activities.
3. *Bargaining* is an attempt to postpone dying until certain tasks are complete (e.g., birth of a grandchild, a relative's graduation). These requests are usually made to God and provide a way for the patient to deal with the situation in small increments.
4. *Depression* occurs with the realization that many losses are imminent (e.g., family, job, control, lifestyle, life itself) and produces a profound sadness and depression.
5. *Acceptance* is a time of acknowledgement and recognition that death is inevitable, and the patient accepts it after having gone through all the other stages. S/he may become increasingly disengaged and project an attitude of "It is all right." Some patients never reach this stage and die in denial, with anger or sorrow.

The nurse's responsibilities include giving support, empathy, and compassion so as to facilitate dignity, growth, and peace in the process of dying. Support groups and/or professional supervision from specialists in thanatology are helpful to assist with appropriate management of grief and mourning.

Nursing Assessment

☐ PERTINENT HISTORY

Type of illness (e.g., length, character, progression), previous serious illnesses, previous experiences with losses and death

☐ PHYSICAL FINDINGS

Amount of pain or discomfort, confusion, level of consciousness, vital signs, ability to participate in self-care and activities of daily living (ADL), alterations in body image, fatigue, nausea and vomiting, alopecia, insomnia, restlessness

☐ PSYCHOSOCIAL CONCERNS/ DEVELOPMENTAL FACTORS

Past and present support system, patient's/family's previous responses to crises, cultural and ethnic beliefs and practices, religious requirements and preferences, personality characteristics (e.g., pessimism, optimism), usual coping mechanisms, psychiatric problems or diagnoses, suicidal ideation or attempts, symptoms of anxiety

☐ PATIENT AND FAMILY KNOWLEDGE

Disease entity and probable course of progression, options regarding treatment, acceptance of diagnosis and prognosis, intellectual capacity, alternatives to hospitalization, support or bereavement groups, community resources

Nursing Care

☐ LONG-TERM GOAL

The patient will experience physical comfort during the terminal process; the patient will die in a manner appropriate to and consistent with his/her values, beliefs, and philosophy of life. The family will assist in meeting the final needs of the patient; the family will progress toward acceptance of loss and toward adaptive grieving.

NURSING DIAGNOSIS #1

a. **Powerlessness** related to poor prognosis, inevitable death, loss of control/function
b. **Ineffective individual coping** related to inability to face death
c. **Anxiety** related to an unknown future

Rationale: *Fear of the unknown, of pain, mutilation, rejection, being alone at time of death, dependency, loss of control, identity, self-esteem, and loss of the physical body contribute to decreased stamina and effectiveness of coping mechanisms. High anxiety and fear narrow perceptions and interfere with learning and coping. Usual coping mechanisms may not work during this time of crisis and the patient may resort to maladaptive coping strategies.*

☐ GOAL

The patient will identify and develop effective and adaptive coping mechanisms to reduce anxiety and fear and facilitate normal grief.

☐ IMPLEMENTATION

- Identify the stages of the grieving and dying process on a continuing basis; remember that more than one stage may be evident at the same time, progression is not necessarily sequential and may arrest at any stage; coping will change with each stage and with the passage of time.
- Determine what the MD has told patient/family (it is MD's responsibility to inform patient/family of probable death); be present when diagnosis and prognosis are discussed with patient/family if possible to help in planning for future care.
- Allow patient to experience denial as needed without reinforcing denial; do not force the acceptance of truths patient is not yet ready to deal with; discuss the reality of the situation without stripping patient of all hope.
- Monitor presence of mutual avoidance between patient and family (pretending dying is not occurring in order to protect each other); this may persist until death occurs and could keep the patient isolated and unable to express wishes and feelings.
- Be alert for displacement of anger onto family/staff; assist to express feelings more directly by use of reflection (e.g., "It must be very hard for you to not be out of bed today.").
- Provide privacy for and encourage the expression of crying, screaming; provide alternative outlets to express anger (e.g., an extra pillow for punching) if energy permits.
- Assist patient to verbalize feelings regarding fears of the unknown, abandonment, etc.; explore their meaning; be alert for spiritual needs and possibly psychiatric referral.
- Allow control of own care and ADL as possible to minimize fears of dependence and shame over decreased functioning.
- Be flexible with schedules to assist patient in accepting additional care required with less stress.
- Accept irritability and do not take personally or act defensively; be aware of own nonverbal behavior in communicating to patient.
- Demonstrate concern and caring by giving empathy and reflecting your observations (e.g., "You seem upset today.").
- Monitor the degree of hope present; do not encourage false or unrealistic hopes but allow patient's faith and hope to sustain him/her throughout the dying process.
- Show interest in patient's plans for the future and help adjust to the future as being "a day" or "a week" from now rather than longer periods of time.
- Assist patient to deal with guilt feelings by identifying what they feel guilty about; correct distorted perceptions; encourage making amends if possible (e.g., writing a letter, asking for forgiveness) and forgiving themselves so that peace and acceptance can occur.
- Encourage verbalization of feelings of depression and fears regarding the many losses associated with the loss of life; refer to *The Patient Experiencing Grief and Loss,* page 272

- Watch for clues to suicidal ideation (e.g., "It would be better to end this quickly."); provide a safe environment at all times and institute precautions as necessary.
- Allow grief to be expressed in any way that is not detrimental to patient; know that silence may signify the beginning of acceptance and disengagement, and is normal.
- Use touch judiciously; know that some patients need to be held and touched and are unable to ask for it; other patients may prefer not to be touched.
- Show receptivity to what patient may be trying to explain (e.g., visions or conversations experienced in altered states of consciousness preceding death); question carefully to gain understanding of meanings but do not pry into the experience.
- Assist patient with life review; identify tangible and intangible legacies and fulfillments that have been achieved; encourage reminiscing with family/friends.
- Lend perspective that it is good to have others' lives go on even though his/hers is ending, that death is part of life and can be faced with courage to attain a sense of completion.
- Allow for individual differences in dying process as dictated by culture and lifelong patterns of living; know that people face death in a manner similar to how they deal with other life crises.
- Be aware of patient/family wishes regarding death and assist with their being carried out; inform physician and other members of the health care team.

☐ EVALUATION CRITERIA/DESIRED OUTCOMES

The Patient

- Does not despair
- Has a reduced level of anxiety and fear
- Copes adaptively with the dying process
- Expresses feelings constructively

NURSING DIAGNOSIS #2

Alteration in comfort: pain related to trauma, advanced disease, dying process

Rationale: *During the process of dying, many physical and psychologic changes occur that may produce pain and discomfort. These vary in severity, intensity, and duration but are a source of concern to the patient and to the family, and require attention by the nurse to provide comfort and peace at the end of life.*

☐ GOAL

The patient will verbalize when discomfort, pain, and feelings of anxiety occur so they can be minimized and comfort provided.

☐ IMPLEMENTATION

- Ask patient to tell you when discomfort, pain, or anxiety is felt; ask family to watch for signs and report these as they develop; refer to *The Patient Experiencing Pain,* page 180, and *The Patient Experiencing Anxiety,* page 250.
- Keep patient dry, clean, and in comfortable surroundings; provide light, loose bed covers and circulating air; reposition patient frequently for comfort but do not move unnecessarily.
- Provide sufficient indirect light; do not draw shades as patient has decreased vision in darkness and can see only what is near; encourage visitors to sit near the head of the bed for better vision.
- Keep in mind that patients are often very anxious about going to sleep at night because they fear dying alone in the darkness; check on patient frequently and leave soft light on at all times.
- Monitor for elevated temperature; know that internal temperature may be elevated even though patient is cool to the touch.
- Speak in normal voice rather than a whisper; encourage family to continue talking to patient even though comatose; do not discuss patient within his/her hearing.
- Use noninvasive measures (e.g., backrubs, soothing music) in conjunction with pain medications to increase comfort and therapeutic effects of the analgesics.
- Administer oral care as needed, suction gently; elevate head of the bed to 30°-45° to ease respirations if necessary.
- Inform family when analgesics are allowed and how they will be administered; know that maintaining a pain-free state is a goal for terminal patients though not all experience pain.

EVALUATION CRITERIA/DESIRED OUTCOMES

The Patient

- Verbalizes occurrence of discomfort
- Accepts noninvasive comfort measures
- Responds to analgesics when administered
- Achieves adequate rest and sleep
- Remains pain-free as much as possible

NURSING DIAGNOSIS #3

Self-care deficit: feeding, bathing/hygiene, dressing/grooming, toileting related to decrease in physical and emotional strength

Rationale: *The progression of the dying process creates increased fatigue and decreased interest and ability to perform self-care activities. There is also an increased need for physical care related to possible immobility, incontinence, fever, dehydration, and other manifestations of severe illness.*

GOAL

The patient will maintain as much control as physical condition permits over ADL for as long as possible; the family will contribute to the care of the patient whenever appropriate.

IMPLEMENTATION

- Encourage participation in self-care as long as possible; ask for preferences (e.g., best time for bathing) to sustain patient interest in maintaining functioning; do not ask patient/family to perform tasks they are unable or unwilling to do.
- Protect from embarrassment over incontinence, altered body image, inability to eat neatly; provide privacy during times when shame over decreased abilities might upset patient.
- Provide accepting, nonjudgmental, concerned care; make sure patient knows s/he is still considered a part of the living and not "in limbo" or unimportant in the eyes of the care givers.
- Allow to wear own clothes if possible; encourage family to bring favorite clothing from home.
- Encourage family to assist with feeding, grooming, etc., to decrease isolation and occupy visiting time; teach as necessary to facilitate any care giving.
- Provide cosmetics, wigs, ribbons, etc. to encourage cheerfulness in patient's life and improve appearance and self-esteem.
- Monitor skin condition; encourage patient to participate with grooming as much as possible; provide for shaving and hair care regularly as patient/family desire.
- Refer to *The Patient Experiencing a Body-Image Disturbance,* page 253.
- Maintain a neat, comfortable environment for patient/family; allow presence of personal articles that are pleasing and meaningful to patient.

EVALUATION CRITERIA/DESIRED OUTCOMES

The Patient

- Participates in ADL as strength allows
- Expresses personal preferences regarding grooming and environment

The Family

- Participates appropriately in patient care

NURSING DIAGNOSIS #4

a. **Social isolation** related to separation from family, friends, and confinement to hospital environment

b. **Diversional activity deficit** related to fatigue, immobility, withdrawal

Rationale: *The patient who is terminal conserves failing strength and energy for the dying process and may be unwilling and/or unable to show interest in outside activities. Required occupations of family may prevent frequent visits, and the awkward feelings of friends regarding death may decrease social contacts. The increasing disengagement also contributes to feelings of abandonment.*

GOAL

The patient will participate in visits from others; will enjoy activities as strength permits.

IMPLEMENTATION

- Arrange to spend time with patient even when care is not needed to promote feelings of acknowledgement and prevent feelings of abandonment and alienation.

- Discuss interests and activities that patient has enjoyed; determine what physical strength is available for diversion; make allowances for unscheduled pleasurable times when patient is able to participate.
- Encourage family/friends to visit; explore their feelings of discomfort regarding patient's terminal illness.
- Explain to family that the patient's silence does not necessarily mean rejection and that the presence of a loved one is helpful even if conversation is not continuous.
- Involve occupational/adjunctive therapist as appropriate to provide ideas and supervision for acceptable diversions.
- Discuss how much contact patient desires with others; consider possibility of appropriate roommate to help decrease the sense of isolation that is often felt.
- Remember loneliness is the greatest pain of all and that patients may not want to be removed from unit activities even though unable or unwilling to participate.

☐ EVALUATION CRITERIA/DESIRED OUTCOMES

The Patient

- Participates in activities as strength allows
- Anticipates and acknowledges visitors
- Has minimal level of withdrawal

NURSING DIAGNOSIS #5

Alteration in family process related to anticipatory grieving

Rationale: *Family members experience the same stages of response to the dying process as the patient as defined by Kübler-Ross. These do not occur at the same time in all family members or simultaneously with the patient. If the spouse or another member of the family remains fixated at the denial stage, it may be difficult for meaningful communication regarding dying to occur. The family may experience ambivalence and guilt related to partial acceptance of the anticipated death.*

☐ GOAL

The family will progress through stages of adaptation to impending death; will resolve feelings that may prevent expressions of timely grieving.

☐ IMPLEMENTATION

- Establish a trusting relationship with family members; encourage ventilation of feelings regarding patient's condition on an ongoing basis.
- Assess information given to family; determine whether it is the same as what patient knows; answer questions; ask what they do not understand and clarify as needed; refer to other members of the health care team as appropriate.
- Listen carefully to what family members say; observe what information is imparted through nonverbal behavior; encourage them to share feelings with members of health care team.
- Monitor for destructive or inappropriate behavior caused by tension, anxiety, anger, or fear; do not argue with family but remain supportive and nonjudgmental; remember family is sensitive to implied criticism due to feelings of guilt and anger; use empathic statements (e.g., "This must be very painful for you.").
- Assess dysfunction in family caused by imminent death (e.g., patterns of ineffective communication, lack of problem-solving abilities); encourage to function (e.g., "What will you do about . . .?").
- Monitor for development of pathologic grieving reactions; intervene with appropriate referrals as indicated.
- Utilize all health care team members in meeting needs of family (e.g., social worker, nurse therapist).
- Assist to obtain outside assistance as needed for financial problems, supplies (e.g., social service agencies, American Cancer Society).
- Explore role strain; assist family in changing roles as needed to minimize stress and maintain family cohesiveness.
- Encourage open communication and the sharing of feelings, concerns with each other; respect that some people do not wish to discuss grieving and feelings.
- Support progress of grieving through each stage; reassure that feelings are normal and resolve with appropriate expression and the passage of time.
- Encourage review of patient's life with family; help to integrate past into the present for increased acceptance of the dying process.

- Encourage normalcy in family life as much as possible to provide and maintain mutual support.
- Encourage family to maintain social relationships as much as possible to facilitate reinvolvement in usual activities following successful grieving.

EVALUATION CRITERIA/DESIRED OUTCOMES

The Family

- Demonstrates progress in adapting to impending death
- Expresses feelings of grief
- Shows cohesiveness, tolerance, and support of each other
- Functions adequately in stressful situations
- Expresses knowledge regarding use of appropriate community resources

NURSING DIAGNOSIS #6

Spiritual distress related to a disturbance in belief system, hopelessness, or inability to participate in services

Rationale: *The patient's religious beliefs and philosophy of life provide a source of strength, hope, and faith in life. A terminal illness can produce profound disturbances in the belief and value systems of patients and families that may result in feelings of anger, guilt, and fear. When a patient begins to question "Why me?" and "What have I done to deserve this?", spiritual distress may result.*

GOAL

The patient will express increased understanding and acceptance of death; will participate in religious practices as desired and as strength permits.

IMPLEMENTATION

- Determine wishes of patient/family regarding pastoral care and services; remember that the actual offering of spiritual counseling may verify to patient/family that illness is terminal; obtain MD's order if required; contact spiritual advisor when requested.
- Respect right of patient/family to refuse participation of spiritual leader in dying process.
- Assess influence of cultural beliefs related to spiritual needs; become as knowledgeable as possible about the practices and requirements of various religions in care of the dying.
- Show acceptance of spiritual needs; remain nonjudgmental and understanding about patient's/family's search for meaning in suffering.
- Permit beneficial rituals as much as possible; provide privacy and seclusion as necessary.
- Consult health care team members to provide requested services; allow diet restrictions according to beliefs without endangering physical condition.
- Permit possession of religious or spiritual articles (e.g., Bible, rosary beads, clothing).
- Encourage spiritual rituals not damaging to physical condition; assist as necessary with positioning and provision of articles required for participation.
- Determine ritual care and arrangements required for the dying, dead, and for burial; involve physician and other staff as indicated.
- Respond with concern and empathy when patient/family discuss spiritual beliefs; do not attempt to change or influence religious affiliations.
- Continue to offer services of a spiritual leader if initially refused.
- Know that strong feelings of anger toward God, ambivalence toward the dying person, and guilt for having these feelings are natural (although usually temporary) in family members, and that intervention by a religious professional may diminish these feelings.

EVALUATION CRITERIA/DESIRED OUTCOMES

The Patient

- Expresses increased acceptance of death
- States increased spiritual peace
- Accepts and practices spiritual rituals indicated for specific beliefs

The Family

- Discusses concerns and feelings with appropriate spiritual leader
- Expresses understanding of guilt and ambivalence toward ill member

NURSING DIAGNOSIS #7

Knowledge deficit regarding terminal care in nonacute setting and resocialization of family following death of member

Rationale: *As an alternative to death in an acute hospital, it may be possible to provide home or hospice care for the terminally ill. Utilization of community services and family members can provide more personal attention and allows family to experience less guilt and more positive adjustments to their grief.*

☐ GOAL

The patient will accept nonacute care if indicated; the family will provide care in an outpatient setting that meets needs of patient; will utilize community services when needed to adjust to loss of member.

☐ IMPLEMENTATION

- Inform patient/family of options to acute hospital care (e.g., hospice, private home, own home).
- Ensure complete understanding of physical and psychologic requirements of the patient and the willingness and ability of the family to meet those needs.
- Refer to home health agency for predischarge visit; work with discharge planner to teach necessary skills to family and provide information regarding medications, and physical and emotional care.
- Refer to social worker for information regarding financial difficulties caused by extended illness; assist family to utilize social service agencies as needed.
- Inform care givers of available mental health services and how to set up an appointment.
- Provide family with phone numbers of agencies and people for questions and emergencies.
- Identify agencies which may be of value to family in coping with loss (e.g., support, bereavement, spouse groups) if indicated.
- Refer to appropriate community resources for assistance in terminal care in outpatient settings (e.g., American Cancer Society, Alzheimer's Disease Association).

☐ EVALUATION CRITERIA/DESIRED OUTCOMES

The Patient

- Indicates acceptance of nonacute care without anxiety

The Family

- Demonstrates understanding of requirements for care and abilities to provide it
- Expresses knowledge regarding community resources and appropriate support persons and groups available

The Patient Experiencing Fear

Definition/Discussion

Fear is an emotional response to a consciously recognized internal/external source that is perceived as dangerous.

Nursing Assessment

☐ PERTINENT HISTORY

Precipitating factors, length and severity of response, degree of restriction of life-style, usual methods of coping

☐ PHYSICAL FINDINGS

Changes in vital signs, sweating, pupillary dilations, trembling, tension, restlessness, insomnia, decreased ability to concentrate, crying, demanding behavior, somatic complaints

☐ PSYCHOSOCIAL CONCERNS/ DEVELOPMENTAL FACTORS

Childhood fears, nightmares, past experiences and memories, patterns of pessimism/persistent worry

☐ PATIENT AND FAMILY KNOWLEDGE

Previously learned responses and management, degree of disruption, perception and interpretation of fear-producing event(s), readiness and willingness to learn

Nursing Care

☐ LONG-TERM GOAL

The patient will interact with the environment in such a way that factors and situations that cause fearfulness are recognized and managed in an adaptive way.

NURSING DIAGNOSIS #1

Ineffective individual coping related to fearful response

Rationale: *A decrease in control, objectivity, and judgment occurs when fear is experienced resulting in personality disorganization and impaired ability to maintain activities of daily living (ADL).*

☐ GOAL

The patient will identify the fear, its cause, and methods of effective coping.

☐ IMPLEMENTATION

- Attempt to identify the specific source of the fear.
- Use indirect, open-ended questions (e.g., "What is it about being in the hospital that concerns you most?").
- Go slowly in exploring fears; wait in silence; show willingness to get involved; remember the patient may not discuss the greatest fears as readily as those of less importance.
- Reassure that emotions felt are manageable.
- Give careful explanation of all that is to occur; following explanations, have patient tell you in own words what you said and what it means to him/her; repeat this procedure as often as needed to ensure understanding.
- Encourage, when tolerated, the examination of the fears and different ways they can be managed; do not make decisions for the patient.
- If you are unable to reduce the fear (e.g., of dying during surgery) prior to the event, notify physician so appropriate corrective action can be taken (surgery may be cancelled).

☐ EVALUATION CRITERIA/DESIRED OUTCOMES

The Patient

- Identifies fear-promoting sources
- Verbalizes responses to fear
- Corrects distorted perceptions
- Defines alternative coping techniques

NURSING DIAGNOSIS #2

Alteration in comfort related to physical indicators of fear

Rationale: *Physiologic changes that may cause discomfort occur during the emotional response of fear. The experience of pain is heightened when accompanied by fear.*

☐ GOAL

The patient will discuss fears; will participate in measures to relieve fear and discomfort; will demonstrate increased relaxation and decreased physiologic behaviors of fear.

☐ IMPLEMENTATION

- Provide serene and safe environment; decrease disturbing stimuli.
- Encourage identification of specific discomforts and use indicated methods of alleviation (e.g., medication, back rub, bathing).
- Minimize muscle tension by proper alignment, positioning, and support.
- Encourage ambulation and exercise as indicated as a constructive use of energy.
- Teach relaxation techniques appropriate to age and condition (e.g., deep breathing, visualization).
- Use touch as indicated; be aware of individual variations in acceptance.
- Provide diversionary activities (e.g., music, books, TV, games, visitors).

☐ EVALUATION CRITERIA/DESIRED OUTCOMES

The Patient

- Has no complaints of physical discomfort
- Uses calm verbal communication
- Is free from visible muscle tension
- Utilizes diversionary activities

The Patient Experiencing Grief and Loss

Definition/Discussion

Loss is the removal of something/someone of great value to the person. Grief is the emotional responses that follow the perception, or anticipation, of a loss. Mourning is the psychologic process that results from a loss. The grief and mourning process is the process of coping with and adapting to the loss. There are three categories of loss

- *nurturing:* loss of a significant other through death, divorce
- *self-image:* loss of one or more aspects of usual self-image (e.g., self-respect; also includes loss of a body part or function such as a leg, bowel function),
- *sexual role identity:* loss of usual roles (e.g., family role, career role, sexual functioning, control over one's life)

An actual or anticipated loss in any of these categories will trigger the grief and mourning process. Although grief, loss, and mourning are most frequently associated with a death, they are present with all losses—such as the loss associated with a mastectomy (body part), with a colostomy (normal bowel function), or with paraplegia (normal body function plus usual role functions). According to Engel (1965), the grief and mourning process involves three stages: 1) shock and disbelief, 2) developing awareness of the loss, and 3) restitution. Full restitution may take a year or more and some people never completely recover. Each stage has its own adaptive responses and time frame.

Nursing Assessment

☐ PERTINENT HISTORY

Recency, causative or contributing factors of current loss(es); past experiences with loss and its successful/unsuccessful resolution

☐ PHYSICAL FINDINGS

Loss of body part/function; chronic pain; changes in physical status as response to loss (e.g., appetite, bowel habits, nausea, sleeplessness, fatigue, headaches, general malaise)

☐ PSYCHOSOCIAL CONCERNS/ DEVELOPMENTAL FACTORS

Developmental stage and tasks; recent change in life-style (e.g., childbirth, marriage, loss of significant other, change in economic state); social support system or lack of; multiple losses; category of loss (sexual role, self-image, nurturing); stage of grieving (Engel), individual's responses to loss

☐ PATIENT AND FAMILY KNOWLEDGE

Adaptation to loss, plans for the future; self-help groups; professional counseling to enhance grief work or resolve past losses

Nursing Care

☐ LONG-TERM GOAL

The patient will cope with the loss experienced by completing each stage of the grief and mourning process.

NURSING DIAGNOSIS #1

Grieving related to shock and disbelief over loss

Rationale: *Shock and disbelief comprise the first stage of the grieving process. The individual must work thorough denial of what is occurring. This is difficult to do in an unanticipated loss such as occurs in an auto or plane crash. Common behaviors are deny-*

ing what is happening, crying, screaming, and anger; these are considered adaptive behaviors. Almost any behavior is adaptive in this stage except homocidal or suicidal behavior. This stage usually lasts 1-7 days.

☐ GOAL

The patient will use nondestructive coping mechanisms to being to deal with the loss.

☐ IMPLEMENTATION

- Accept any behavior that is not physically destructive; allow patient to cry, scream, pound fists, etc.; do not try to cut it off or limit it.
- Reinforce the occurrence of the loss while encouraging the patient to talk about it; do not support denial but elicit feelings (e.g., "It must be difficult to believe this is happening.")
- Spend at least 15 minutes/shift talking or just sitting and listening to the patient; allow the patient to direct the conversation.

☐ EVALUATION CRITERIA/DESIRED OUTCOMES

The Patient

- Demonstrates adaptive first-stage grieving behaviors

NURSING DIAGNOSIS #2

Grieving related to developing awareness of the stated loss

Rationale: *In the second stage of grief, loss is acknowledged ("Maybe I'll look OK with a prosthesis." "Do you think I'll be able to work with this?" "I'll never be able to cope."). Mood swings are common. Self-blame is a part of this stage (e.g., "If only I'd done . . ."). Adaptive behaviors of stage 1 may be interspersed with these new behaviors. This behavior can last from several weeks to months. When a loved one is lost, the length of this stage and the next seem to be dependent on the length and importance of the relationship. Reminiscing is an important part of this stage as is reliving the actual loss event.*

☐ GOAL

The patient will express an awareness of the loss and its impact.

☐ IMPLEMENTATION

- Incorporate a discussion of the loss into your daily conversations with patient/family; appropriate questions might be "How do you see the effect of what has happened to you?" or "How is your family coping with what has occurred?"
- When patient begins to share feelings (e.g., anger, guilt, depression, sadness), encourage to do so; sit and listen.
- Reiterate that grieving is normal for this situation.
- When appropriate, tell the patient s/he is doing a good job of dealing with the loss.
- Involve in planning and doing some aspects of self-care.
- Restate questions the patient has asked so that s/he can explore the answers with your assistance.
- Ensure the patient has ongoing situational supports to help deal with the loss (e.g., friends, family, clergy).
- Adjust visiting hours for family/friends to stay as necessary; try to fulfill any patient requests.

☐ EVALUATION CRITERIA/DESIRED OUTCOMES

The Patient

- Talks about loss and its impact on life-style (e.g., wearing a prosthesis)
- Expresses feelings of anger, guilt, depression, sadness
- Develops/increases situational supports

NURSING DIAGNOSIS #3

Grieving related to restitution

Rationale: *In the final stage of the grief process, the patient deals with the loss, structures new habits, and goes on with the business of living. Typical behaviors include making plans for the future, remembering both positive and negative aspects of life before the loss. Full restitution can take up to a year or more and some people never complete this stage. Be-*

haviors from stage 2 may be observed periodically in this stage but lessen in frequency as time passes.

☐ GOAL

The patient will be able to talk about the positive and negative aspects of the loss; will make plans for the future.

☐ IMPLEMENTATION

- Praise efforts to adapt to changed life-style; give positive reinforcement for making future plans.
- Allow the patient control over as much of own care and method of resolving the loss as possible.
- Refer for ongoing counseling, to community agencies as appropriate.

☐ EVALUATION CRITERIA/DESIRED OUTCOMES

The Patient

- Expresses both positive and negative impact of loss
- Makes plans for the future
- Increases situational supports over what was established in stage of developing awareness
- Resumes preloss roles and functions or modifications thereof.

NURSING DIAGNOSIS #4

Knowledge deficit regarding the process of loss resolution

Rationale: *Many responses that the individual has to the loss may be frightening or confusing; simple information giving provides reassurance and structure.*

☐ GOAL

The patient will understand typical grief responses.

☐ IMPLEMENTATION

- Discuss patient's response to grief with patient; point out how response is common and necessary, that others experiencing a loss have many of the same responses.
- Tell what to expect next in the grieving process.
- Give positive reinforcement for all attempts to adapt to the loss.
- Explain that restitution will eventually occur and that frightening feelings/responses will diminish over time.

☐ EVALUATION CRITERIA/DESIRED OUTCOMES

The Patient

- Verbalizes adequate knowledge of grief process
- States expectations for the future
- Explains that responses to grief are limited in time

The Patient Experiencing Sensory Alteration

Definition/Discussion

Sensory alteration occurs when environmental stimulation (input) is inadequate, overwhelming (overload), meaningless, or monotonous to the individual. Typical responses to inadequate, meaningless, or monotonous stimuli are daytime sleeping, confusion, and hallucinatory behaviors. Responses to overload are increased anxiety, confusion, and "ICU syndrome," simulating psychosis. Sensory alteration occurs in all acute care settings. With the advent of critical care units, life-saving equipment, protective environments, and medical and nursing specialization, the intrusion on a person's environment and/or lack of stimuli has increased and even contributed to morbidity rates.

Sensory disturbances can occur through any or all senses (touch, smell, visualization, hearing). Causes can include confinement in a small room; lack of or excessive touching; no verbal input or too much verbalization around the patient; confinement in a windowless room; lack of new or meaningful stimuli; placement in isolation; change in external environment (e.g., new room, change in placement of equipment, personal supplies); semiconsciousness/movement through different levels of consciousness causing a distortion (misperception) of what is heard, felt, seen, or touched; separation from family; sleep deprivation; the approach of the evening/night hours.

Nursing Assessment

☐ **PERTINENT HISTORY**

Past experiences with sensory disturbances

☐ **PHYSICAL FINDINGS**

Acuity of all senses, level of activity, age, response to approach of evening and night, amount/type of sensory input used to at home, present pathophysiology, metabolic state, oxygen deprivation, mobility restrictions

☐ **PSYCHOSOCIAL CONCERNS/ DEVELOPMENTAL FACTORS**

Support system; availability of family; hobbies and interests; personal toiletries, pajamas, robe, pictures, and other belongings; coping strategies for dealing with confinement; layout of immediate environment and stimulation offered; social isolation; pain; stress

☐ **PATIENT AND FAMILY KNOWLEDGE**

Hospital routine; sounds, sights experienced and meaning of them; need for visitors and personal belongings, definition of sensory disturbance and ways of coping with it; medical regimen/treatment plan, diagnosis and prognosis, nursing treatment plan; level of knowledge, readiness and willingness to learn

Nursing Care

☐ **LONG-TERM GOAL**

The patient will regain and maintain sensory equilibrium.

NURSING DIAGNOSIS #1

Sensory-perceptual alteration related to amount (e.g., overload, monotony) and meaningfulness of environmental stimuli

Rationale: *Patients are at risk for sensory-perceptual alteration when they are out of their usual, known environment or are not able to use their coping mechanisms for controlling and changing stimuli. The aged are especially vulnerable. A frequent response is confusion.*

Sufficient and meaningful sensory input must be introduced.

GOAL

The patient will be able to perceive and describe the components of the environment in an oriented, nondisturbed manner; will demonstrate optimal contact with reality.

IMPLEMENTATION

- Assess at least once every shift for sensory status.
- Talk directly to patient; make eye contact.
- Use touch; give back rubs, massages, change position, stroke hair, etc.
- Give frequent, intermittent attention; do not isolate patient physically or emotionally; speak to patient each time you enter or leave the room.
- Be aware of environmental monotony; use clocks, calendars, books, newspapers, television, radio, pictures, patient's personal possessions to stimulate and encourage patient to explore surroundings and maintain orientation.
- Give the patient several periods of rest intermixed with stimulation throughout the day.
- Identify what you are going to do each time you see the patient; consider and utilize safety precautions as needed.
- Provide opportunities for the patient to sit, stand, or be partially upright; give passive or active exercises (some disturbances are caused by recumbent position alone).
- Approach patient often and reassure; do not increase fear and confusion by avoiding the patient; know that confusion that is physiologic in nature cannot be controlled by behavioral approaches.
- Control light, noise, odors, sights to tolerable levels; provide change of scenery, walks, rides, conversations with other patients, recreational or occupational therapy, and social activities as appropriate and possible.
- Have staff observe how patient is responding to them and the care they are giving (remember, the patient's response is a mirror of needs, not a response to take personally).
- Ensure that staff/family are aware of the patient's need for intermittent rest and stimulation; sensory overload mixed with sleep deprivation does not allow the patient to cope adequately with the hospitalization.
- Provide stimuli in quiet forms (e.g., conversation, playing games, reading to patient).
- Ensure that blind/deaf patients have the opportunity to express their special needs and have them met; communicate to all staff the sensory facilities the patient may be lacking (e.g., blind or without glasses; deaf and without a hearing aid); increase input to other senses if one is nonfunctional.
- Refer patients with long-term sensory impairments to the appropriate community resources (e.g., Society for the Blind).

EVALUATION CRITERIA/DESIRED OUTCOMES

The Patient

- Is oriented to environment, self
- Participates in plan of care to the extent possible

NURSING DIAGNOSIS #2

Knowledge deficit related to sensory status (overload/monotony)

Rationale: *Most individuals are unaware of the importance of receiving optimal level of stimulation for orientation and a sense of well-being. The patient must know that s/he has a responsibility to identify and communicate when meaningful stimuli are absent, or if there is overload or sensory restriction. Giving the patient responsibility aids greatly in supplying meaningful stimuli.*

GOAL

The patient will be able to identify stimuli conducive to treatment and recovery; will identify risk factors or stimuli that increase fear, anxiety, and restlessness; will devise a plan to make incoming stimuli optimal and meaningful.

IMPLEMENTATION

- Inform patient that being away from familiar surroundings will tend to produce feelings of isolation and monotony resulting in sensory alterations; it is helpful to bring in familiar pictures, radios, tapes and other items from home to facilitate orientation.
- Explain that the patient also has a responsi-

bility for maintaining sensory equilibrium, and how to facilitate this specifically.

- Ask the patient to tell you when the stimulus is too little or too much (e.g., "It's so noisy." "I would like to rest."); attempt to reduce or increase the stimuli to meet the patient's needs.
- Instruct to vary activities frequently during the day (e.g., read, watch television, listen to radio); help devise a written plan to be kept at bedside as a guide/reminder.
- Involve family in the plan for introducing meaningful stimuli; educate family to the hazards of sensory deprivation, overstimulation, etc., and how to minimize factors that cause disturbances.

☐ EVALUATION CRITERIA/DESIRED OUTCOMES

The Patient

- States importance of optimal sensory input
- Assumes responsibility as possible for level and type of stimuli
- Identifies and utilizes sources of support to deal with sensory overload/deprivation

NURSING DIAGNOSIS #3

Sleep pattern disturbance related to inability to fall asleep within 20 minutes of bedtime, sleeping during day and staying awake at night

Rationale: *The individual experiencing a sensory alteration may experience a sleep disturbance manifested by inability to fall asleep at bedtime or a reversal of sleep time, such as sleeping during the day and staying awake at night. This first pattern may occur as a result of too much input; the second pattern occurs when sensory input during the day is insufficient to maintain the patient at an alert, awake level of consciousness.*

☐ GOAL

The patient will discuss feelings and concerns about sleep pattern; will experience a balance of rest and activity during day; will sleep 6-7 hours (or specific time) at night.

☐ IMPLEMENTATION

For the individual with an inability to fall asleep within 20 minutes at bedtime

- Provide comfort measures such as back rub, positioning; medicate for pain.
- Determine patient's usual bedtime routine and establish it as much as possible during hospitalization.
- Provide periods of rest during the day to control buildup of effects of sensory overload as the day progresses.
- Intervene to reduce stress and anxiety (refer to *The Patient Experiencing Anxiety*, page 250.
- Allow patient to engage in interesting but nonstimulating activity during periods of restlessness.
- Increase physical exercise during the day as much as possible.

For the individual who sleeps during the day

- Provide an increase of stimulation during the day so that the patient remains alert and awake
  - visits from family members or hospital volunteers
  - physical exercise within reasonable limits
  - making or receiving phone calls
  - engaging in hobbies/activities of interest
- Monitor the fatigue level of the patient during the day and provide short rest periods when necessary.
- Awaken the individual who is sleeping except during arranged rest periods.

☐ EVALUATION CRITERIA/DESIRED OUTCOMES

The Patient

- Falls asleep and continues to sleep during the night for a specified amount of time
- Remains alert and awake during the day

NURSING DIAGNOSIS #4

Potential for injury related to sensory defects, reduced ability to protect self from hazards

Rationale: *Perceptual or physiologic defects that reduce the ability to protect oneself may include kinesthetic deficits resulting in paralysis or weakness, visual or auditory deficits, decreased hearing, tactile deficits (e.g., numbness or lack of ability to discriminate*

pain and/or extremes of heat or cold), or problems with balance. These deficits tend to increase with age. Patients with perceptual/physiologic defects are at risk for accident and injury and need preventive nursing measures to assure safety.

GOAL

The patient will remain free from injury; will acknowledge specific sensory defects and assistance needed; will utilize specific assistive devices.

IMPLEMENTATION

- Determine effect of deficit on patient's ability to function safely, type of assistance needed from the nursing staff or family, teaching needed regarding the deficit, safety measures.
- Ensure that prescribed aids (e.g., hearing aids, eye glasses, braces, orthopedic shoes, walkers, canes) are utilized and in good working condition.
- Control hazards in the environment
  - keep the furniture and other items in the same place all of the time
  - keep the bed at the lowest position with wheels locked
  - answer the call light promptly when the patient requests help
  - provide description of the environment and remind patient of safety measures and hazards as needed

EVALUATION CRITERIA/DESIRED OUTCOMES

The Patient

- Remains free from injury
- Utilizes specific aids/appliances
- Requests assistance with activities of daily living or ambulation as needed

Appendix
Nursing Diagnoses: Accepted List

Activity intolerance
Adjustment, impaired
Airway clearance, ineffective
Anxiety: mild, moderate, severe, panic
Body temperature, alteration in: potential
Bowel elimination, alteration in: constipation
Bowel elimination, alteration in: diarrhea
Bowel elimination, alteration in: incontinence
Breathing pattern, ineffective
Cardiac output, alteration in: decreased
Comfort, alteration in: pain
Comfort, alteration in: chronic pain
Communication, impaired: verbal
Coping, family: potential for growth
Coping, ineffective family: compromised
Coping, ineffective family: disabling
Coping, ineffective individual
Diversional activity, deficit
Family process, alteration in
Fear
Fluid volume, alteration in: excess
Fluid volume deficit
Gas exchange, impaired
Grieving, anticipatory
Grieving, dysfunctional
Growth and development, alteration in
Health maintenance, alteration in
Home maintenance management, impaired
Hyperthermia
Hypothermia
Incontinence, functional
Incontinence, reflex
Incontinence, stress
Incontinence, total
Incontinence, urge
Infection, potential for
Injury, potential for: (poisoning, potential for; suffocation, potential for; trauma, potential for)
Knowledge deficit (specify)
Mobility, impaired physical
Noncompliance (specify)
Nutrition, alteration in: less than body requirements
Nutrition, alteration in: more than body requirements
Oral mucous membrane, alteration in
Parenting, alteration in
Post trauma response
Powerlessness
Rape trauma syndrome
Self-care deficit: feeding, bathing/hygiene, dressing/grooming, toileting
Self-concept, disturbance in: body image, self-esteem, role performance, personal identity
Sensory-perceptual alteration: visual, auditory, kinesthetic, gustatory, tactile, olfactory
Sexual dysfunction
Sexuality patterns, alteration in
Skin integrity, impairment of
Sleep pattern disturbance
Social interaction, impaired
Social isolation
Spiritual distress (distress of the human spirit)
Swallowing, impaired
Thermoregulation, ineffective
Thought processes, alteration in
Tissue integrity, impaired
Tissue perfusion, alteration in: cerebral, cardiopulmonary, renal, gastrointestinal, peripheral
Unilateral neglect
Urinary elimination, alteration in patterns of
Urinary retention
Violence, potential for: self-directed or directed at others

Bibliography

General

Alspach, J., & Williams, S. (1985). *Core curriculum for critical care nursing* (3rd ed.). Philadelphia: Saunders.

Brunner, L., & Suddarth, D. (1984). *Textbook of medical-surgical nursing* (5th ed.). Philadelphia: Lippincott.

Carpenito, L. (1984). *Handbook of nursing diagnosis.* Philadelphia: Lippincott.

Carpenito, L. (1983). *Nursing diagnosis: Application to clinical practice.* Philadelphia: Lippincott.

Duesphol, A. (1986). *Nursing diagnosis handbook.* Philadelphia: Saunders.

Fardy, P., Bennett, J., Reits, N., & Williams, M. (1980). *Cardiac rehabilitation.* St. Louis: Mosby.

Fletcher, B. (1983). *Quick reference to critical care nursing.* Philadelphia: Lippincott.

Gordon, M. (1982). *Nursing diagnosis—Process and application.* New York: McGraw-Hill.

Gordon, M. (1982). *Manual of nursing diagnoses.* New York: McGraw-Hill.

Iyer, P., Taptic, B., & Bernocchi-Losey, D. (1986). *Nursing process and nursing diagnosis.* Philadelphia: Saunders.

Johnson, B., Dungca, C., Hoffmeister, D., & Wells, S. (1981). *Standards for critical care.* St. Louis: Mosby.

Kenner, C., Guzzetta, C., & Dossey, B. (1985). *Critical care nursing* (2nd ed.). Boston: Little, Brown.

Kim, M., McFarland, G., & McLane, A. (1984). *A pocket guide to nursing diagnosis.* St. Louis: Mosby.

Kinney, M., Dear, C., Packa, D., & Voorman, D. (1981). *AACN's Clinical reference for critical care nurses.* New York: McGraw-Hill.

Long, B., & Phipps, W. (1985). *Essentials of medical-surgical nursing.* St. Louis: Mosby.

Price, S., & Wilson, L. (1982). *Pathophysiology: Clinical concepts of disease processes* (2nd ed.). New York: McGraw-Hill.

Porth, C. (1986). *Pathophysiology: Concepts of altered health states* (2nd ed.). Philadelphia: Lippincott.

Thompson, J., McFarland, G., Hirsch, J., Tucker, S., & Bowers, A. (1986). *Clinical nursing.* St. Louis: Mosby.

Tucker, S., Breeding, M., Canobbio, M., Paquett, E., Wells, M., & William, M. (1984). *Patient care standards.* St. Louis: Mosby.

Underhill, S., Woods, S., Sivarajan, E., & Halpenny, C. (1982). *Cardiac nursing.* Philadelphia: Lippincott.

Acquired Immune Deficiency Syndrome (AIDS)

Acquired immune deficiency syndrome (AIDS): Precautions for health care workers and allied health professionals. (1983). *Public Health Letter,* November.

Acquired immunodeficiency syndrome (AIDS) update—United States. (1983). *Morbidity & Mortality Weekly Review, 32,* 450-451.

Allen, J., & Mellin, G. (1982). The new epidemic. *American Journal of Nursing, 82,* 1718-1722.

Bennett, J. (1985). AIDS epidemiology update. *American Journal of Nursing, 85,* 968-972.

Irish, A. (1983). Straight talks about gay patients. *American Journal of Nursing, 83,* 1169-1170.

Lillard, J., Lotsperch, P., Gurich, J., & Jesse, J. (1984). Acquired immunodeficiency syndrome (AIDS) in home care—maximizing helpfulness and minimizing hysteria. *Home Healthcare Nurse, 2*(6), 11-16.

Popkin, J., et al. (1983). Caring for the AIDS patient. *Nursing83, 13*(9), 50-55.

Questions and answers on acquired immune deficiency syndrome (AIDS). (1982). *California Morbidity Supplement, 12*(10), 48.

Turner, J., et al. (1986). AIDS: a challenge for contemporary nursing. *Focus on Critical Care, 13*(3) 53-61.

Angiography

Marinelli-Miller, D. (1983). What your patient wants to know about angiography—but may not ask. *RN, 46*(11), 52-54.

Radiology in trauma treatment. (1983). *Emergency Medicine, 30*(11), 27-30.

Angioplasty

Bouman, C. (1984). Intracoronary thrombolysis and percutaneous transluminal coronary angioplasty. Nursing implications. *Nursing Clinics of North America, 19*(3), 397-409.

Ng, L. (1983). Percutaneous transluminal coronary recanalization with streptokinase: nursing care and implications. *Cardiovascular Nursing, 19*(6), 25-30.

Sprengel, R. (1981). Exciting new alternatives to coronary bypass surgery. *RN, 44*(12), 24-28.

Aortic Aneurysm

Baum, P. (1982). Abdominal aortic aneurysm. *Nursing82, 12*(12), 34-41.

Asthma

Hudgel, D., & Madsen, L. (1980). Acute and chronic asthma: A guide to intervention. *American Journal of Nursing, 80*, 1791-1795.

Kiriloff, L., & Tibbals, S. (1983). Drugs for asthma: A complete guide. *American Journal of Nursing, 83*, 55-61.

Simkins, R. (1981). Asthma: Reactive airways disease. *American Journal of Nursing, 81*, 522-524.

Stempel, D., & Mellon, M. (1984). Management of acute severe asthma. *Pediatric Clinics of North America, 31*, 879-890.

Automatic Implantable Cardioverter-Defibrillator (AICD)

Flores, B., & Hildebrandt, M. (1984). The automatic implantable defibrillator. *Heart and Lung, 13*, 608-613.

Flores, B. (1987). The automatic implantable defibrillator. In *1987 NTI proceedings book*. Newport Beach, CA: American Association of Critical Nurses.

Nuel, D., et al. (1986). Challenging concerns for patients with automatic implantable cardioverter defibrillators. *Focus on Critical Care, 13*, 50-58.

Wilson, L., & Miller, P. (1986). The automatic implantable cardioverter defibrillator: A lifesaving device. *American Journal of Nursing, 86*, 1004-1008.

Blood and Blood Product Transfusions

Blood transfusions today: What you should know and should do. (1978). *Nursing78, 8*, 68-72.

Committee on Transfusion Practices, American Association of Blood Banks. (1986). The latest protocols for blood transfusions. *Nursing86, 16*(11), 34-42.

Professional Guide to Drugs (2nd ed.). (1982). Horsham, PA: Intermed.

Putnam, R., et al. (1979). Blood therapy. *American Journal of Nursing, 79*, 926-948.

Smith, L. (1984). Protocols for handling transfusion reactions. *American Journal of Nursing, 84*, 1096-1101.

Burns

Hurt, R. (1985). More than skin deep: Guidelines for caring for the burn patient. *Nursing85, 15*(6), 52-57.

Johnson, C., & Cain, V. (1985). CE burn care: The rehab guide. *American Journal of Nursing, 85*, 48-51.

Luterman, A., & Curreri, P. (1984). Emergency protocol for the severely burned patient. *Hospital Medicine, 20*(10), 131-146.

Robertson, K., et al. (1985). CE burn care: The crucial first days. *American Journal of Nursing, 85*, 29-45.

Rosequist, C., & Shepp, P. (1985). CE burn care: The nutrition factor. *American Journal of Nursing, 85*, 45-47.

Surveyor, J., & Cougherty, D. (1983). Burn scars: Fighting the effects. *American Journal of Nursing, 83*, 746-751.

Winkler, J. (Ed.). (1984). Burn care update. *Critical Care Quarterly,7*(3), 1-84.

Cardiac Conditions

Brannon, P. (1986). Ventricular failure: New therapy using the mechanical assist device. *Critical Care Nurse, 6*(2), 70-85.

Burke, C., et al. (1986). Perfusion scans and pulmonary angiography. *Heart and Lung, 15*, 357-360.

Burrows, S., & Gassert, C. (1984). *Moving right along after open heart surgery*. Atlanta: Pritchett and Hull.

Conti, C. (1986). Unstable angina before and after infarction: Thoughts on pathogenesis and therapeutic strategies. *Heart and Lung, 15*, 361-368.

Cromwell, V., et al. (1980). Understanding the needs of your coronary bypass patient. *Nursing81, 11*(3), 34-41.

DeGroot, K., et al. (1986). Monitoring intra-arterial pressure. *Critical Care Nurse, 6*(1), 74-78.

Estes, M. (1985). Management of cardiac tamponade: A nursing framework. *Critical Care Nurse, 5*(5), 17-16.

Johanson, B., et al. (1985). *Standards for critical care*, (2nd ed.). St. Louis: Mosby.

Klein, D. (1984). Physiology of angina. *Nursing84, 14*(2), 44-46.

Kleinhenz, T. (1985). Preload/afterload. *Nursing85, 15*(5), 50-54.

McCauley, K., & Burke, K. (1984). CHF drugs. *Nursing84, 14*(5), 46-50.

McGuran, W. (1981). *People with cardiac problems: Nursing concepts*. Philadelphia: Lippincott.

Norsen, L., & Fox, G. (1985). Cardiac output. *Nursing85, 15*(4), 34-42.

Owen, P. (1984). Defibrillating pacemaker patients. *American Journal of Nursing, 84*, 1129-1132.

Peters, R. (1986). Temporary transcutaneous pacing: New indications for an old technique. *AORN Journal, 44*, 245-246, 248-249.

Porterfield, J., et al. (1986). Understanding electrophysiologic studies. *Focus on Critical Care, 13*(3), 30.

Purcell, J., & Burrows, S. (1985). A pacemaker primer. *American Journal of Nursing, 85*, 553-568.

Rodgers, C. (1983). Needs of relatives of cardiac surgery patients during the acute phase. *Focus on Critical Care, 10*(5), 50-55.

Sadler, P. (1978). Nursing assessment of postcardiotomy delirium. *Heart and Lung, 7*(4) , 987-994.

Scordo, K. (1982). This procedure called PTCA: Your patient's CABG substitute? *Nursing82, 12*(2), 50-55.

Sprengel, R. (1981). Exciting new alternatives to coronary by-pass surgery. *RN, 44*(12), 24-47.

Thorpe, C. (1979). A nursing care plan—The adult cardiac surgery patient. *Heart and Lung, 8*(4), 690-698.

Wadsworth, L., et al. (1982). Intracoronary streptokinase infusion. *Nursing82, 12*(5), 58-65.

White, S. (1984). *The sensuous heart*. Atlanta: Pritchett and Hull.

Cardiac Catheterization

Alspach, J., & Williams, S. (1985). *Core curriculum for critical care nursing*. Philadelphia: Saunders.

Bauman, C. (1984). Intracoronary thrombolysis and

percutaneous transluminal coronary angioplasty: Nursing implications. *Nursing Clinics of North America, 19,* 397-409.

Chrzanowski, A. (1984). Cardiac coronary angiography. *Occupational Health Nursing, 32,*(2), 81-5, 112-7.

Johanson, B., et al. (1985). *Standards for critical care* (2nd ed.). St. Louis: Mosby.

Purcell, J. (1982). *Cardiac catheterization* (A patient teaching book). Atlanta: Pritchett and Hull.

Teasley, D. (1982). Don't let cardiac catheterization strike fear in your patient's heart. *Nursing82, 12*(3) 53-55.

Ventura, B. (1984). What you need to know about cardiac catheterization. *RN, 47*(9) 24-30.

Yacone, L., (1984). Cardiac diagnostic studies: Nuclear scanning and cardiac catheterization. *RN, 47*(5) 129-130.

Cardiac Surgery

Borders, C. (1985). *Patient Care, 19*(9), entire issue.

Borders, C. Bypass: Patient's perceptions and fears. *Patient Care,19*(11), entire issue.

Gassert, C., & Burrows, S. (1985). *Going for heart surgery.* Atlanta: Pritchett and Hull.

Mayer, R., et al. (1979). What open-heart surgery patients want to know. *American Journal of Nursing, 79,* 1558-1560.

Cerebral Aneurysm

Chase, M., & Whelan-Decker, E. (1984). Nursing management of a patient with subarachnoid hemorrhage. *Journal of Neurosurgical Nursing, 16,* 23-29.

Finch, K. (1980). Vasospasm secondary to subarachnoid haemorrhage: The current controversy, research, and nursing dilemmas. *Journal of Neurosurgical Nursing, 12,* 199-202.

Gray, R. (1981). Cerebral vasospasm: Process, trends, and interventions. *Journal of Neurosurgical Nursing, 13,* 258-264.

Kim, L., & Tew, J. (1985). Saccular aneurysms, subarachnoid hemorrhage, and the timing of surgery. *Heart and Lung, 14*(1), 68-74.

Morris, D. (1982). Intraoperative aneurysm clipping. *Journal of Neurosurgical Nursing, 14,* 150-153.

Oertel, L. (1985). The dilemma of cerebral vasospasm treatment. *Journal of Neurosurgical Nursing, 17,* 7-13.

Stanley, M. (1984). Cerebral vasospasm: Pathphysiology and nursing care. *Critical Care Nurse, 4*(6), 39-42.

Cerebral-Vascular Accident

O'Brien, M., & Pallett, P. (1978). *Total care of the stroke patient.* Boston: Little, Brown.

Snyder, M. (Ed.). (1983). *A guide to neurological and neurosurgical nursing.* New York: Wiley.

Taylor, J. (1985). Nursing management of stroke: Acute care: Part I. *Cardiovascular Nursing, 21*(1), 1-5.

Taylor, J. (1985). Nursing management of stroke: Acute care: Part II, *Cardiovascular Nursing, 21*(2), 7-12.

Cirrhosis

Brodsley, T. (1982). Avoiding a crisis: The assessment. *American Journal of Nursing, 82,* 1865-1873.

Joyce, C. (1982). The hospitalized alcoholic. *American Journal of Nursing, 82,* 1861.

Kinney, M. (1981). *AACN's clinical reference for critical care nursing.* New York: McGraw-Hill.

La Fortune, F. (1984). When the liver fails. *American Journal of Nursing, 82,* 64-67.

Thompson, M. (1981). Managing the patient with liver dysfunction. *Nursing81, 11*(11), 101-107.

Diabetes

Bille, D. (1986). Tailoring your diabetic patient's careplan to fit his life-style. *Nursing86, 16*(2), 54-57.

Crigler-Meringola, E. (1984). Making life sweet again for the elderly diabetic. *Nursing84, 14*(4), 61-64.

Essig, M. (1983). Update your knowledge of oral antidiabetic agents. *Nursing83, 13*(10), 58-64.

Forbes, K., & Stokes, S. (1984). Saving the diabetic foot. *American Journal of Nursing, 84,* 884-888.

Fredholm, N., et al. (1984). Insulin pumps: The patients' verdict. *American Journal of Nursing, 84,* 36-38.

Graham, S., & Morely, M. (1984). What 'foot care' really means. *American Journal of Nursing, 84,* 889-891.

Jackson, C. (1981). Diabetes: How your patient looks at it. *Nursing81, 11*(5), 82-83.

McCarthy, J. (1985). The continuum of diabetic coma. *American Journal of Nursing, 84,* 878-882.

Miller, V. (1986). Diabetes: Let's stop testing urine. *American Journal of Nursing, 86,* 54.

Pelczynski, L., & Reilly, A. (1981). Helping your diabetic patients help themselves. *Nursing81, 11*(5), 76-81.

Robertson, C. (1986). Interpreting blood glucose studies. *Nursing86, 16*(8), 64.

Snyder, J. (1980). Diabetes in pregnancy. *Nursing80, 10*(11), 44-49.

Stock-Barkman, P. (1983). Confusing concepts: Is it diabetic shock or diabetic coma? *Nursing83, 13*(6), 33-41.

Surr, C. (1983). Teaching patients to use the new blood-glucose monitoring products, part I. *Nursing83, 13*(1), 42-45.

Surr, C. (1983). Teaching patients to use the new blood-glucose monitoring products, part II. *Nursing83, 13*(2), 58-62.

Thatcher, G. (1985). Insulin injections: The case against random rotation. *American Journal of Nursing, 85,* 690-692.

Epilepsy

Beniak, J., & Beniak, T. (1983). Social isolation. M. Snyder (Ed.). In *A guide to neurological and neurosurgical nursing.* New York: Wiley.

Tucker, C. (1985). Safety assessment for the postictal confusional phase following complex partial seizures. *Journal of Neurosurgical Nursing, 17,* 201-209.

Esophageal Varices

Gruber, M., & Nuever, N. (1982). Treating esophageal varices with injection sclerotherapy. *American Journal of Nursing, 82,* 1214-1217.

Kenney, M. (1981). *AACN's clinical reference for critical care nursing.* New York: McGraw-Hill.

Lamphier, T., & Lamphier, R. (1981). Upper GI hemorrhage: Emergency evaluation and management. *American Journal of Nursing, 81,* 1817-1821.

Fluid and Electrolyte Disturbances

Baer, C. (1982). *Fluid and electrolyte problems in the critically ill patient.* Nation Teaching Institute: American Association of Critical Care Nurses.

Folk-Lightly, M. (1984). Solving the puzzles of patients' fluid imbalances. *Nursing84, 14,*(2), 34-41.

Hakki, A., et al. (1986). A simple formula for monitoring parenteral infusion/medication. *Critical Care Nurse, 6*(3), 57-62.

Kee, J. (1982). *Fluids and electrolytes with clinical applications: A programmed approach* (3rd ed.). New York: Wiley.

Kuthley, J., & Fraulini, K. (1982). What's behind that IV line? *Nursing82, 12*(3), 32-42.

Lowe, J., et al. (1986). Nomograms: Shortcuts to accuracy. *Focus on Critical Care, 13*(3), 36-40.

Metheny, N. (1984). *Quick reference to fluids and electrolytes.* Philadelphia: Lippincott.

Miller, P. (1985). Assessing CVP. *Nursing85, 15*(9), 44-46.

Guillain-Barré Syndrome

Blanco, K., & Cuomo, N. (1983). From the other side of the bedrail: A personal experience with Guillain-Barré syndrome. *Journal of Neurosurgical Nursing, 15,* 355-359.

Prydun, M. (1983). Guillain-Barré syndrome: disease process. *Journal of Neurosurgical Nursing, 15,* 27-32.

Samonds, R. (1981). Guillain-Barré syndrome: The acute stage. *Critical Care Update, 8*(11), 38-44.

Tikkanen, P. (1982). Landry-Guillain-Barré-Strohl syndrome. *Journal of Neurosurgical Nursing, 14,* 74-81.

Head Injury

Bowers, S., & Marshall, L. (1982). Severe head injury: Current treatment and research. *Journal of Neurosurgical Nursing, 14,* 210-219.

Rogers, P., & Kreutzer, J. (1984). Family crises following head injury: A network intervention strategy. *Journal of Neurosurgical Nursing, 16,* 343-346.

Stevens, M. (1982). Post concussion syndrome. *Journal of Neurosurgical Nursing, 14,* 239-244.

Hemodynamic Monitoring

Daily, E., & Schroeder, J. (1985). *Techniques in bedside hemodynamic monitoring* (3rd ed.). St. Louis: Mosby.

Fletcher, B. (1983). *Quick reference to critical care nursing.* Philadelphia: Lippincott.

Fraulini, K., & Kleinhenz, T. (1985). Action stat! dislodged PA catheter. *Nursing85, 15*(10), 33.

Guzzetta, C., & Dossey, B. (1984). *Cardiovascular nursing: Bodymind tapestry.* St. Louis: Mosby.

Hathaway, R. (1978). The Swan-Ganz catheter: A review. *Nursing Clinics of North America, 13,* 389-407.

Morra, L. (1987). Troubleshooting pulmonary artery catheters. *RN, 50*(2), 46-52.

Murray, J., & Smallwood, J. (1977). CVP monitoring. *Nursing77, 7*(1), 42-47.

Niemczura, J. (1985). Eight rules to remember when caring for the patient with a Swan-Ganz catheter. *Nursing85, 15*(3), 38-41.

Schakenbach, L., & Dennis, M. (1985). And now, a quad-lumen IV catheter. *Nursing85, 15*(11), 50-51.

Scordo, K. (1985). Hemodynamic monitoring—learning to read the waves. *Nursing85, 15*(7), 40-42.

Smith, S., & Duell, D. (1982). *Nursing skills and evaluation: A nursing process approach.* St. Louis: Mosby.

Spangler, R. (1985). Update on pulmonary artery catherization. *Nursing85, 15*(8), 42-45.

Intraaortic Balloon Pump

Bregman, D. (1985). Intra-aortic balloon: New developments, techniques, complications, and results. In S. Atarr (Ed.), *New developments in cardiac assist devices.* New York: Praeger Scientific.

Guzzetta, C., & Dossey, B. (1984). *Cardiovascular nursing: Bodymind tapestry.* St. Louis: Mosby.

Quaal, S. (1984). *Comprehensive intra-aortic balloon pumping.* St. Louis: Mosby.

Quaal, S. (1987). State of the art: Methods of mechanical assistance for the failing heart. *NTI Proceedings Book.* American Association of Critical Care Nurses.

Roberts, S. (1985). *Physiological concepts and the critically ill patient.* Englewood Cliffs, NJ: Prentice-Hall.

Whitman, G. (1978). Intra-aortic balloon pumping and cardiac mechanics: A programmed lesson. *Heart and Lung, 7,* 1034-1050.

Intracranial Pressure

Burgess, K. (1985). Recognizing and responding to increased ICP. *Nursing Life,* March/April, 33-48.

Fear of floating to neurology. (1982). *Nursing82, 12*(1), 48-49.

Johnson, L. (1983). If your patient has increased intracranial pressure, your goal should be: No surprises. *Nursing83, 13*(6), 58-64.

Johnson, M., & Quinn, J. (1977). The subarachnoid screw. *American Journal of Nursing, 77,* 448-450.

Jones, C., & Cayard, C. (1982). Care of ICP monitoring devices: A nursing responsibility. *Journal of Neurosurgical nursing, 14,* 255-261.

Lipe, H., & Mitchell, P. (1980). Positioning the patient with intracranial hypertension: How turning and head rotation affect the internal jugular vein. *Heart and Lung, 9,* 1031-1037.

Mitchell, P., Ozuna, J., & Lipe, H. (1981). Moving the patient in bed: Effects on intracranial pressure. *Nursing Research, 30,* 212-218.

Price, M. (1981). Significance of intracranial pressure waveform. *Journal of Neurosurgical Nursing, 13,* 202-206.

Robinet, K. (1985). Increased intracranial pressure: Management with an intraventricular catheter. *Journal of Neurosurgical Nursing, 17,* 95-104.

Laryngectomy

Blues, K. (1978). A framework for nurses providing care to laryngectomy patients. *Cancer Nursing, 1,* 441-445.

Dietz, J. (1981). *Rehabilitation oncology.* New York: Wiley.

Harris, L., et al. (1986). After T-E puncture: Re-learning to speak...the Bloom-Singer voice prosthesis. *American Journal of Nursing, 86,* 55-58.

Patry-Lahey, R. (1985). Helping your laryngectomy patient go home. *Nursing85, 15*(3), 63-64.

Speese-Owens, N. (1981). Nursing care of patients with head and neck tumors. In R. Bouchard (Ed.), *Nursing care of the cancer patient* (5th ed.). St. Louis: Mosby.

Meningitis

Gaddy, D. (1980). Meningitis in the pediatric population. *Nursing Clinics of North America, 15,* 83-97.

Medical staff conference. (1984). Meningitis. *The Western Journal of Medicine, 140,* 433-436.

Muwaswes, M. (1985). Increased intracranial pressure and its systemic effects. *Journal of Neurosurgical Nursing, 17,* 238-243.

Nebens, I., & Jackson, B. (1982). A case of acute fulminating meningococcemia. *American Journal of Nursing, 82,* 1390-1393.

Wing, S. (1981). Brain abscess. *Journal of Neurosurgical Nursing, 13,* 123-126.

Wink, D. (1984). Bacterial meningitis in children. *American Journal of Nursing, 84*(4), 456-460.

Yoshikawa, T., & Norma, D. (1981). Bacterial meningitis—disease of young and old. *Consultant, 21*(11), 219-231.

Pacemaker: Temporary—External/Noninvasive

Clinton, J., Zoll, P., Zoll, R., & Ruiz, E. (1985). Emergency noninvasive cardiac pacing. *Journal of Emergency Medicine 2,* 155-162.

Falk, R., Zoll, P., & Zoll, R. (1983). Safety and efficacy of noninvasive cardiac pacing. *New England Journal of Medicine, 309,* 1166-1168.

Mickus, D., Monohan, K., & Brown, C. (1986). Exciting external pacemaker. *American Journal of Nursing, 86,* 403-405.

National Conference on Cardiopulmonary Resuscitation (CPR) and Emergency Cardiac Care (ECC). 1986). Standards and Guidelines of CPR and ECC. *JAMA, 255*(21), 2905-2984.

Voorhees, W., Foster, K., Geddes, L., & Babbs, C. (1984). Safety factor for precordial pacing: Minimum current thresholds for pacing and for ventricular fibrillation by vulnerable-period stimulation. *PACE, 7*(3), 356-360.

Zoll, P., Zoll, R., Falk, R., Clinton, J., Eitel, D., & Antman, E. (1985). External noninvasive temporary cardiac pacing. *Circulation, 71*(5), 937-944.

Pancreatitis

Cooperman, A.M., (1981). Chronic pancreatitis. *Surgical Clinics of North America, 61,* 71-83.

Dickerman, R., & Dunn, E. (1981). Splenic, pancreatic and hepatic injuries. *Surgical Clinics of North America, 61,* 3-15.

Gotch, P. (1981). Are you ready for a total pancreatectomy patient? *RN, 44*(11), 54-57.

Ranson, J. (1981). Acute pancreatitis: Where are we? *Surgical Clinics of North America, 61,* 55-70.

Rudick, J. (1981). Physiology of pancreatic secretion. *Surgical Clinics of North America, 61,* 47-54.

Renal Conditions

Bauer, D. (1980). Preventing the spread of hepatitis B in dialysis units. *American Journal of Nursing, 80,* 260-261.

Binkley, L. (1984). Keeping up with peritoneal dialysis. *American Journal of Nursing, 84,* 729-733.

Binkley, L. (Ed.). (1981). Transplantation. *Nephrology Nurse, 3*(6), whole issue.

Cairoli, O., & Voyce, P. (1982). *Memory bank for hemodialysis.* Baltimore: Williams & Wilkins.

Chambers, J. (1981). Assessing the dialysis patient at home. *American Journal of Nursing, 81,* 750-754.

Cianci, J., Lamp, J., & Ryan, R. (1981). Renal transplantation. *American Journal of Nursing, 81,* 354-355.

David-Kasdan, J. (1984). Alteration in body image in the hemodialysis population. *Journal of Nephrology Nursing, 1,* 25-28.

Davis, V., & Lavandero, R. (1980). Caring for the catheter carefully, part I. *Nursing 80, 10*(12), 67-71.

Faris, M. (1980). *When your kidneys fail.* San Diego: National Kidney Foundation.

Fleming, L. (1984). Step by step guide to safe peritoneal dialysis. *RN, 47*(2), 44-47.

Hekleman, F. (1985). A framework for organizing a CAPD training program. *Journal of Nephrology Nursing, 2,* 56-60.

Hughes, C. (1985). Stabilizing catheters—Tenckhoff catheter placement. *American Nephrology Nurses Association Journal, 12*(3), 204.

Irwin, B. (1981). Now—peritoneal dialysis for chronic patients, too. *RN, 44*(6), 49-52.

Lane, T. (1983). Standards of care for the CAPD patient. *Home Health Care Nurse, 4*(5), 34, 36, 41-45.

Levi, M. (1984). Learning to live with dialysis. *Journal of Nephrology Nursing, 1,* 153-154.

Levi, M. (1985). Learning to live with dialysis—dialysis or transplant. *Journal of Nephrology Nursing, 2,* 27.

Moncrief, J., & Popovich, R. (1981). *CAPD update.* New York: Masson.

Montefusco, C. (1984). Cyclosporin immunosuppression in organ transplant recipients—nursing complications. *Critical Care Nursing, 4*(2), 117-119.

Payne, G. (1984). Reducing stress in renal patients and their families. *Journal of Nephrology Nursing, 1* 138-140.

Peterson, L. (1984). Home dialysis training. *American Nephrology Nurses Association Journal, 11*(4), 27-29.

Pitman, N. (1982). *Nephrology nursing standards of clinical practice.* American Association of Nephrology Nurses and Technicians.

Plaweski, H. (1985). Counseling the sexually dysfunctioning hemodialysis patient. *Journal of Nephrology Nursing, 2,* 166-168.

Powers, A. (1981). Renal transplantation: The patient's choice. *Nursing Clinics of North America, 16,* 551-564.

Rambaks, I. (1985). Post-transplant hypertension and the renal transplant. *Journal of Nephrology Nursing, 2,* 115-118.

Rhodes, V. (1985). Monthly home patient checklist—a dialysis assessment tool. *Journal of Nephrology Nursing, 2* 28-29.

Richard, A. (1985). Renal transplantation—nursing management of the recipient. *JOARN, 41,* 1022-1036, 1038, 40, 41.

Sandeval, M., & Parks, C. (1981). The evolution to CAPD. *Nephrology Nurse, 3*(5), 27-30,32.

Sorrels, P. (1981). Peritoneal dialysis: A rediscovery. *Nursing Clinics of North American, 16,* 515-530.

Stevenson, J. (1984). Health related problems of patients on hemodialysis. *Journal of Nephrology Nursing, 1,* 101-105.

Topor, M. (1981). Chronic renal disease in children. *Nursing Clinics of North America, 16,* 587-598.

Weiss, M. (1981). Evaluation of a home hemodialysis instruction program. *Nephrology Nurse, 3*(4), 8, 10-12, 42-43.

Respiratory Conditions

Callahan, M. (1985). A prudent pulmonary rehab program. *American Journal of Nursing, 85,* 1368-1369.

Cooper, D. (1986). Sexual counseling of the patient with chronic lung disease. *Focus on Critical Care, 13*(3), 18-20.

Humbrecht, B., & Van Parys, E. (1982). From assessment to intervention. *Nursing 82, 12*(4), 34-42.

Irwin, M., & Openbrier, D. (1985). A delicate balance: Strategies for feeding ventilated COPD patients. *American Journal of Nursing, 85,* 274-280.

Irwin, M., & Openbrier, D. (1985). Feeding ventilated patients safely. *American Journal of Nursing, 85,* 544-546.

McDonald, B. (1985). Validation of three respiratory nursing diagnoses. *Nursing Clinics of North America, 20,* 697-710.

Montanari, J., et al. (1986). The fine art of measuring tracheal cuff pressure. *Nursing86, 16*(7), 46-49.

Sjoberg, E. (1983). Nursing diagnosis and the COPD patient. *American Journal of Nursing, 83,* 244-248.

Westra, B. (1984). I can't breathe. *Nursing84, 14*(5), 34-40.

York, K. (1985). Clinical validation of two respiratory nursing diagnoses. *Nursing Clinics of North America, 20,* 657-667.

Spinal Cord Injury

Aadalen, S., & Stroebel-Kahn, F. (1981). Coping with quadriplegia. *American Journal of Nursing, 81,* 1471-1478.

Agee, B., & Herman, C. (1984). Cervical logrolling on a standard hospital bed. *American Journal of Nursing, 84,* 315-318.

Benda, S. (Ed.). (1983). *Spinal cord injury nursing education—suggested content.* Chicago: American Spinal Injury Foundation.

Friedman, M., Campbell, M., & Hart, C. (1984). Theoretical strategies and nursing interventions to promote psychosocial adaptation to spinal cord injuries and disability. *Journal of Neurosurgical Nursing, 16,* 335-342.

Giubilato, R. (1982). Acute care of the high-level quadreplegia patient. *Journal of Neurosurgical Nursing, 14,* 128-132.

Howard, M., & Corbo-Pelaia, S. (1982). The psychological aftereffects of halo traction and a review of acute care. *American Journal of Nursing, 82,* 1839-1843.

Hummelgard, A., & Martin, E. (1982). Management of the patient in a halo brace. *Journal of Neurosurgical Nursing, 14,* 113-119.

Kaiser, C. (1985). *Patient education: process and product.* Rancho Los Amigos Medical Center, Nursing Department, Downey, CA.

Larrabee, J. (1977). The person with a spinal cord injury—physical care during early recovery. *American Journal of Nursing, 77,* 1320-1329.

Parkinson, J. (1977). The spinal cord-injured patient—autonomic hyperreflexia. *Journal of Neurosurgical Nursing, 9,* 1-4.

Pepper, G. (1977). The person with a spinal cord injury—psychological care. *American Journal of Nursing, 77,* 1330-1336.

Richmond, T. (1985). A critical care challenge—The patient with a cervical spinal cord injury. *Focus on Critical Care, 12*(2), 23-33.

Snyder, M. (Ed.). (1983). *A guide to neurological and neurosurgical nursing.* New York: Wiley.

Solomon, J. (1982). Sex and the spinal cord injured patient. *Journal of Neurosurgical Nursing, 14,* 125-127.

Stanton, G. (1984). A needs assessment of significant others following the patient's spinal cord injury. *Journal of Neurosurgical Nursing, 16,* 253-256.

Starck, P. (1980). Maslow's needs and the spinal cord injured client. *Rehabilitation Nursing, 5*(5), 17-20.

Taylor, T., & Ballenger, S. (1980). *Neurological dysfunctions and nursing interventions.* New York: McGraw-Hill.

Total Hip Replacement

Adair, F. (1984). Hip replacement. *Nursing Mirror, 158*(3), 19-20.

Total Parenteral Nutrition (TPN)

Fox, B., & Stegall, B. (1985). Take precautions now. *Nursing85, 15*(5), 48-49.

Jeejeebhoy, K. (1984). Food for the critically ill. *Emergency Medicine, 152,* 156-159, 162-164.

Munro-Black, J. (1984). The ABC's of total parenteral nutrition. *Nursing84, 14*(2), 50-56.

Rodgers, B. (1984). Home parenteral nutrition: Principles and management. *Nurse Practitioner, 9*(3), 42, 47-48, 50 52.

Smith, S., & Duell, D. (1982). *Nursing skills and evaluation: A nursing process approach,* St. Louis: Mosby.

Wilhelm, L. (1985). Helping your patient "settle in" with TPN, *Nursing85, 15*(4), 60-64.

Tracheostomy

Fuchs, P. (1984). Streamlining your suctioning technique—tracheostomy suctioning. *Nursing84, 14*(7), 39-43.

Nursing photobook: providing respiratory care. (1980). Horsham, Pa: Intermed Communications.